How to access the supplemental online video

We are pleased to provide access to online video that supplements your textbook, *Sport Therapy for the Shoulder.* This resource offers 21 video clips that demonstrate the application of the 21 tests for clinical evaluation of the shoulder presented in chapter 3.

Accessing the online video is easy!
Follow these steps if you purchased a new book:

1. Visit **www.HumanKinetics.com/SportTherapyForTheShoulder**.

2. Click the <u>first edition</u> link next to the book cover.

3. Click the Sign In link on the left or top of the page. If you do not have an account with Human Kinetics, you will be prompted to create one.

4. If the online product you purchased does not appear in the Ancillary Items box on the left of the page, click the Enter Key Code option in that box. Enter the key code that is printed at the right, including all hyphens. Click the Submit button to unlock your online product.

5. After you have entered your key code the first time, you will never have to enter it again to access this product. Once unlocked, a link to your product will permanently appear in the menu on the left. For future visits, all you need to do is sign in to the textbook's website and follow the link that appears in the left menu!

→ Click the Need Help? button on the textbook's website if you need assistance along the way.

How to access the online video if you purchased a used book:

You may purchase access to the online video by visiting the text's website, **www.HumanKinetics.com/SportTherapyForTheShoulder**, or by calling the following:

800-747-4457 . . . . .U.S. customers
800-465-7301 . . . . .Canadian customers
+44 (0) 113 255 5665 . . . . European customers
08 8372 0999 . . . . Australian customers
0800 222 062 . . . . .New Zealand customers
217-351-5076 . . . . .International customers

For technical support, send an e-mail to:
support@hkusa.com . . . . U.S. and international customers
info@hkcanada.com . . . . Canadian customers
academic@hkeurope.com . . . . European customers
keycodesupport@hkaustralia.com . . . . . Australian and New Zealand customers

HUMAN KINETICS
The Information Leader in Physical Activity & Health

Product: Sport Therapy for the Shoulder online video

Key code: ELLENBECKER-7IZ7H3-COURSE

This unique code allows you access to the online video.

Access is provided if you have purchased a new book. Once submitted, the code may not be entered for any other user.

SPORT THERAPY

FOR THE

SHOULDER

SPORT THERAPY

FOR THE

SHOULDER

Evaluation, Rehabilitation, and Return to Sport

SPORT THERAPY SERIES

Todd S. Ellenbecker, DPT, MS, SCS, OCS, CSCS
Physiotherapy Associates
Scottsdale Sports Clinic, A Select Medical Company
Scottsdale, AZ

Kevin E. Wilk, PT, DPT, FAPTA
Champion Sports Medicine
Birmingham, AL

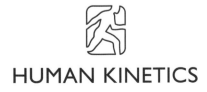

HUMAN KINETICS

Library of Congress Cataloging-in-Publication Data

Names: Ellenbecker, Todd S., 1962- , author. | Wilk, Kevin E., author.
Title: Sport therapy for the shoulder : evaluation, rehabilitation, and
   return to sport / Todd S. Ellenbecker, Kevin E. Wilk.
Other titles: Sport therapy series.
Description: Champaign : Human Kinetics, [2017] | Series: Sport therapy
   series | Includes bibliographical references and index.
Identifiers: LCCN 2016002959 | ISBN 9781450431644 (print)
Subjects: | MESH: Shoulder--injuries | Athletic Injuries--rehabilitation |
   Shoulder Joint--injuries | Joint Diseases--rehabilitation | Return to Sport
Classification: LCC RD557.5 | NLM WE 810 | DDC 617.5/72044--dc23 LC record available at http://lccn.loc
.gov/2016002959

ISBN: 978-1-4504-3164-4 (print)

Acquisitions Editor: Roger W. Earle; **Developmental Editor:** Melissa J. Zavala; **Senior Managing Editor:** Carly S. O'Connor; **Copyeditor:** Joyce Sexton; **Indexer:** Michael Ferreira; **Permissions Manager:** Dalene Reeder; **Senior Graphic Designer:** Keri Evans; **Cover Designer:** Keith Blomberg; **Photograph (cover):** © Human Kinetics; anatomical illustration by Heidi Richter; **Photographs (interior):** Neil Bernstein, unless otherwise noted; © Human Kinetics, unless otherwise noted; **Photo Asset Manager:** Laura Fitch; **Visual Production Assistant:** Joyce Brumfield; **Photo Production Manager:** Jason Allen; **Senior Art Manager:** Kelly Hendren **Illustrations:** © Human Kinetics, unless otherwise noted; **Printer:** Walsworth

We thank Physiotherapy Associates Scottsdale Sports Clinic in Scottsdale, Arizona, for assistance in providing the location for the photo shoot for this book.

The video contents of this product are licensed for private home use and traditional, face-to-face classroom instruction only. For public performance licensing, please contact a sales representative at **www.HumanKinetics.com/ SalesRepresentatives**.

Printed in the United States of America   10   9   8   7   6   5   4   3   2   1

The paper in this book is certified under a sustainable forestry program.

Human Kinetics
Website: www.HumanKinetics.com

United States: Human Kinetics
P.O. Box 5076
Champaign, IL 61825-5076
800-747-4457
e-mail: info@hkusa.com

Canada: Human Kinetics
475 Devonshire Road Unit 100
Windsor, ON N8Y 2L5
800-465-7301 (in Canada only)
e-mail: info@hkcanada.com

Europe: Human Kinetics
107 Bradford Road
Stanningley
Leeds LS28 6AT, United Kingdom
+44 (0) 113 255 5665
e-mail: hk@hkeurope.com

Australia: Human Kinetics
57A Price Avenue
Lower Mitcham, South Australia 5062
08 8372 0999
e-mail: info@hkaustralia.com

New Zealand: Human Kinetics
P.O. Box 80
Mitcham Shopping Centre, South Australia 5062
0800 222 062
e-mail: info@hknewzealand.com

E5729

Contents

Preface

The *Sport Therapy Series* brings together leading clinicians specializing in regional musculoskeletal conditions to develop highly focused, visually attractive, and evidence-based books that describe anatomical structures and biomechanical attributes of a specific joint; provide directions of evaluation techniques; and prescriptively recommend therapeutic activities with return-to-sport exercise progressions. *Sport Therapy for the Shoulder: Evaluation, Rehabilitation, and Return to Sport* is the first book in this series.

The shoulder is a very complex joint, affording massive amounts of mobility to allow for terrific functional range of motion and enabling humans to perform amazing sport-specific movement patterns. However, this mobility must be balanced by the appropriate amount of stability to ensure optimal performance and prevent injury. This complex joint provides clinicians in physical rehabilitation settings with an opportunity to truly affect and improve function. It is this ability afforded to clinicians that drives the need for evidence-based evaluation and treatment, which is ultimately the primary focus of this book.

As authors, we have assembled chapters to first provide a platform for the evaluation and treatment of the shoulder through a detailed review of clinical pertinent anatomy and biomechanics of the shoulder girdle. Within this overview of anatomy and biomechanics are key descriptions of sport-specific mechanics, both proper and improper, that can lead to the overuse injuries so common in overhead athletes. Chapter 3 provides a comprehensive approach to evaluation of the shoulder. Anatomical photos and an accompanying online video of 21 video clips, demonstrating special tests and procedures needed to properly evaluate an individual with shoulder dysfunction, are aimed at helping clinicians develop this critical skill. The ability to review and observe the patient position, clinician contact, and movement patterns recommended during the performance of these clinical tests is a feature we hope will assist clinicians in applying the optimal evaluation techniques to their patients.

Following the discussion and presentation of the clinical examination, the book focuses on treatment, both in nonoperative rehabilitation of shoulder pathologies and in specific postoperative conditions. This section of the book also has copious photos to fully depict the exercise progressions and treatment techniques used by the authors to treat patients with shoulder injuries. The inclusion of protocols will provide progression guidance for clinicians after common surgical procedures used to treat shoulder pathology. The appendix contains two helpful and widely used programs for injured athletes, the Thrower's Ten and the Advanced Thrower's Ten programs, originally developed by Kevin Wilk. These programs are illustrated with photos and accompanied by instructions. The Advanced Thrower's Ten program may be reproduced and used as a handout for patients.

Finally, one area that is perhaps most overlooked during standard shoulder rehabilitation is the return to play phase. To address this, we have included interval sport return programs

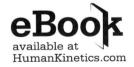

available at HumanKinetics.com

as well as specific criteria that can be used to objectively evaluate the patient before starting a functional return program. The step-by-step programs, coupled with the earlier portions of the book detailing the biomechanical demands of sport-specific movement patterns, will provide the clinician with the information needed to successfully progress the patient through this vitally important final stage of rehabilitation.

This compilation of chapters on shoulder evaluation and treatment offers the clinician an evidence-based resource providing clinically applicable information to enable comprehensive evaluations as well as the design of evaluation-based treatment programming. The inclusion of photos, online video, an image bank, and exhaustive references from the existing literature on shoulder injuries makes for a key resource for rehabilitation specialists who treat the shoulder. The image bank is available to instructors at www.HumanKinetics.com/SportTherapy ForTheShoulder.

The online video is also available at www .HumanKinetics.com/SportTherapyForThe Shoulder. See Accessing the Online Video for more information.

It is the authors' hope that this book will assist clinicians in providing the highest level of evaluation and treatment progressions to optimally treat shoulder pathology and return patients to full activity.

Acknowledgments

Like many authors, I have so many people to acknowledge who enabled me to write this book. First, my physical therapy mentors, George Davies, Janet Sobel, Gary Derscheid, and Bill Norris, trained me and provided an unbelievable example of excellence throughout my career. My physician mentors, Drs. Robert Nirschl, Ben Kibler, Per Renstrom, David Dines, David Altchek, Gary Windler, Marc Safran, Giovanni DiGiacomo, Brian Hainline, Babette Pluim, David Bailie, Angelo Mattalino, and James Andrews, provided me with opportunities, support, and the privilege of learning from and working with each of them. Also my respected colleagues have and continue to challenge and motivate me through their amazing work, prolific publishing, and gifts of friendship and support: Rob Manske, Ann Cools, Terry Malone, Kevin Wilk, Mark Paterno, Ellen Shanley, Chuck Thigpen, Phil Page, Mark DeCarlo, Kathleen Stroia, Masa Tsuruike, and Tim Tyler. And last but certainly not least are the sport scientists who have provided exceptional collaboration and mentorship: Paul Roetert, Mark Kovacs, Jack Groppel, Jim Loehr, Paul Lubbers, and Dan Gould. Without all of these amazing individuals' involvement in my life, I would never have had the many opportunities in my career, and I will be forever in debt and thankful for the contribution and support they have provided. Specific to this book, the concept was vetted in New Orleans at a meeting with Loarn Robertson who developed the idea and guided the initial project. Thanks to the great team at HK that followed, including Roger Earle, Melissa Zavala, Carly O'Connor, Neil Bernstein, and Doug Fink. Their professionalism and dedication produced this fine product.

—TSE

Accessing the Online Video

High-definition online streaming video accompanies this book. The video clips demonstrate the application of the 21 tests for clinical evaluation of the shoulder presented in chapter 3. Each clip is referenced in the book with this icon:

VIDEO 1 demonstrates the scapular assistance test.

You can access the online video by visiting www.HumanKinetics.com/Sport TherapyForTheShoulder. If you purchased a new print book, follow the directions included on the orange-framed page at the front of your book. That page includes access steps and the unique key code that you'll need the first time you visit the *Sport Therapy for the Shoulder* website. If you purchased an e-book from HumanKinetics .com, follow the access instructions that were e-mailed to you following your purchase.

Once at the *Sport Therapy for the Shoulder* website, select Online Video in the upper left corner of the screen. Use the link on the Online Video page to access the videos. Note that the numbers under the thumbnail images along the right side of the video player correspond with video number cross-references in the book, and the title under the player corresponds with the exercise title in the book. Scroll through the list of clips until you find the video you want to watch. Select that clip and the full video will play.

I

ANATOMY AND BIOMECHANICS OF THE SHOULDER COMPLEX

The shoulder is one of the most complex joints in the human body, with perhaps the greatest overall range of motion used in human function. Clinicians must thoroughly understand both the key anatomical structures and the biomechanical function of the shoulder complex to optimally design evaluation sequences and evidence-based treatment progressions. Part I provides this key baseline information on anatomy and biomechanics of the shoulder complex, as well as an overview of some key sport biomechanics and pathomechanics, to facilitate high-level understanding of the demands of sport activity patterns on the shoulder that produce injuries in overhead athletes particularly. Understanding the information in part I will prepare the reader for the examination and treatment sections that form parts II through IV.

Functional Anatomy of the Shoulder Complex

The glenohumeral joint is commonly dislocated (Kazar & Relouszky 1969, Rowe & Zarins 1981, Simonet & Cofield 1981), especially in contact and collision sports (Hovelius et al. 2008, Mazocca et al. 2005). The fact that the shoulder is frequently dislocated and frequently injured could be partially attributed to the unique anatomy of the glenohumeral joint, which is more suited for mobility than stability. Additionally, shoulder injuries are common in overhead sports. Conte and colleagues (2001) reported that 28% of all injuries occurred to the glenohumeral joint in professional baseball players. Posner and colleagues (2011) stated that 31% of days on the disabled list in professional baseball were due to shoulder joint injuries in the pitcher. Kovacs and colleagues (2014) surveyed over 800 elite junior tennis players and found that the shoulder was the most injured joint or area in players in the 12- and 14-year-old competitive divisions (23-25%) and was the second most frequently injured area among players in the 16-year-old division (11%), second only to lower back injuries. The anatomy of the glenohumeral joint is unique and worth detailed discussion.

JOINT STRUCTURE

The glenohumeral joint is the most complex joint in the human body. The glenohumeral joint combined with the scapulothoracic, sternoclavicular, and acromioclavicular joints composes the shoulder joint complex. All these joints are critical to normal pain-free function. The glenohumeral joint has the greatest amount of motion of any joint in the human body.

The overall function of the upper extremity is related to the shoulder complex, with the ultimate purpose of this mechanism being the placement and full use of the hand. The joint mechanisms of the limb permit the placement, functioning, and control of the hand directly in front of the body, where the functions can be observed (Kelley 1971). Some movements of the hand are controlled by the shoulder complex, which positions and directs the humerus; the elbow, which positions the hand in relation to the trunk; and the radioulnar joints, which determine the position of the palm (Dempster 1965, DePalma 1973). Sports that involve actions such as throwing, using a racket, and swimming require excessive glenohumeral joint motion. For example, the excessive motion required to throw a baseball is accomplished through the integrated and synchronized motion of the various joints in the upper quadrant, most significantly the glenohumeral and scapulothoracic joints, with the thoracic and lumbar spine contributing to the motion (Fleisig et al. 1995).

The shoulder complex provides the upper limb with a range of motion exceeding that of any other joint mechanism (Bateman 1971). This range of motion is greater than that required for most daily functional activities. For example, use of the hand in limited activities of daily living is possible when the shoulder complex is immobilized with the humerus held by the side. Compensation for absent shoulder motion is provided by the cervical spine, elbow, wrist, and finger joint mechanisms (Bateman 1971, Bechtol 1980).

The shoulder complex consists of four joints that function in a precise, coordinated, synchronous manner. Position changes of the arm involve movements of the clavicle, scapula, and humerus. These movements are the direct result of the complex mechanism composed of the sternoclavicular, acromioclavicular, and glenohumeral joints and the scapulothoracic gliding mechanism (Bechtol 1980, Inman et al. 1944, Warwick & Williams 1973).

Sternoclavicular Joint

The sternoclavicular joint is the only joint connecting the shoulder complex to the axial skeleton (Moore 1980, Perry 1973). Although the structure of this synovial joint is classified as a plane, its function most closely resembles a ball-and-socket articulation (Abbott & Lucas 1954, Warwick & Williams 1973). The articular surfaces lack congruity. Approximately one-half of the large, rounded medial end of the clavicle protrudes above the shallow sternal socket. An intra-articular disc is attached to the upper portion of this nonarticular segment of the clavicle. The articular surface is saddle-shaped, anteroposteriorly concave, and downwardly convex (Dempster 1965, Ljungren 1979, Warwick & Williams 1973).

The medial end of the clavicle is bound to the sternum, the first rib, and its costal cartilage. Ligaments strengthen the capsule anteriorly, posteriorly, superiorly, and inferiorly. The main structures stabilizing the joint, resisting the tendency for medial displacement of the clavicle and limiting clavicular movement, are the articular disc and the costoclavicular ligament (figure 1.1) (Bearn 1967, Warwick & Williams 1973).

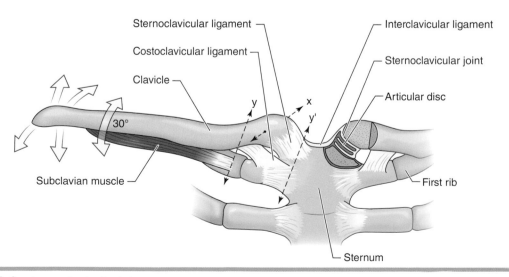

Sternoclavicular ligament

Costoclavicular ligament

Clavicle

Subclavian muscle

Interclavicular ligament

Sternoclavicular joint

Articular disc

First rib

Sternum

Figure 1.1 Sternoclavicular joint.

The articular disc is a strong, almost circular fibrocartilage that completely divides the joint cavity (Moseley 1968). The disc is attached superiorly to the upper medial end of the clavicle and passes downward between the articular surfaces to the sternum and first costal cartilage (Warwick & Williams 1973). This arrangement permits the disc to function as a hinge, a mechanism that contributes to the total range of joint movement. The areas of compression between the articular surfaces and intra-articular disc vary with movements of the clavicle. During elevation and depression, most motion occurs between the clavicle and articular disc. During protraction and retraction, the greatest movement occurs between the articular disc and the sternal articular surface (Dempster 1965). The combination of taut ligaments, pressure on the disc, and articular surfaces is important for maintaining stability in the plane of motion.

The articular disc also stabilizes the joint against forces applied to the shoulder, which are transmitted medially through the clavicle to the sternum. Without this attachment, the clavicle would tend to override the sternum, resulting in medial dislocation. Forces acting on the clavicle are most likely to cause fractures of the bone medial to the attachment of the coracoclavicular ligament but rarely cause dislocation of the sternoclavicular joint (Bateman 1971).

The costoclavicular ligament is a strong bilaminar structure attached to the inferior surface of the medial end of the clavicle and first rib. The anterior component of the ligament passes upward and laterally, the posterior aspect upward and medially. The ligament is a major stabilizing structure and strongly binds the medial end of the clavicle to the first rib. The ligament becomes taut when the arm is elevated or when the scapula is protracted (Warwick & Williams 1973).

The joint capsule is supported by oblique anterior and posterior sternoclavicular ligaments. Both ligaments pass downward and medially from the sternal end of the clavicle to the anterior and posterior surfaces of the manubrium and limit anteroposterior movement of the clavicle. An interclavicular ligament runs across the superior aspect of the sternoclavicular joint, joining the medial ends of the clavicles. This ligament, with deep fibers attached to the upper margin of the manubrium, provides stability to the superior aspect of the joint (Moore 1980, Warwick & Williams 1973).

The sternoclavicular joint allows elevation and depression, protraction and retraction, and long-axis rotation of the clavicle. The axis for both angular movements lies close to the clavicular attachment of the costoclavicular ligament (Moore 1980).

Acromioclavicular Joint

The acromioclavicular joint is a synovial plane joint between the small, convex, oval facet on the lateral end of the clavicle and a concave area on the anterior part of the medial border of the acromion process of the scapula (Moore 1980, Warwick & Williams 1973). The joint line is oblique and slightly curved. The curvature of the joint permits the acromion, and thus the scapula, to glide forward or backward over the lateral end of the clavicle. This movement keeps the glenoid fossa continually facing the humeral head. The oblique nature of the joint is such that forces transmitted through the arm tend to drive the acromion process under the lateral end of the clavicle, with the clavicle overriding the acromion (figure 1.2). The joint also contains a fibrocartilaginous disc that is variable in size and does not completely separate the joint into two compartments (Moore 1980, Moseley 1968). The acromioclavicular joint is important because it contributes to total arm movement in addition to transmitting forces between the clavicle and acromion (Kent 1971, Warwick & Williams 1973).

The acromioclavicular joint has a capsule and superior acromioclavicular ligament that strengthen the upper aspect of the joint (Abbott & Lucas 1954, Warwick & Williams 1973). The main ligamentous structure stabilizing the joint and binding the clavicle to the scapula is the coracoclavicular ligament.

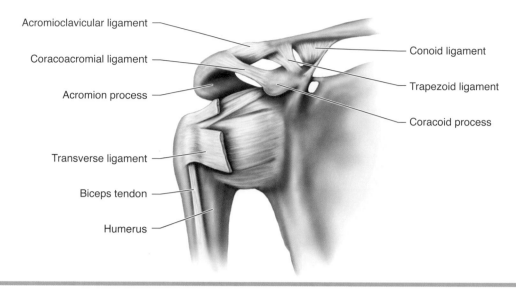

Acromioclavicular ligament

Coracoacromial ligament

Acromion process

Conoid ligament

Trapezoid ligament

Coracoid process

Transverse ligament

Biceps tendon

Humerus

Figure 1.2 Acromioclavicular joint.

Although this ligament is placed medially and is separate from the joint, it forms the most efficient means of preventing the clavicle from losing contact with the acromion (Bateman 1971, Frankel & Nordin 1980, Inman et al. 1944, Kent 1971, Moore 1980, Warwick & Williams 1973).

The coracoclavicular ligament consists of two parts, the trapezoid and the conoid. These two components, functionally and anatomically distinct, are united at their corresponding borders. Anteriorly, the space between the ligaments is filled with adipose tissue and, frequently, a bursa. A bursa also lies between the medial end of the coracoid process and the inferior surface of the clavicle. In up to 30% of subjects, these bony components may be opposed closely and may form a coracoclavicular joint (Dempster 1965, Frankel & Nordin 1980). The coracoclavicular ligament suspends the scapula from the clavicle and transmits the force of the upper fibers of the trapezius to the scapula (Dempster 1965).

The trapezoid ligament, the anterolateral component of the coracoclavicular ligament, is broad, thin, and quadrilateral. It is attached from below to the superior surface of the coracoid process. The ligament passes laterally almost horizontally in the frontal plane and is attached to the trapezoid

line on the inferior surface of the clavicle (Moore 1980, Warwick & Williams 1973). The primary function of this ligament is to prevent overriding of the clavicle on the acromion (Bateman 1971, Kessler & Hertling 1983). The conoid ligament is located partly posteriorly and medially to the trapezoid ligament. It is thick and triangular, with its base attached from above to the conoid tubercle on the inferior surface of the clavicle. The apex, which is directed downward, is attached to the "knuckle" of the coracoid process (i.e., medial and posterior edge of the root of the process). The conoid ligament is oriented vertically and twisted on itself (Kessler & Hertling 1983, Warwick & Williams 1973). The ligament limits upward movement of the clavicle on the acromion. When the arm is elevated, the rotation of the scapula causes the coracoid process to move and increases the distance between the clavicle and coracoid process. This movement increases the tension on the conoid ligament, resulting in dorsal (posterior) axial rotation of the clavicle. Viewed from above, the clavicle has a shape resembling a crank. The taut coracoclavicular ligament acts on the outer curvature of the crank-like clavicle and effects a rotation of the clavicle on its long axis (Abbott & Lucas 1954, Dvir & Berme 1978). This clavicular rotation allows the scapula to continue to rotate and increase the degree of arm elevation. During full elevation of the arm, the clavicle rotates 50° axially (Abbott & Lucas 1954). When the clavicle is prevented from rotating, the arm can be abducted actively to only 120° (Inman et al. 1944, Warwick & Williams 1973).

Movement of the acromioclavicular joint is an important component of total arm movement. A principal role of the joint in the elevation of the arm is to permit continued lateral rotation of the scapula after about 100° of abduction when sternoclavicular movement is restrained by the sternoclavicular joint ligaments. The acromioclavicular joint has three degrees of freedom. Movement can occur between the acromion and lateral end of the clavicle about a vertical axis, around a frontal axis, or about a sagittal axis. Functionally, the two main movements at the acromioclavicular joint, however, are a gliding movement as the shoulder joint flexes and extends and an elevation and depression movement to conform to changes in the relation between the scapula and humerus during abduction (Bateman 1971, Frankel & Nordin 1980, Moore 1980).

Glenohumeral Joint

The glenohumeral joint is a multiaxial ball-and-socket synovial joint. This type of joint geometry permits a tremendous amount of motion; however, the inherent stability is minimal (figure 1.3). The articular surfaces, head of the humerus, and glenoid fossa of the scapula, although reciprocally curved, are oval and are not sections of true spheres (Warwick & Williams 1973). Because the head of the humerus is larger than the glenoid fossa, only part of the humeral head can be in articulation with the glenoid fossa in any position of the joint. At any given time, only 25% to 30% of the humeral head is in contact with the glenoid fossa (Bost & Inman 1942, Codman 1934, Steindler 1955). The surfaces are not congruent, and the joint is loose-packed. Full congruence and the close-packed position are obtained when the humerus is in full elevation (Gagey et al. 1987, Johnston 1937).

The design characteristics of the joint are typical of an incongruous joint. The surfaces are asymmetrical; the joint has a movable axis of rotation; and muscles related to the

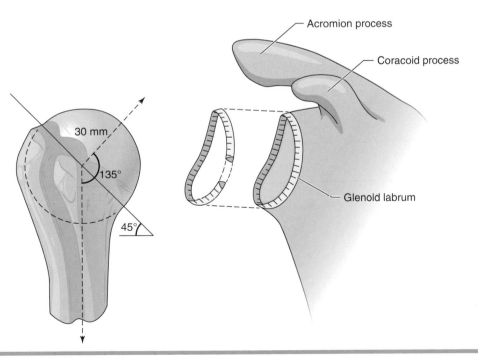

Figure 1.3 Glenohumeral joint.

joint are essential in maintaining stability of the articulation (Moore 1980). The humeral articular surface has a radius of curvature of 35 to 55 mm. The humeral head and neck make an angle of 130° to 150° with the shaft and are retroverted about 20° to 30° with respect to the transverse axis of the elbow (Norkin & Levangie 1983, Sarrafian 1983).

The topic of retroversion has received increased attention because of the implications of its effect on glenohumeral joint motion. Nowhere is this point more evident than with the overhead athlete, who exhibits excessive external rotation and a limitation of internal rotation. Crockett and colleagues (2002) have studied professional baseball pitchers and noted a bilateral difference in humeral retroversion. The investigators noted a 17° difference, with the throwing shoulder exhibiting greater external rotation and loss of internal rotation. This difference was not observed in the control group of non–overhead throwing athletes. Other investigators have also reported bilateral differences in retroversion in overhead athletes, in whom the throwing side exhibits greater retroversion (Osbahr et al. 2002, Pieper 1998, Reagan et al. 2002).

The glenoid fossa is somewhat pear-shaped and resembles an inverted comma (figure 1.4). The surface area is 25% to 33%, the vertical diameter 75%, and the transverse diameter 55% of that of the humeral head (Sarrafian 1983). In 75% of subjects, the glenoid fossa is retroverted an average of 7.4° in relation to the plane of the scapula (Saha 1971, 1973). Furthermore, the glenoid fossa has a slight upward tilt of about 5° with reference to the medial border of the scapula (Basmajian & Bazant 1959); this is referred to as the **inclination angle**. It was suggested that this relation is important in maintaining horizontal stability of the joint and counteracting any tendency toward anterior displacement of the humeral head (Saha 1971, 1973, Sarrafian 1983). However, this concept has not been supported by subsequent studies (Cyprien et al. 1983, Randelli & Gambrioli 1986). The articular cartilage lining the glenoid fossa is thickest in the periphery and thinnest in the central region.

Because of the amount of pathology involving the acromion and head of the humerus, the acromion has been studied extensively. Bigliani and colleagues (1986) have classified the shapes of the acromion into three categories. Type I acromions are those with a flat undersurface and have the lowest risk for impingement syndrome and its sequelae. Type II acromions have a curved undersurface, and type III acromions have a hooked undersurface (figure 1.5). Type III has the highest correlation with impingement syndromes, rotator cuff pathologies, or both. Nicholson and associates

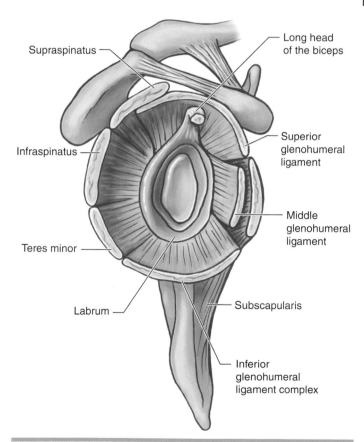

Figure 1.4 Glenoid fossa with labrum and surrounding capsular ligaments and tendons.

Supraspinatus

Long head of the biceps

Infraspinatus

Superior glenohumeral ligament

Teres minor

Middle glenohumeral ligament

Labrum

Subscapularis

Inferior glenohumeral ligament complex

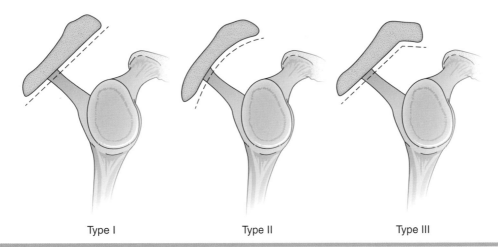

| Type I | Type II | Type III |

Figure 1.5 Acromial morphology.

(1996) have reported that the shape of the acromion is congenital and does not develop over time. The acromions have epiphyses and occasionally may not fuse, leading to acromion deformity, often referred to as os acromiale (Lieberson 1937).

Scapulothoracic Joint

The resting position of the scapula in reference to the trunk is anteriorly rotated about 30° to 40° (Laumann 1987, Saha 1983, Steindler 1955) with respect to the frontal plane as viewed from above. This has been referred to as the scapular plane. The scapula is also rotated upward about 3° and tilted forward approximately 20° (Laumann 1987, Morrey & An 1990). The position of the scapula is significantly influenced by posture, soft tissue tightness, muscle activity, and fatigue. These concepts are discussed in detail later (chapter 2). It is important to note here that the ideal movements of the scapula with arm elevation are posterior tilt, external rotation, and upward rotation.

The scapula plays a vital role in normal shoulder function and serves as the attachment site of critically important muscular structures that govern and dictate both glenohumeral and scapulothoracic joint function. These muscles are discussed in detail later in this chapter, as a complete understanding of both normal and abnormal scapulothoracic joint motion and rhythm is critical to the comprehensive evaluation of the patient with shoulder pathology. Normal scapulohumeral motion and rhythm are required for pain-free normal shoulder function.

MUSCLE ANATOMY

Unique to the shoulder is a large dependence on muscular or dynamic stabilization. It is important that the clinician fully understand the key muscular structures and their function and role in the force couples of the glenohumeral and scapulothoracic joints.

Rotator Cuff

The rotator cuff is the musculotendinous complex formed by the attachment to the capsule of the supraspinatus muscle superiorly, the subscapularis muscle anteriorly, and the teres minor and infraspinatus muscles posteriorly. These tendons blend intricately with the fibrous capsule and the adjacent rotator cuff tendon (Clark & Harryman 1992). They provide active support for the joint and can be considered true dynamic ligaments that provide dynamic stability (Inman et al. 1944). The capsule is less well protected inferiorly because the tendon of the long head of the triceps brachii muscle is separated from the capsule by the axillary nerve and posterior circumflex humeral artery (Warwick & Williams 1973).

The rotator cuff tendons insert into a large contact point onto the greater and lesser tuberosities of the humerus and not a small insertion point, as was once thought. Dugas and associates (2002) reported that the rotator cuff inserts less than 1 mm from the articular margin. Curtis and coworkers (2006) later reported that the insertional anatomy in cadaveric shoulders exhibits a consistent pattern and noted interdigitation of the muscles, particularly between the supraspinatus and infraspinatus. The average insertional lengths and widths for the rotator cuff muscles were as follows: supraspinatus 23 ± 16 mm, subscapularis 40 ± 20 mm, infraspinatus 29 ± 19 mm, and teres minor 29 ± 11 mm. Bassett and colleagues (1990) have studied the cross-sectional area of the rotator cuff muscles as they cross the glenohumeral joint capsule. They found that the larger the cross-sectional area, the more significant the contribution to shoulder stability. Miller and associates (2003) described a space between the supraspinatus and infraspinatus and referred to this area as the posterior rotator cuff interval. They went on to discuss the importance of releasing this area when rotator cuff repairs are performed in specific types of patients who exhibit supraspinatus retraction and scarring.

It is generally accepted that the deltoid and the rotator cuff muscles are prime movers of glenohumeral abduction (Comtet et al. 1989, DeLuca & Forrest 1973, Howell et al. 1986). These muscles have been found to contribute equally to torque production in functional planes of motion (Howell et al. 1986). With the arm at the side, the directional force of the deltoid muscle is almost vertical (Lucas 1973, Sarrafian 1983). Thus, most of the deltoid force causes a superior shear force of the humeral head that, if unopposed, would cause the humeral head to contact the coracoacromial arch, resulting in impingement of soft tissues (Poppen & Walker 1978). The force vectors of the infraspinatus, subscapularis, and teres minor muscles are such that each tends to have a compressive component as well as a rotational force (Morrey & An 1990, Poppen & Walker 1978). Each muscle's compressive force offsets the superior shear force of the deltoid (Morrey & An 1990). The infraspinatus, teres minor, and subscapularis thus form a force couple with the deltoid and act to stabilize the humeral head on the glenoid fossa, allowing the deltoid and supraspinatus to act as abductors of the humerus (Saha 1983) (figure 1.6). As a result, the rotator cuff muscles are often called the **compressive cuff**. In studies on a mechanical model, Comtet and coworkers (1989) have determined that the depressor forces are at their maximum between 60° and 80° of elevation and disappear beyond 120°. The supraspinatus has a small superior shear component, but its main function is compression because of the horizontal orientation of the muscle fibers (Morrey & An 1990); thus, it opposes the upward superior shear action of the deltoid.

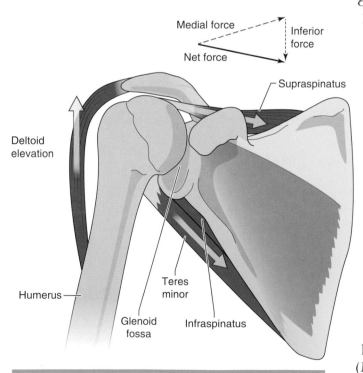

Figure 1.6 The rotator cuff and deltoid force couple.

Lesions of the rotator cuff mechanism can occur as a response to repetitious activity over time or to overload activity that causes a spontaneous lesion (Brewer 1979). Stress applied to a previously degenerated rotator cuff may cause the cuff to rupture. Often, this stress also tears the articular capsule, resulting in a communication between the joint cavity and subacromial bursa. Rotator cuff tears result in considerably reduced force of elevation of the glenohumeral joint. In attempting to elevate the arm, the patient shrugs the shoulder. If the arm is abducted passively to 90°, the patient should be able to maintain the arm in the abducted position (Moore 1980).

The space between the supraspinatus and superior border of subscapularis has been termed the **rotator interval**. This space is triangular, with its base located medially at the coracoid process. The rotator interval contains the coracohumeral ligament, superior glenohumeral ligament, glenohumeral capsule, and biceps tendon (Fitzpatrick et al. 2003, Harryman et al. 1992, Hunt et al. 2007, Nobuhara & Ikeda 1987). The medial aspect consists of two layers, and the lateral portion is composed of four layers. The superficial layer of the medial rotator interval is composed of the coracohumeral ligament, and the deep layer consists of the superior glenohumeral ligament and joint capsule. The coracohumeral ligament also represents the superficial layer of the lateral portion of the rotator interval. The second layer is composed of the fibers of the supraspinatus and subscapularis. The third layer consists of the deep fibers of the coracohumeral ligament, and the fourth layer is the superior glenohumeral ligament and lateral capsule (Hunt et al. 2007, Jost et al. 2000). The size of the rotator cuff interval varies. The larger the interval, the greater the inferior and posterior laxity (Harryman et al. 1992).

The function of the long head of the biceps is controversial. Some believe that it contributes to the stability of the glenohumeral joint by preventing upward migration of the head of the humerus during powerful elbow flexion and forearm supination. Lesions of the long head of the biceps, therefore, may produce instability and shoulder dysfunction (Kumar et al. 1989). Conversely, other physicians (Boileau et al. 2007, Kelly et al. 2005, Walch et al. 2005) have reported performing biceps tenotomy in patients with refractory biceps pain. Once the biceps was released, pain was eliminated in over 70% of patients and no functional limitations, instability, or weakness was reported. Thus, the function of the proximal long head of the biceps brachii is still being debated.

Scapular Stabilizers

Numerous muscles about the scapula play a critical role in accomplishing a stabilizing function (figure 1.7). The trapezius muscle is the largest and most superficial scapulothoracic muscle. This muscle originates from the medial superior nuchal line, external protuberance of the occiput, and ligamentum nuchae as well as the spinous processes of the C7 through T12 vertebrae. The muscle is classified into upper, middle, and lower fibers. Insertion of the upper fibers is over the distal third of the clavicle. The lower cervical and upper thorax fibers insert over the acromion and spine of the scapula. The lower portion of the trapezius inserts into the base of the spine of the scapula.

The rhomboids function similarly to the midportion of the trapezius (Inman et al. 1944). The origin of the rhomboids is from the lower ligamentum nuchae, C7 and T1 for the rhomboid minor, and T2 through T5 for the rhomboid major. The rhomboid minor inserts onto the posterior portion of the medial base of the spine of the scapula. The rhomboid major inserts onto the medial border of the scapula. The levator scapulae muscle proceeds from its origin on the transverse processes from C1 through C3 (and sometimes C4) and inserts onto the superior angle of the scapula.

The serratus anterior takes its origin from the ribs on the lateral wall of the thoracic cage. The serratus has three divisions: upper, middle, and lower. The upper fibers originate from ribs 1 and 2, the middle fibers from

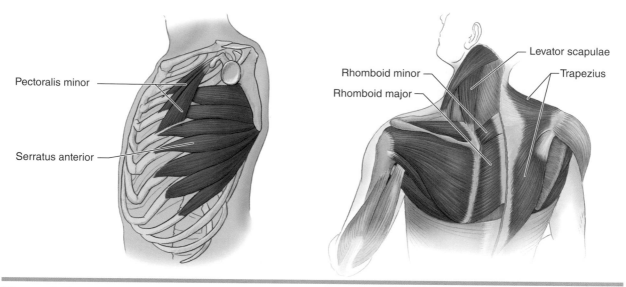

Figure 1.7 Scapular musculature.

ribs 2 through 4, and the lower from ribs 5 through 9. The serratus anterior muscle orientation is in individual slips from each rib. The serratus inserts onto the superior angle, medial border, and inferior angle of the scapula, respectively.

The pectoralis minor runs from the second through fifth ribs upward to the medial base of the coracoid. Somewhat frequently (approximately 15% incidence), there is an aberrant slip from the pectoralis minor to the humerus, glenoid, clavicle, or scapula (Lambert 1925, Vare & Indurak 1965). The subclavius muscle is a small muscle that originates from the first rib and inserts as a muscle onto the inferior surface of the medial third of the clavicle. This muscle stabilizes the sternoclavicular joint.

ADDITIONAL ANATOMICAL STRUCTURES

Several anatomical structures that play a vital role in shoulder function and structure are now discussed to allow the clinician to have a deeper understanding of the role these structures play in both abnormal and pathologic shoulder conditions.

Glenoid Labrum

The total surface of the humeral head is approximately four times larger than that of the glenoid, contributing to the tremendous joint mobility available at the glenohumeral joint. Glenohumeral stability is the result of the interplay between multiple anatomical structures that include the capsule, ligaments, muscles, tendons, osseous configuration, and glenoid labrum. Each of these elements contributes in controlling glenohumeral joint translation via a sophisticated biomechanical system that allows the shoulder to function successfully as the most mobile joint of the human body. The glenoid labrum plays an important role in this process (O'Brien et al. 1998, Resch et al. 1993, Wilk & Arrigo 1993). Perry (1973) demonstrated that the depth of the glenoid fossa across its equatorial line is doubled, from 2.5 to 5 mm, by the presence of the labrum.

The labrum is a fibrous structure strongly attached around the edge of the glenoid that serves to increase the contact surface area between the glenoid and the humeral head (Cooper et al. 1992). Although it is commonly stated that the glenoid labrum consists mainly of fibrous cartilage (Bost

& Inman 1942, Codman 1934, DePalma et al. 1949), some studies have shown that it is composed of dense fibrous collagen tissue (Cooper et al. 1992, Moseley & Overgaard 1962). Moseley and Overgaard (1962) also noted that the superior and inferior labrum exhibit significantly different anatomy and that the labrum changes appearance in varying degrees of humeral rotation. The superior labrum is rather loose and mobile and has a "meniscal" aspect, while the inferior labrum appears rounded and more tightly attached to the glenoid rim. Histologically, the attachment of the labrum to the glenoid rim consists of loose connective fibers above the equator of the glenoid, while the inferior portion of the labral attachment is fixed by inelastic fibrous tissue (Cooper et al. 1992). The labrum is attached to the lateral portion of the biceps anchor superiorly. Additionally, approximately 50% of the fibers of the long head of the biceps brachii originate from the superior labrum, and the remaining fibers originate from the supraglenoid tubercle of the glenoid (Cooper et al. 1992). The fibers of the biceps tendon blend with the superior labrum continuing posteriorly to become a periarticular fiber bundle, making up the bulk of the labrum (Huber & Putz 1997). The anterosuperior labral fibers appear to be attached more to the middle and inferior glenohumeral ligaments rather than directly to the glenoid rim itself.

Vascular supply to the labrum arises mostly from its peripheral attachment to the capsule and is from a combination of the suprascapular, circumflex scapular branch of the subscapular, and the posterior circumflex humeral arteries (Cooper et al. 1992). The anterosuperior labrum appears to generally have poor blood supply, whereas the inferior labrum exhibits significant blood flow (Cooper et al. 1992). Vascularity of the labrum decreases with increasing age (Cooper et al. 1992).

The glenoid labrum enhances shoulder stability by

- producing a "chock-block" effect between the glenoid and the humeral head that serves to limit humeral head translation (Cooper et al. 1992, O'Brien et al. 1998, Wilk 1999, Wilk & Arrigo 1993),

- increasing the "concavity–compression" effect between the humeral head and the glenoid (Cooper et al. 1992, Mileski & Snyder 1998, O'Brien et al. 1998, Wilk 1999, Wilk & Arrigo 1993),

- contributing to the stabilizing effect of the long head of the biceps anchor (Resch et al. 1993, Wilk 1999, Wilk & Arrigo 1993), and

- increasing the overall depth of the glenoid fossa (Cooper et al. 1992, Wilk 1999, Wilk & Arrigo 1993).

The inner surface of the labrum is covered with synovium; the outer surface attaches to the capsule and is continuous with the periosteum of the scapular neck. The shape of the labrum adapts to accommodate rotation of the humeral head, adding flexibility to the edges of the glenoid fossa. The tendons of the long head of the biceps brachii muscle contribute to the structure and reinforcement of the labrum. The long head of the biceps brachii attaches to the superior region of the labrum. The width and thickness of the glenoid labrum vary. The anterior labrum appears thicker and at times larger than the posterior labrum.

It has been suggested (Moseley & Overgaard 1962) that the labrum protects the edges of the glenoid, assists in lubrication of the joint, and deepens the glenoid cavity, thus contributing to stability of the joint (Bateman 1971, Moore 1980, Perry 1983, Warwick & Williams 1973). Others have stated that the labrum does not increase the depth of the concave surface substantially, and that the glenoid labrum is no more than a fold of capsule composed of dense fibrous connective tissue that stretches out anteriorly with external rotation and posteriorly with internal rotation of the humerus (Moseley & Overgaard 1962). The main function of the labrum may be to serve as an attachment for the glenohumeral ligaments (Moseley & Overgaard 1962, Warwick & Williams 1973). When that attachment is compromised, it represents a Bankart lesion, in which the capsular–labral complex is detached from the glenoid rim (see figure 4.6 in chapter 4).

Coracohumeral Ligament

The coracohumeral ligament is an important ligamentous structure in the shoulder complex (Basmajian & Bazant 1959). The ligament is attached to the base and lateral border of the coracoid process and passes obliquely downward and laterally to the humerus, blending with the supraspinatus muscle and the capsule. Laterally, the ligament separates into two components that insert into the greater and lesser tuberosities, creating a tunnel through which the biceps tendon passes (Ferrari 1990). Inferiorly, the coracohumeral ligament blends with the superior glenohumeral ligament. The anterior border of the ligament is distinct medially and merges with the capsule laterally. The posterior border is indistinct and blends with the capsule (Moore 1980, Warwick & Williams 1973).

It has been suggested that the downward pull of gravity on an adducted arm is counteracted largely by the superior capsule, coracohumeral ligament, and inferior glenohumeral ligament (Ferrari 1990, Turkel et al. 1981). As the arm is abducted, the restraining force is shifted to the inferior structures and the primary restraining force is the inferior glenohumeral ligament (Brown & Warren 1991). Because the coracohumeral ligament is located anteriorly to the vertical axis about which the humerus rotates axially, the ligament checks lateral rotation during arm elevation between 0° and 60°. When the humerus, in a position of neutral rotation, is elevated in the sagittal plane, the movement is limited to approximately 75° by the coracohumeral ligament. For elevation to continue, the humerus is medially rotated and moves toward the scapular plane by the dynamic tension in this ligament (Gagey et al. 1987).

Glenohumeral Ligaments

The three glenohumeral ligaments lie on the anterior and inferior aspect of the joint. They are described as thickened parts of the capsule (figure 1.8). The superior gleno-

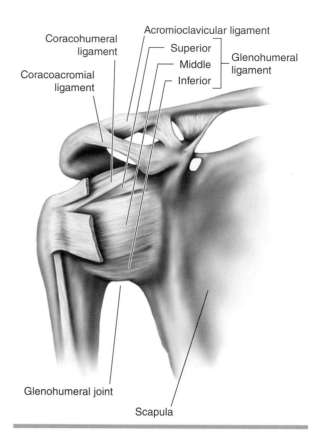

Figure 1.8 Anterior view of the glenohumeral ligaments.

humeral ligament passes laterally from the superior glenoid tubercle, upper part of the glenoid labrum, and base of the coracoid process to the humerus, between the upper part of the lesser tuberosity and anatomic neck (Ferrari 1990, Turkel et al. 1981). The ligament lies anterior to and partly under the coracohumeral ligament. The superior glenohumeral ligament, together with the superior joint capsule and rotator cuff muscles, assists in preventing downward displacement of the humeral head (Schwartz et al. 1987, Turkel et al. 1981).

The middle glenohumeral ligament has a wide attachment, extending from the superior glenohumeral ligament along the anterior margin of the glenoid fossa down as far as the junction of the middle and inferior thirds of the glenoid rim (Turkel et al. 1981). From this attachment, the ligament passes laterally, gradually enlarges, and attaches to the anterior aspect of the anatomic neck and lesser tuberosity of the humerus. The ligament lies under the tendon of the subscapularis muscle and is intimately attached to it (Ferrari 1990, Sarrafian 1983). Note the large variation in size of the middle glenohumeral ligament; it can be 2 cm wide but is absent in some individuals. This structure exhibits the greatest amount of structural variation of the glenohumeral ligaments. The middle glenohumeral ligament and subscapularis tendon limit lateral rotation from 45° to 75° of abduction and are important anterior stabilizers of the glenohumeral joint, particularly effective in the lower to middle ranges of abduction.

The inferior glenohumeral ligament is the thickest of the glenohumeral structures and is the most important stabilizing structure of the shoulder in the overhead athlete. The ligament attaches to the anterior, inferior, and posterior margins of the glenoid labrum and passes laterally to the inferior aspects of the anatomic and surgical necks of the humerus (Sarrafian 1983, Warwick & Williams 1973). The ligament can be divided into three distinct portions—the anterior band, axillary pouch, and posterior band (figure 1.9) (O'Brien et al. 1990). The inferior part is thinner and broader and is termed the **axillary pouch**. The anterior band strengthens the capsule anteriorly and supports the joint most effectively in the upper ranges (more than 75°) of abduction (O'Brien et al. 1990). The anterior band of the inferior glenohumeral ligament provides a broad buttress-like support for the anterior and inferior aspects of the joint, preventing subluxation in the upper part of the range (Turkel et al. 1981).

O'Brien and associates (1990) have demonstrated that with the arm abducted to 90° and externally rotated, the anterior band of the inferior glenohumeral ligament complex wraps around the humeral head like a hammock to prevent anterior humeral head migration. This structure provides stability during the throwing motion, tennis serve motion, freestyle stroke, or any overhead arm position.

Tightening of the inferior glenohumeral ligament during coronal plane abduction limits elevation to an average of 90°. To continue to elevate, the humerus must move toward the scapular plane and laterally

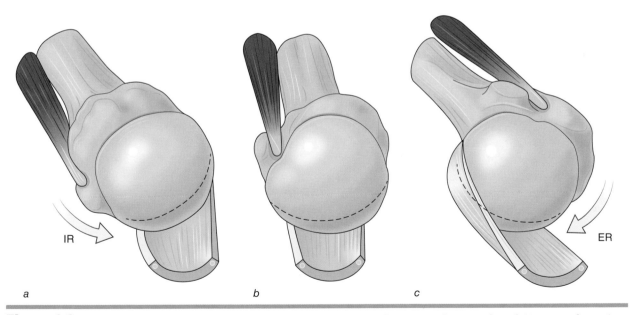

IR   ER

a   b   c

Figure 1.9 The inferior glenohumeral ligament complex: *(a)* internal rotation, *(b)* neutral, and *(c)* external rotation.

From O'Brien, S. J., Neves, M. C., Arnoczky, S. P., Rozbruck, S. R., Dicarlo, E. F., Warren, R. F., Schwartz, R., Wickiewica, T. L. (1990). The anatomy and histology of the inferior glenohumeral ligament complex of the shoulder. *The American Journal of Sports Medicine* Vol. 18(5) pp. 449-456. Copyright © 1990 by American Orthopaedic Society for Sports Medicine. Adapted by permission of SAGE Publications, Inc.

(externally) rotate. Gagey and coworkers (1987) have stated that both movements occur because of dynamic tension in the inferior glenohumeral ligament.

The coracohumeral and glenohumeral ligaments viewed from the front form a Z pattern. This arrangement creates potential areas of capsular weakness above and below the middle glenohumeral ligament. The subscapularis bursa communicates with the joint cavity through the superior opening, or foramen of Weitbrecht, between the superior and middle glenohumeral ligaments. Ferrari (1990) has also reported the presence of an inferior subscapular bursa, between the middle and inferior glenohumeral ligaments. This bursa was present in all 14 specimens in those younger than 55 years and could be seen up to the age of 75 years. When the middle glenohumeral ligament is attenuated or absent, this anterior defect is enhanced and may contribute to anterior instability of the joint (Ferrari 1990).

Inside the glenohumeral joint capsule is negative pressure in comparison with outside the joint capsule. This is referred to as negative intra-articular pressure and provides a stabilizing effect on the shoulder joint (Hurchler et al. 2000). Wulker and colleagues (1995) have demonstrated that venting the capsule (creating a cut into the capsule, thus eliminating the negative intra-articular pressure) may increase translation of the humerus on the glenoid by 19% to 50%.

Capsule

The capsule itself surrounds the joint and is attached medially to the margin of the glenoid fossa beyond the labrum. Laterally, it is attached to the circumference of the anatomic neck, and the attachment descends about 1/2 inch (1.3 cm) onto the shaft of the humerus. The capsule is loose-fitting, allowing the joint surfaces to be separated 2 to 3 mm by a distractive force (Warwick & Williams 1973). Matsen and colleagues (1991) have shown 22 mm inferior, 6 mm anterior, and 7 mm posterior translation in normal subjects. The capsule is relatively thin and, by itself, would contribute little to the stability of the joint. The integrity of the capsule and maintenance of the normal glenohumeral relationship depend on the reinforcement of the capsule by ligaments and attachment of the muscle tendons of the rotator cuff mechanism (Frankel & Nordin 1980, Moore 1980, Warwick & Williams 1973).

The superior part of the capsule, together with the superior glenohumeral ligament, is important in strengthening the superior aspect of the joint and resisting the effect of gravity on the dependent limb (Basmajian & Bazant 1959, Warwick & Williams 1973). Anteriorly, the capsule is strengthened by the anterior glenohumeral ligaments and attachment of the subscapularis tendon (Ovesen & Nielsen 1986a). Posteriorly, the capsule is strengthened by the attachment of the teres minor and infraspinatus tendons (Ovesen & Nielsen 1986b). Inferiorly, the capsule is relatively thin and weak and contributes little to the stability of the joint. The inferior part of the capsule is subjected to considerable strain because it is stretched tightly across the head of the humerus when the arm is elevated.

The inferior part of the capsule, the weakest area, is lax and lies in folds when the arm is adducted. Kaltsas (1983) has compared the collagen structure of the shoulder joint capsule with that of the elbow and hip. When the joint capsules were subjected to a mechanical force, the shoulder joint capsule showed a greater capacity to stretch than to rupture. When the capsule was tested to failure, the structure ruptured anteroinferiorly (Kaltsas 1983, Reeves 1968). Also, Reeves (1968) has demonstrated that the force required to cause glenohumeral joint dislocation is less in those younger than 20 years and greater in those older than 50 years.

Fealy and colleagues (2000) examined the glenohumeral joint in 51 fetal shoulders ranging from 9 to 40 weeks of gestation. The authors noted distinct capsules with ligaments present, especially a prominent inferior glenohumeral ligament complex. A coracohumeral ligament and rotator cuff interval were also present.

Johnston (1937) stated that, with the arm by the side, the capsular fibers are oriented with a forward and medial twist. This twist increases in abduction and decreases in flexion. The capsular tension in abduction compresses the humeral head into the glenoid fossa. As abduction progresses, the capsular tension exerts an external rotation moment. This external rotation untwists the capsule and allows further abduction. The external rotation of the humerus that occurs during coronal plane abduction may therefore be assisted by the configuration of the joint capsule (Johnston 1937).

The capsule is lined by a synovial membrane attached to the glenoid rim and anatomic neck inside the capsular attachments (Warwick & Williams 1973). The tendon of the long head of the biceps brachii muscle passes from the supraglenoid tubercle over the superior aspect of the head of the humerus and lies within the capsule, emerging from the joint at the intertubercular groove. The tendon is covered by a synovial sheath to facilitate movement of the tendon within the joint. The structure is susceptible to injury at the point at which the tendon arches over the humeral head and the surface on which it glides changes from bony cortex to articular cartilage (Bateman 1971).

Coracoacromial Arch

The coracoacromial ligament is triangular, with the base attached to the lateral border of the coracoid process (figure 1.10). The ligament passes upward, laterally, and slightly posteriorly to the superior aspect of the acromion process (Rothman et al. 1975, Warwick & Williams

1973). Superiorly, the ligament is covered by the deltoid muscle. Posteriorly, the ligament is continuous with the fascia that covers the supraspinatus muscle. Anteriorly, the coracoacromial ligament has a sharp, well-defined, free border. Together with the acromion and the coracoid processes, the ligament forms an important protective arch over the glenohumeral joint (Moore 1980). The arch forms a secondary restraining socket for the humeral head, protecting the joint from trauma from above and preventing upward dislocation of the humeral head. The supraspinatus muscle passes under the coracoacromial arch, lies between the deltoid muscle and the capsule of the glenohumeral joint, and blends with the capsule. The supraspinatus tendon is separated from the arch by the subacromial bursa (Moore 1980).

The space between the inferior acromion and head of the humerus (subacromial distance) has been measured on radiographs and is used as an indicator of proximal humeral subluxation (Petersson & Redlund-Johnell 1984, Weiner & Macnab 1970). The distance was found to be between 9 and 10 mm in 175 asymptomatic shoulders and was greater in men than in women

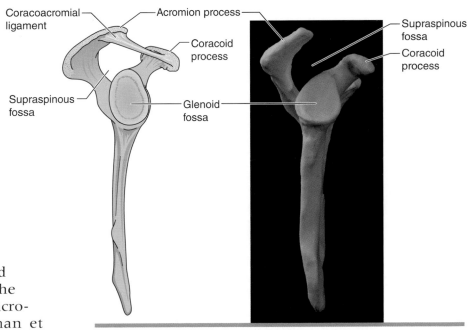

Figure 1.10   Coracoacromial arch.

(Petersson & Redlund-Johnell 1984). A distance of less than 6 mm was considered pathologic and was thought to be indicative of supraspinatus tendon attenuation or rupture (Petersson & Redlund-Johnell 1984).

During elevation, with internal rotation of the arm in abduction and flexion, the greater tuberosity (the supraspinatus tendon) of the humerus may apply pressure against the anterior edge and inferior surface of the anterior third of the acromion and coracoacromial ligament. This is in part because of the anterior orientation of the supraspinatus tendon. In some cases, the impingement also may occur against the acromioclavicular joint. This often occurs when the acromioclavicular joint exhibits degenerative joint disease or spurring or both. Most upper extremity functions are performed with the hand placed in front of the body, not lateral to it. When the arm is raised forward in flexion, the supraspinatus tendon passes under the anterior edge of the acromion and acromioclavicular joint. For this movement, the critical area for wear is centered on the supraspinatus tendon and also may involve the long head of the biceps brachii muscle.

Flatow and colleagues (1994) have examined the concept of impingement, compression between the supraspinatus and acromion. The investigators measured the distance between the undersurface of the acromion and humeral head at various degrees of abduction. At 0° adduction (arm at the side), the acromiohumeral space or interval was approximately 11 mm; at 90° of abduction it was 5.7 mm, and at 120° of abduction it was less than 5 mm (4.8 mm). Furthermore, the investigators placed Fuji contact film, which measures pressure per square area, on the acromion and humeral head. They found that with arm abduction from 60° to full elevation, there was contact between the acromion and humeral head. Therefore, Flatow and associates (1994) reported that contact between the humeral head and acromion is normal.

Bursae

Several bursae are found in the shoulder region (Warwick & Williams 1973). Two bursae particularly important to the clinician are the subacromial and subscapular bursae (Kent 1971). Other bursae located in relation to the glenohumeral joint structures are between the infraspinatus muscle and capsule, on the superior surface of the acromion, between the coracoid process and capsule, under the coracobrachialis muscle, between the teres major and long head of the triceps brachii muscles, and in front of and behind the tendon of the latissimus dorsi muscle. Because bursae are located where motion is required between adjacent structures, they have a major function in the shoulder mechanism. The subacromial bursa (figure 1.11) is located between the deltoid muscle and capsule, extending under the acromion and coracoacromial ligament and between them and the supraspinatus muscle. The bursa adheres to the coracoacromial ligament and to the acromion above and rotator cuff below. The bursa does not frequently communicate with the joint; however, a communication may develop if the rotator cuff is ruptured (Rothman et al. 1975). The subacromial bursa is important for allowing gliding between the acromion and deltoid muscle and rotator cuff. It also reduces friction on the supraspinatus tendon as it passes under the coracoacromial arch (Moore 1980, Rothman et al. 1975). Often, with repetitive overhead motion, the bursae may become inflamed and thickened, which may decrease the critical space in the subacromial region.

The subscapular bursa lies between the subscapularis tendon and neck of the scapula. It protects this tendon where it passes under the base of the coracoid process and over the neck of the scapula. The bursa communicates with the joint cavity between the superior and middle glenohumeral ligaments (Moore 1980, Turkel et al. 1981) and often between the middle and inferior glenohumeral ligaments (Ferrari 1990, Moseley & Overgaard 1962).

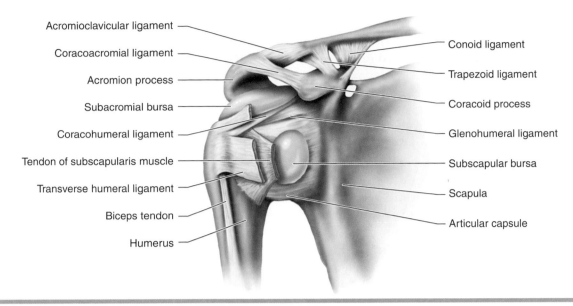

Figure 1.11 Bursae and ligaments of the shoulder complex.

NEUROVASCULAR ANATOMY

The rotator cuff is a frequent site of pathologic conditions, usually degenerative and often in response to fatigue stress (Kessler & Hertling 1983). Because degeneration may occur even with normal activity levels, the nutritional status of the glenohumeral structures is of great importance.

Vascular Supply

The blood supply to portions of the rotator cuff is from the circumflex scapular and suprascapular arteries (Warwick & Williams 1973). These arteries supply principally the infraspinatus and teres minor muscle areas of the cuff. The anterior aspect of the capsular ligamentous cuff is supplied by the anterior humeral circumflex artery and occasionally by the thoracoacromial, suprahumeral, and subscapular arteries. Superiorly, the supraspinatus muscle is supplied by the thoracoacromial artery. The supraspinatus tendon has a region of relative avascularity 1 cm proximal to the humeral insertion, often including its insertion into the humerus (Rathbun & Macnab 1970, Rothman & Parke 1965). Rothman and Parke (1965) have reported hypovascularity in the tendon in 63% of 72 shoulders studied. In a study by Rathbun and Macnab (1970), an avascular area was found in all specimens and was unrelated to age. Abduction of the arm resulted in relaxation of the tension on the supraspinatus muscle and complete filling of vessels throughout the tendon. In addition, with increasing age, the area of avascularity also increases (Brewer 1979); thus, the potential for healing decreases with age. The other cuff tendons generally demonstrate good vascularity, except for an occasional zone of hypovascularity in the superior portion of the insertion of the infraspinatus tendon (Rathbun & Macnab 1970, Rothman & Parke 1965).

Articular Neurology

Innervation of the shoulder region is derived from C5, C6, and C7; C4 also may add a minor contribution. The nerves supplying the ligaments, capsule, and synovial membrane are axillary, suprascapular, subscapular, and musculocutaneous nerves. Branches from the posterior cord of the brachial plexus also may supply the joint structures. Occasionally, the shoulder may receive a greater supply from the axillary nerve than from the musculocutaneous nerve; the reverse may also be true. The complex overlapping innervation pattern makes denervation of the joint difficult. The nerve supply follows the small blood vessels into periarticular structures (Bateman 1971, Warwick & Williams 1973).

The skin on the anterior region of the shoulder complex is supplied by the supraclavicular nerves from C3 and C4 and by the terminal branches of the sensory component of the axillary nerve. The articular structures on the anterior aspect of the glenohumeral joint are supplied by the axillary nerve and, to a lesser degree, by the suprascapular nerves. The subscapular nerve and posterior cord of the brachial plexus may also innervate the anterior aspect of the joint after piercing the subscapularis muscle (Bateman 1971, Moore 1980, Warwick & Williams 1973).

The supraclavicular nerves supply the skin on the superior and upper posterior aspects of the shoulder region. The lower, posterior, and lateral aspects of the shoulder are supplied by the posterior branch of the axillary nerve. The periarticular structures on the superior aspect of the joint obtain part of their innervation from the suprascapular nerve. The axillary and musculocutaneous nerves and the lateral pectoral nerve may also contribute to the innervation of the superior aspect of the joint. Posteriorly, the main nerve supply is from the suprascapular nerve, which supplies the proximal part of the joint, and the axillary nerve, which supplies the distal region (Bateman 1971, DePalma 1973, Moore 1980, Warwick &

Williams 1973). The acromioclavicular joint is innervated by the lateral supraclavicular nerve from the cervical plexus (C4) and by the lateral pectoral and suprascapular nerves from the brachial plexus (C5 and C6). The sternoclavicular joint is innervated by branches from the medial supraclavicular nerve from the cervical plexus (C3 and C4) and subclavian nerve from the brachial plexus (C5 and C6) (Moore 1980, Warwick & Williams 1973).

CONCLUSION

The shoulder complex is more mobile than any other joint mechanism of the body because of the combined movement at the glenohumeral and scapulothoracic articulations. This wide range of motion permits positioning of the hand in space, allowing performance of numerous gross and skilled functions. Shoulder complex stability is also required during dynamic activity, particularly when the distal extremity encounters resistance. The glenohumeral joint is inherently unstable because of the shallowness of the glenoid fossa, as well as the disproportionate size and lack of congruency between the articular surfaces. During dynamic activities, stabilization of the humeral head on the glenoid fossa depends on an intact capsule and glenohumeral ligaments, as well as on coordinated and synchronous activity in the deltoid and rotator cuff muscles. Injury or disease of any of these structures can lead to instability and impingement of subacromial structures, resulting in pain and dysfunction in the shoulder region.

Mechanics of the Shoulder

Due to the complex function of the human shoulder, it is imperative that clinicians optimally understand both normal and compromised biomechanics of the entire shoulder complex. This chapter reviews key topics in shoulder biomechanics as well as shoulder-specific biomechanical information from important upper extremity sports that often can produce shoulder injury. Knowledge of these biomechanical principles is very important to any clinician treating the shoulder at a high level.

PRIMARY BIOMECHANICAL PRINCIPLES

Several key biomechanical principles are highly relevant to the shoulder, and gaining an understanding of them will help the material in the evaluation and treatment sections of this book make more sense. These include the scapular plane concept, muscular force couples, scapulohumeral rhythm, and the kinetic chain.

Scapular Plane Concept

One of the key concepts in upper extremity rehabilitation is the scapular plane concept. The scapular plane has ramifications for treatment, evaluation, and even functional activity in sport. According to Saha (1983), the **scapular plane** is defined as being 30° anterior to the coronal or frontal plane of the body. This plane is formed by the retroversion of the humeral head, which averages 30° relative to the shaft of the humerus coupled with the native anteversion of the glenoid, which is also 30° (Kapandji 1985, Neumann 2002). It is important for clinicians to realize this relationship during humeral head translation testing and exercise positioning due to the inherent advantages of the position. With the glenohumeral joint placed in the scapular plane, bony impingement of the greater tuberosity against the acromion does not occur, owing to the alignment of the tuberosity and acromion in this orientation (Saha 1983). In addition to the optimal bony congruency afforded in the scapular plane, this position also decreases stress on the anterior capsular components of the glenohumeral joint, and enhances activation of the posterior rotator cuff due to a length–tension enhancement compared to function in the coronal plane (Neumann 2002, Saha 1983). Placement of the glenohumeral joint in the scapular plane optimizes the osseous congruity between the humeral head and the glenoid and is widely recommended as an optimal position for the performance of various evaluation techniques, as well as during many rehabilitation exercises recommended throughout this book (Ellenbecker 2006, Saha 1983).

Muscular Force Couples

Another important general concept of relevance for this chapter is that of muscular force couples. One of the most important biomechanical principles in shoulder function is the deltoid rotator cuff force couple (Inman et al. 1944) (see figure 1.6 in the previous chapter). The phenomenon known as a **force couple** can be defined as two opposing muscular forces working together to enable a particular motion to occur, with these muscular forces being synergists, or agonist–antagonist pairs (Inman et al. 1944). The deltoid muscle provides force primarily in a superior direction when contracting unopposed during arm elevation (Weiner & MacNab 1970). The muscle–tendon units of the rotator cuff must provide both a compressive force and an inferiorly or caudally directed force to minimize superior migration and minimize contact or impingement of the rotator cuff tendons against the overlying acromion (Inman et al. 1944). Failure of the rotator cuff to maintain humeral congruency leads to glenohumeral joint instability, rotator cuff tendon pathology, and labral injury (Burkhart et al. 2003). Imbalances in the deltoid rotator cuff force couple, which primarily occur during inappropriate and unbalanced strength training, as well as through repetitive overhead sport activities, can lead to development of the deltoid without concomitant increases in the rotator cuff strength and also increase

the superior migration of the humeral head provided by the deltoid, leading to rotator cuff impingement.

Additionally, the serratus anterior and trapezius force couple is the primary muscular stabilizer and prime mover of upward rotation of the scapula during arm elevation (figure 2.1). Bagg and Forrest (1988) have shown how the upper trapezius and serratus anterior function during the initial 0° to 80° of arm elevation, providing upward scapular rotation and stabilization. Due to a change

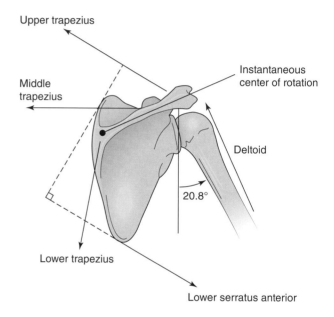

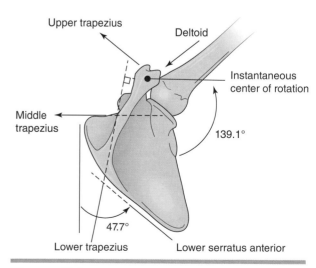

Figure 2.1 Trapezius and serratus anterior force couple.

in the lever arm of the lower trapezius that occurs during the lateral shift of the scapulothoracic instantaneous center of rotation with arm elevation, the lower trapezius and serratus anterior function as the primary scapular stabilizer in phases II and III (80° to 140°) of elevation (Bagg & Forrest 1988). Analysis of the serratus anterior and lower trapezius force couple in this elevated (90°) position is of particular importance due to the inherent demands and stabilization of the scapula needed during throwing and serving activities in overhead athletes. This book emphasizes increasing scapular stabilization through the use of specific exercises targeting the serratus anterior and lower trapezius; these are concepts needed for shoulder rehabilitation and are predicated on a firm understanding and knowledge of the important muscular force couples in the human shoulder.

Scapulohumeral Rhythm

Inman and colleagues (1944) described scapulohumeral rhythm as contributions made by multiple joints (glenohumeral joint and scapulothoracic joint) to create shoulder elevation. His original rhythm, "2 to 1," composed of 2° of glenohumeral motion for every 1° of scapulothoracic joint motion, has been classically referenced, although other researchers have reported ratios that range from 1.25:1 to 4:1 depending on the ranges of motion studied and the method used to quantify the motion. Based on the Inman model of scapulohumeral rhythm, it is generally accepted that to achieve a full 180° of shoulder elevation, 120° will be contributed by humeral elevation from the glenohumeral joint and an additional 60° will be due to scapular upward rotation.

Kinetic Chain

The term **kinetic chain** refers to energy being created by the larger segments and muscles and the transfer of that energy up through the legs and trunk and out to the throwing arm, wrist, and ultimately the ball (Fleisig et al. 1993). The motion of each of the segments in the chain helps not only to maintain the energy transferred but also to build on it (Dillman 1990, Feltner & Dapena 1989a, 1989b). The more body segments that sequentially contribute to the total force output, the greater the potential velocity at the distal end where the object is released. Proper execution of the kinetic chain in the overhead motion increases the efficiency of the movements by requiring less energy. Additionally, the performance of the throw or serve (i.e., velocity or distance) should be enhanced as well. During the throwing motion, movements are initiated from the larger muscles of the base segments and are transferred to the core of the body, then terminating with the smaller distal segments. There appear to be primarily seven segments that have both angular and linear movements during the overhead throwing motion: (1) lower extremity, (2) pelvis, (3) spine, (4) shoulder girdle, (5) upper arm, (6) forearm, and (7) hand (Atwater 1979, Dillman 1990, Dillman et al. 1993, Feltner & Dapena 1989a, 1989b). A practical drill used by many baseball coaches to illustrate the importance of the legs and trunk in throwing is the following. First, kneel on the ground and throw a baseball as far as possible. Next, stand and use your whole body and throw. The ball will go at least twice as far. Thus, the muscles of the shoulder complex alone cannot generate sufficient energy to produce such a throw, nor can they dissipate the energy after the throw is completed.

The kinetic chain concept describes how the body can be considered a series of interrelated links or segments, with movement of one segment affecting other segments both proximally and distally. Kibler (1998) has described the kinetic link system as a series of sequentially activated body segments. Understanding the upper extremity kinetic chain is predicated on knowledge of how the shoulder (glenohumeral articulation) functions with direct links to the trunk and scapulothoracic and distal arm segments, both in rehabilitation and in sport and functional movement patterns (Davies

1992). It is also important to appreciate the prevalence of sequential segmental rotations in the kinetic chain concept. This applies to virtually all human movements and particularly to the overhead throwing motion and tennis serve. Groppel (1992) applied the kinetic chain system to the analysis and description of optimal upper extremity sport biomechanics (figure 2.2). The description of optimal kinetic chain utilization demonstrated in figure 2.2a starts with sequential activation of the links initiated by ground reaction forces and proceeds up the chain to the hips, trunk, shoulder, and ultimately the hand–racket interface to ball contact, to use this example applied to a tennis player. Figure 2.2b shows the effects of a missing link in the kinetic chain such as when a hip injury occurs; nonoptimal progression of forces from the lower body to trunk ensues,

ultimately affecting shoulder and upper extremity function. Additionally, nonoptimal timing of sequential segmental activation is shown in figure 2.2c, also affecting the kinetic chain. These theoretical concepts provide a basic framework for more specific discussions on throwing and other upper extremity techniques in this chapter.

THROWING MECHANICS

A thorough review of throwing mechanics is needed in order for clinicians to truly appreciate the demands placed on the shoulder during repetitive overhead activity. This detailed review provides a platform for both the evaluation and treatment concepts outlined in future sections of this book.

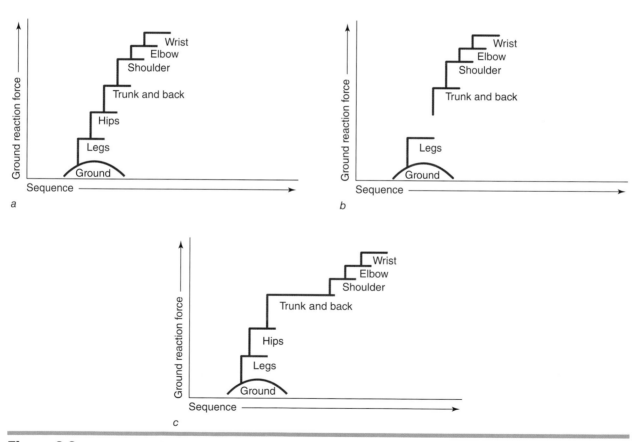

Figure 2.2 *(a)* Kinetic link system, *(b)* nonoptimal use of the kinetic chain system because of a missing link, and *(c)* nonoptimal use of the kinetic link system due to improper timing.

Reprinted, by permission, from T.S. Ellenbecker and G. Davies, 2001, *Closed kinetic chain exercise* (Champaign, IL: Human Kinetics), 21; Adapted from Groppel 1992.

Baseball Pitching and Throwing Motion

The throwing motion is a complex movement pattern that requires flexibility, muscular strength, coordination, synchronicity of muscular firing, and neuromuscular efficiency. The overhead throwing athlete appears to be in fine balance and is a highly skilled individual. The thrower's shoulder must be flexible enough to allow the excessive external rotation required to throw a baseball. However, the shoulder must also be stable enough to prevent symptomatic subluxations in the shoulder joint. Therefore, the thrower's shoulder exhibits significant adaptations described in this book to assist the clinician during the evaluation process. Specifically, one must know which adaptations are considered normal or in response to repetitive sport participation and which may be considered abnormal or may increase injury risk. The thrower's shoulder must be loose enough to throw, but stable enough to prevent humeral head subluxation and to maintain control during the entire throwing motion (acceleration and deceleration phases). Hence the thrower's shoulder is in delicate balance between mobility and stability. The overhead throwing motion places tremendous demands on the shoulder joint complex musculature to produce functional stability. The surrounding musculature must be strong enough to assist in arm acceleration but must exhibit neuromuscular efficiency to produce dynamic functional stability. During the act of pitching, the angular velocity at the shoulder joint exceeds 7000°/sec and has been referred to as the fastest human movement (Fleisig et al. 1993, 2011b). Furthermore, tremendous forces are generated at the shoulder joint, sometimes up to one times body weight. Because of these tremendous demands, at incredible angular velocities, various shoulder injuries may occur. Rehabilitative and preventive rotator cuff and scapular exercise plays a key role in preventing injury to the overhead thrower and is imperative for both performance enhancement and injury prevention.

To best study the throwing motion, most research has broken down this complex motion into a series of phases. Description of the phases of throwing is complicated by the lack of consistency in terminology and division of phases in the literature (Blackburn 1991, Fleisig et al. 1995, 2011b, McLeod 1985, Michaud 1990, Perry & Gousman 1990, Tullos & King 1972, Werner et al. 1993). For the purposes of the discussion in this book, the throwing motion is divided into six phases: windup, stride, arm cocking, arm acceleration, arm deceleration, and follow-through. Figure 2.3 shows the arm and body position during the late cocking and early acceleration phase of the pitching motion. The following subsections discuss each phase in some detail to enable better understanding of the muscular activity

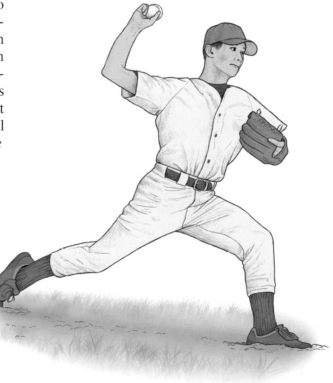

Figure 2.3 Arm and body position of the throwing motion during the early portion of the acceleration phase.

and joint positions inherent in each phase (Dillman et al. 1993, Fleisig et al. 1995, 2000).

Windup

The windup is the initial phase of the throwing motion, when the pitcher begins the pitching motion. The muscular forces and loads on the body are minimal during this phase, and the termination of this phase occurs when the stride leg maximally flexes at the hip joint. It is important to note that at the termination of the windup phase, the pitcher has achieved a balanced position for progression into the next phase of pitching. Failure to do so may negatively affect performance and also set the pitcher up for possible injury and compensation (Fleisig et al. 2011a, 2011b). This phase occurs during a relatively short period of time (typically 0.5 second to 1 second in duration). The weight should be evenly distributed between the two feet, and the phase starts with the stance leg limb's foot pivoting to a position that is parallel with the pitching rubber. The lead leg is elevated by concentric contractions of the hip flexors. The stance leg, which supports the pitcher's body weight, flexes slightly, and is controlled by eccentric contractions from the quadriceps muscles. High reliance on core stabilization for successful performance occurs with the gluteus medius, gluteus minimus, and tensor fascia latae functioning as stabilizers through isometric contraction of the hip of the stance limb (Jacobs 1987). The shoulders are slightly flexed and abducted and held in this position by the anterior and medial deltoids, supraspinatus, and the clavicular portion of the pectoralis major (Jobe et al. 1983, 1984). The windup phase is characterized by low forces, torques, and muscle activity.

Stride

Following the windup phase, the stride phase begins as the lead leg begins to fall and move toward home plate. This is accompanied by simultaneous separation of the hands (ball leaves the glove). The termination of the stride phase occurs when the front (lead foot) touches the ground and becomes weight bearing. The stride phase lasts between 0.5 and 0.75 seconds. Early in the stride phase, eccentric activation of the hip flexors provides a controlled lowering of the lead leg. The stance leg has substantial concentric muscle work from the hip abductors to provide a lengthened stride toward the throwing target. External rotation is a key component of this falling movement of the lead leg, which occurs from contraction of the gluteus maximus, sartorius, and deep rotators. Internal rotation occurs in the stance limb. Detailed study of hip rotation range of motion has been performed clinically by Ellenbecker and colleagues (2007) and McCulloch and colleagues (2014), with the finding of specific patterns of internal rotation, external rotation, and total rotation in the rotation range of motion of the hip.

The length of the stride phase shows significant individual variability, but averages 70% to 80% of the pitcher's height. This measurement of stride length is taken from ankle to ankle at the moment of front foot contact during the terminal portion of the stride phase. When one compares the stride length of pitching to that of a quarterback throwing a football, the quarterback's stride length is only 55% to 65% of his height. The trunk is held in slight lateral flexion during the stride phase. At front foot contact, the foot should be pointed slightly inward in a closed manner, which would involve the foot's pointing to the left (toward third base). The angle of closed-foot position is typically between a 5° and 25° deviation relative to home plate. This position helps the lead leg to act as a stable platform over which the rest of the body can rotate. Landing in a position that is too closed (too rotated) can decrease the ability of the body to rotate over the landing limb and decrease performance (Fleisig et al. 2011b). The knee of the lead leg is flexed approximately 45° to 55° at foot contact. The placement and position of the lead foot are very important in throwing. The lead foot should land directly in front of the rear foot toward the direction of the throw, or a few centimeters closed (lead foot to the right [third base side] of stance foot in right-handed throwing) or open (lead foot to the left [first base side] of stance foot in right-handed throwing). However, if the lead foot is positioned excessively closed, pelvis rotation can be blocked or impeded, and the resulting compensation finds the athlete "throwing across the body." This will decrease the contribution of the lower body to the force and velocity of the throw. During this portion of the stride phase, however, if the foot is positioned excessively "open," pelvis rotation occurs too early (Fleisig et al. 2011b). An open-foot position results in improper timing, causing energy from pelvis rotation to be applied to the upper trunk too early. When this occurs, the thrower often ends up throwing with "too much arm," because the energy generated from the pelvis rotation is dissipated instead of being applied to the arm (Fleisig et al. 2011b). The elastic energy generated in the legs, trunk, and arms during the stride phase is transferred to subsequent phases of the throw, demonstrating how the kinetic chain principle is very relevant to the mechanics of the throwing motion.

From an upper extremity standpoint during the stride, both shoulders undergo abduction and external rotation and horizontally abduct due to concentric muscle action from the rotator cuff, deltoids, and scapular stabilizers. At lead foot contact, the amount of abduction in the dominant throwing shoulder ranges between 80° and 100°. The deltoid and supraspinatus muscles are responsible for both abducting and maintaining arm positioning while maintaining the humeral head in the glenoid fossa (DiGiovine 1992). The upper trapezius and serratus anterior function as a force couple and upwardly rotate and position the scapula (glenoid fossa) for the humeral head. This scapular position is imperative, as an improperly positioned scapula can lead to impingement and shoulder functional control problems (Bradley 1991). During the stride phase, the throwing arm is positioned in horizontal abduction (slightly behind the trunk). This differs from the horizontal

abduction position during football, which finds the shoulder slightly in front of the trunk during passing. The posterior deltoid, latissimus dorsi, teres major, and posterior rotator cuff muscles (infraspinatus and teres minor) are responsible for horizontally abducting the shoulder, and the rhomboids and middle trapezius retract the scapula to ensure optimal joint arthrokinematics (DiGiovine 1992). There should be about 80° to 100° of elbow flexion in the throwing arm at the point of foot contact. Distally, the forearm is in a position of rotation approaching vertical. In comparison to pitchers, quarterbacks have slightly greater elbow flexion at lead foot contact (Fleisig et al. 2011b).

Arm Cocking

The phase termed arm cocking starts when the lead foot contacts the ground, and ends at maximum external rotation of the shoulder. Arm cocking is also a very brief phase, lasting between 0.1 and 0.15 seconds (see figure 2.4). The quadriceps muscle of the lead leg initially contracts eccentrically to decelerate and control knee flexion. The quadriceps also functions isometrically to stabilize the lead leg throughout the arm cocking phase (Fleisig et al. 2011b). During pitching, the ankle of the stance leg plantar flexes as it contacts and subsequently leaves the pitching rubber. This ankle plantar flexion motion occurs with simultaneous pelvis rotation, just after lead foot contact. The pelvis continues to rotate in the transverse plane through bilateral hip internal rotation. Pelvic rotation occurs at a maximum rotation of approximately 400°/sec to 700°/sec, which is why throwing requires both precise and explosive core stabilization to achieve optimal performance. Maximal pelvis rotation has been reported to occur at approximately 0.03 to 0.05 seconds after foot contact. This pelvic rotation occurs approximately 30% into the arm cocking phase (Fleisig et al. 2011b).

During the later stages of the cocking phase, the pelvis rotates to face home plate such that the trunk rotators are placed on stretch, which ultimately produces recoil effect for the subsequent shoulder rotation.

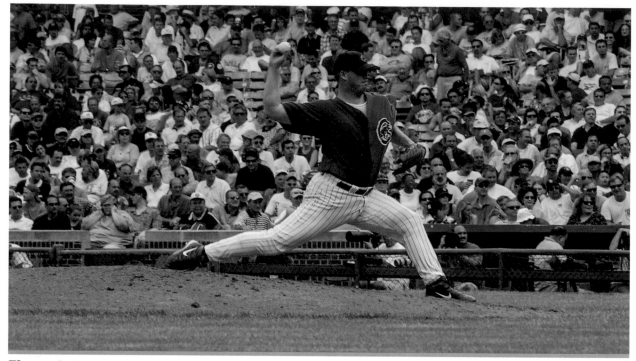

Figure 2.4 Dominant arm external rotation and abduction position during the cocking phase of the pitching motion.

Just after the pelvis rotation begins to occur, the upper torso undergoes transverse rotation relative to the spinal column (Fleisig et al. 2011b). The maximum upper torso angular velocity occurs very rapidly and has been reported to be approximately 900°/sec to 1300°/sec (approximately twice as large as pelvis angular velocity). This action occurs approximately 50% into the arm cocking phase. As the larger base segments of the pelvis and upper torso rotate about the longitudinal vertebral axis, a great deal of energy is imparted to the system through the segmental rotation inherent in a kinetic chain motion. The kinetic chain sequence of attaining maximal pelvic rotation before maximal upper torso rotation is important in establishing proper timing and coordination for subsequent portions of the throw to produce optimal velocities and ultimately optimal throwing performance.

As the trunk rotates to face the home plate, the throwing shoulder starts from a horizontally adducted position of 20° to 30° of horizontal abduction at lead foot contact to a position of 15° to 20° of horizontal

adduction once the shoulder attains maximum shoulder external rotation. Mihata and associates (2015) have shown increases in undersurface impingement (contact) between the supraspinatus tendon and the posterior superior glenoid during the arm cocking position of abduction and external rotation, which increases in intensity with greater amounts of horizontal abduction or what has been termed "hyperangulation" during this critical phase of the throwing motion from a shoulder perspective. The timing of lower body and trunk rotation relative to shoulder horizontal abduction–adduction position is of critical importance to minimize shoulder injury, specifically rotator cuff and labral injury from hyperangulation. Additionally, research by Douoguhi and colleagues (2015) showed that early trunk rotation in professional pitchers was correlated to serious shoulder and elbow injury while also finding that the inverted "W" position did not correlate. Similarly, the presence of arm lag or hyperangulation, which is characterized by excessive horizontal abduction during the cocking phase of throwing, was observed using two-dimensional throwing analysis by Davis and colleagues (2009).

It is important to also note that maximum shoulder horizontal adduction velocity (relative to the trunk) occurs at velocities of 500°/sec to 650°/sec, and is guided by muscular activation of the pectoralis major and the anterior deltoid.

Additional shoulder girdle muscles, including the levator scapulae, serratus anterior, trapezius, rhomboids, and pectoralis minor, are also important during the arm cocking phase, in addition to the rotator cuff. The one with the highest activity, the serratus anterior, is extremely important in that it stabilizes and protracts the scapula (DiGiovine 1992). The muscular force couples of the trapezius and serratus anterior work together in helping to stabilize the scapula and provide optimal positioning of the glenoid for subsequent action of the humeral head. Dysfunction of these scapula muscles may induce additional stress to the anterior shoulder stabilizers as has been proposed by Kibler (1991, 1998). Additionally, during arm cocking, the serratus anterior is important in providing upward rotation and protraction of the scapula, allowing the scapula to move with the horizontally adducting humerus.

From a clinical standpoint, it is imperative to emphasize that throughout the arm cocking phase the shoulder remains abducted approximately 80° to 100°. The forearm and distal hand segments lag behind the rapidly rotating trunk and shoulder, resulting in a maximum shoulder external rotation of approximately 165° to 180° which is a composite motion (combined shoulder external rotation, scapular motion, and trunk extension) (Bradley 1991). During simple visual observation as well as complex biomechanical analysis, the forearm appears to lie in a nearly horizontal position approximately 90° backward from its vertical position obtained at or just after lead foot contact (Fleisig et al. 2011b).

It is also very important to point out that external rotation of the shoulder as measured in biomechanical research includes hyperextension of the trunk, as well as scapular motion, and that the 165° to 180° of external rotation and apparent horizontal position of the forearm at the end of the cocking phase is not due solely to glenohumeral joint external rotation. This is a composite motion composed of multiple contributions from the trunk, scapula, and glenohumeral joint (Fleisig et al. 2011b).

Throwers with inadequate shoulder flexibility may need to perform various shoulder stretching and strengthening exercises to improve their range of motion and the motion available in their trunk and shoulder in order to prevent injuries and optimize joint mobility and stability. Research has shown that repetitive throwing tends to increase shoulder capsule laxity and shoulder flexibility. It is not unusual for a baseball pitcher to possess 125° to 145° of external rotation and 10° to 15° more external rotation in the throwing shoulder compared with the nonthrowing shoulder (Bigliani et al. 1997, Brown et al. 1988, Ellenbecker et al. 2002). This extra range of motion may help to maximize performance and minimize injury potential at the shoulder by allowing a greater range of motion in which force can be generated. It is important to mention here that having too much shoulder range of motion (too much shoulder flexibility) can be detrimental to the thrower as well. Throughout the next chapters on evaluation and treatment, this book focuses on how to measure and identify optimal levels of shoulder range of motion both for injury prevention and for performance enhancement.

Several key glenohumeral joint torques and forces help one to better understand the demands placed on the shoulder during high-level throwing. A maximum compressive force of approximately 550 to 770 N (approximately 80% body weight) is produced to resist distraction due to centrifugal force generated by rapid pelvis and upper torso rotation (Fleisig et al. 2011b, Michaud 1990). DiGiovine (1992) showed that this compressive force is generated mainly through high activity from the rotator cuff muscles (supraspinatus, infraspinatus, teres minor, and subscapularis). This is imperative to allow for joint congruence, maintaining the humeral head centered within the glenoid fossa. Just as important as the compression force, the posterior rotator cuff muscles apply a posteriorly directed force to the humeral head to resist anterior humeral head translation that occurs as the shoulder externally rotates (Cain 1987, Jobe et al. 1983). Eccentric internal rotation torque is produced to decelerate shoulder external rotation through contraction of the subscapularis (DiGiovine 1992). During pitching, peak shoulder internal rotation torques of 55 to 80 Nm are generated just before maximum shoulder external rotation (Fleisig et al. 1995, 2011b) due to strong eccentric contractions from the shoulder internal rotators (pectoralis major, latissimus dorsi, anterior deltoid, teres major, and subscapularis). Lastly, a maximum shoulder anterior shear force of 290 to 470 N, as well as a shoulder horizontal adduction torque of 80 to 120 Nm, is produced at the shoulder to resist posterior translation at the shoulder (Fleisig et al. 1995, 2011b).

Arm Acceleration

The phase termed arm acceleration begins at the point of maximum shoulder external rotation and ends when the ball is released from the hand. This phase is very rapid and brief, lasting 0.03 to 0.04 seconds (Escamilla et al. 2002, Fleisig et al. 1999). There is moderate to high muscle activity in the shoulder joint complex as the arm is accelerating forward in both a linear and angular manner (DiGiovine 1992, Jobe et al. 1983, 1984). Electromyographic (EMG) data show that the subscapularis is the most active shoulder internal rotator, followed by the latissimus dorsi and pectoralis major during the acceleration phase (DiGiovine 1992, Gowan et al 1987, Moynes et al. 1986).

As maximum external rotation is achieved in the shoulder, elbow extension begins, and is immediately followed by the onset of shoulder internal rotation (Escamilla et al. 1998). Elbow extension just before shoulder internal rotation allows the athlete to reduce rotational inertia, resulting in greater internal rotation velocities. With these velocities occurring in excess of 7000°/sec, the shoulder internal rotators function concentrically (Escamilla et al. 2002, Fleisig et al. 1999).

As the elbow extends and the shoulder internally rotates, the trunk flexes forward to a more neutral position from its hyperextended position at the point of ball release (Escamilla et al. 2002, Fleisig et al. 1999). High muscle activity is present in the rectus abdominis and obliques as the trunk flexes forward during the acceleration phase (Watkins et al. 1989). Forward flexing of the trunk is enhanced by lead knee extension, which provides a stable base around which the trunk rotates (Escamilla et al. 2002). The lead knee extends to approximately 15° to 20° from the point of lead foot contact to ball release during the acceleration phase. If the proper amount of lead knee extension is not met due to decreased trunk flexion, ball velocity can be diminished (Matsuo et al. 2000a, 2000b). At the point of ball release, the trunk should ideally be flexed forward 30° to 40° from the vertical position (Escamilla et al. 2002).

During the acceleration phase of throwing, the rotator cuff, trapezius, serratus anterior, rhomboids, and levator scapulae have all demonstrated high levels of activity (DiGiovine 1992). Differences have been measured and reported regarding rotator cuff activity when one compares professional and amateur-level pitchers. Muscle activity in the infraspinatus, teres minor, supraspinatus, and biceps was shown to be as much as three times higher in amateur pitchers, whereas in professional pitchers, subscapularis, serratus anterior, and latissimus dorsi activity was higher (Gowan et al. 1987). Nonetheless, this does imply that glenohumeral control and scapula stabilization are imperative during the acceleration phase. These findings may suggest that professional pitchers better coordinate segmental motion, therefore enhancing the efficiency of the rotator cuff muscles in the stabilization of the glenohumeral joint during the act of throwing.

A high degree of centrifugal force is present during the acceleration phase, producing rapid elbow extension. High angular velocities of approximately 2400°/sec of elbow extension are produced near the midpoint of the acceleration phase (Escamilla et al. 2002, Werner et al. 1993). This force is most frequently generated by rotatory actions at the hips, trunk, and shoulder (Toyoshima et al. 1974). High levels of concentric triceps brachii and anconeus activity have been documented during this phase; however, research suggests that these muscle groups assist more in the stabilization of the arm rather than acting as accelerators (DiGiovine 1992, Feltner & Dapena 1986, Jobe et al. 1984, Sisto et al. 1987, Werner et al. 1993). At the point of ball release, the elbow is near full extension and is positioned slightly anterior to the trunk.

As the arm begins rotating forward and generating speed through the acceleration phase, shoulder internal rotation and elbow varus torques decrease (Fleisig et al. 1995). Wedging of the olecranon against the medial aspect of the trochlear groove and olecranon fossa can often occur, as a result of the high valgus stresses at the elbow as it extends during the early phases of acceleration. This mechanical wedging can create impingement, which can lead to osteophyte formation at the posteromedial aspect of the olecranon that may further lead to chondromalacia and loose body formation (Wilson et al. 1983). Throughout the arm cocking and acceleration phases of throwing, the elbow extends from approximately 85° to 20° of elbow flexion (Fleisig et al. 1995). Wilson and colleagues (1983) coined the phrase "valgus extension overload" as a result of this rapid combination of extension and valgus stress at the elbow. Further research by Campbell and colleagues (1994) would report that a higher measure of valgus torque was present in youth baseball pitchers at the point of ball release, as compared to professional pitchers, further noting this as a possible contributing factor to "Little League elbow syndrome" in skeletally immature throwers.

Low to moderate activity of the elbow flexors is generated during the acceleration phase of throwing (DiGiovine 1992, Sisto et al. 1987). Contraction of the elbow flexors resists elbow distraction resulting from the centrifugal force acting on the forearm, while also enhancing elbow joint stability and eccentrically controlling the rate of elbow extension.

The hand is the final segment that influences forces on the ball during acceleration as the wrist moves from hyperextension to a neutral position at ball release (Barrentine et al. 1998b). At the beginning of acceleration, there is eccentric activity of the wrist flexors to decelerate the hyperextending wrist; however, as acceleration proceeds, the wrist flexors concentrically contract and flex the wrist at the point of ball release (Barrentine et al. 1998a). The pronator teres is also active during this phase, assisting with forearm pronation (DiGiovine 1992).

Arm Deceleration

This phase starts at the point of ball release and ends at maximal shoulder internal rotation. The arm deceleration phase lasts approximately 0.03 to 0.05 seconds. During this phase, shoulder internal rotation will continue until 0°. Extension of the lead knee and throwing elbow continues until roughly full extension is reached in both. The trunk and hips continue to flex. As a reaction to this progressive flexion, the stance leg now begins moving in an upward manner. Moderate to high levels of lumbar paraspinal, rectus abdominis, oblique, and gluteus maximus activity occur during this phase (Watkins et al. 1989).

The posterior muscles of the shoulder (infraspinatus, supraspinatus, teres major and minor, latissimus dorsi, and posterior deltoid) are very active in the deceleration phase, resisting shoulder distraction and anterior subluxation forces (Escamilla et al. 2002, Fleisig et al. 1995, Jobe et al. 1983, 1984). The teres minor exhibits the highest activity of all glenohumeral muscles during this phase of throwing, restraining against excessive anterior humeral head translation (DiGiovine 1992, Jobe et al. 1983). High levels of activation of the lower trapezius, rhomboids, and serratus anterior are also present during this phase, enhancing stability to the scapula (DiGiovine 1992).

Gowan and colleagues reported more than twice as much muscle activity in the biceps and posterior deltoid in amateur pitchers compared to professional pitchers (Gowan et al. 1987). This may imply that amateur throws exhibit a less efficient throwing pattern, placing greater stress on the posterior shoulder. The biceps brachii and brachialis act to decelerate elbow extension throughout this phase (DiGiovine 1992). Large shoulder and elbow forces and torques are needed to decelerate the arm during this phase (Escamilla et al. 2002, Fleisig et al. 1995). Maximum proximal forces of approximate body weight are needed at both the shoulder and elbow to prevent distraction of these joints (Fleisig et al. 1995, Werner et al. 1993).

Rapid pronation occurs at the radioulnar joint during the deceleration phase with the pronator teres exhibiting moderate concentric activity. In contrast, the biceps brachii and supinator muscles act eccentrically to control deceleration of this joint motion (DiGiovine 1992). The wrist and finger flexors exhibit high levels of muscular activity during the deceleration phase, providing wrist flexion. Moderate levels of wrist and finger extensor muscle activity are present as well, eccentrically acting to decelerate the flexing wrist and fingers during this phase (DiGiovine 1992).

Follow-Through

The final phase of the throwing motion begins at maximum shoulder internal rotation and ends when the arm completes horizontal adduction across the body and the thrower obtains a balanced ending position. The follow-through phase lasts 1 second. A long deceleration arc from the throwing arm, combined with forward tilting of the trunk, allows for the dissipation of energy back into the trunk and lower extremities. This absorption of energy throughout the kinetic chain helps reduce the stresses placed on the throwing shoulder. At this point in the follow-through, the stride leg should be straight, supporting almost all of the body's weight, while the stance leg continues to move upward.

Similarly to what occurs in the deceleration phase, the posterior shoulder musculature continues to act eccentrically to decelerate the horizontally adducting shoulder. During the follow-through, shoulder joint torques are much lower than those generated during the deceleration phase (Fleisig et al. 1995). High serratus anterior muscle activity is present during the follow-through to concentrically upwardly rotate the scapula (DiGiovine 1992). The middle trapezius and rhomboids work synergistically to decelerate scapular protraction through eccentric contractions (DiGiovine 1992). Lastly, in the follow-through phase, low levels of muscular activity are present in the wrist and finger extensors in an effort to decelerate wrist flexion (DiGiovine 1992).

Comparison of Different Pitches

Frequently, clinicians, coaches, and parents ask if throwing breaking balls (e.g., curveballs, sliders) creates greater stresses at the shoulder and elbow joint. To help determine these effects, a series of studies was conducted by Escamilla and colleagues (1998), as well as Fleisig and colleagues (2006), comparing the biomechanics of the four most commonly thrown pitches: fastball, change-up, curveball, and slider. Eighteen collegiate baseball pitchers were studied using the motion analysis methods described earlier in this chapter. Compared with fastball kinematics, the kinematics of the slider were similar, whereas the change-up and curveball demonstrated decreased range of motion and decreased joint velocities. Evaluation of elbow and shoulder kinetics indicates that higher loads are produced in the fastball, curveball, and slider pitches than in the change-up.

Results from these studies suggest that the fastball and slider were the most similar pitches, displaying the greatest segmental angular speeds and overall highest forces and torques at the shoulder and elbow. In fact, elbow and shoulder compression forces exceeded body weight. Although the lowest radar gun speeds were seen for the curveball, this pitch displayed high segmental angular speeds and high forces and torques. An important and interesting observation was that the curveball group recorded the greatest elbow medial force and elbow varus torque. It has long been thought by coaches that the curveball may stress the medial elbow to a greater degree than other pitches. The change-up consistently had the lowest segmental angular speeds and generated the lowest stress at the shoulder and elbow. Although more research is needed, the data suggest that the change-up may be a safer off-speed pitch to throw than the curveball, and perhaps just as effective. The change-up is also an easier pitch to teach than the curveball, which is often taught and performed incorrectly. Improperly thrown pitches may, in fact, generate forces and torques even greater than those reported in studies of pitchers with more optimal technique. This highlights the important need for biomechanical evaluation in patients presenting with shoulder and elbow dysfunction from throwing a baseball.

Adult Versus Youth Baseball Pitchers

Although many investigators have studied pitching biomechanics of adult baseball players, relatively little scientific information is available on younger pitchers. Information about young pitchers may be extrapolated from adult pitching studies, but the accuracy of drawn conclusions is unknown. In a study conducted at the American Sports Medicine Institute, kinematics and kinetics of 13 high school pitchers and 13 college pitchers were compared; the results indicated no statistical differences (Fleisig et al. 1996). Using a similar motion analysis method, Cosgarea and associates (1993) conducted two studies to quantify and compare youth and adult pitching biomechanics.

Results from these studies showed that pitchers grouped into levels of competition and various age groups (9-12 years, 13-16 years, collegiate and professional) (Cosgarea et al. 1993) had no significant differences in the kinematics of the legs and trunk between the different levels of competition except for some significant differences in front foot replacement. Younger pitchers placed their front foot in both a more open position (e.g., the left foot of a right-handed pitcher was closer to first base) and a more closed direction (e.g., the anterior direction of the left foot of a right-handed pitcher was pointing more toward third base). A younger pitcher not only had slower ball velocity, but also generated significantly less angular velocity of the upper torso, elbow extension, and shoulder internal rotation.

In the second study, elbow and shoulder joint kinetics were compared between 10 youth and 10 professional pitchers (Campbell et al. 1994). To compensate for differences in body size, all forces were expressed as percentages of body weight and all torques as percentages of the product of body weight and height. In general, joint forces and torques were greater for the adult pitchers. During arm cocking, the adult pitcher produced greater shoulder anterior force, shoulder internal rotation torque, and elbow varus torque. The adult pitcher also generated greater shoulder posterior force during the follow-through. The youth pitcher, however, produced greater elbow varus torque than the adult pitcher during arm acceleration and at ball release. Campbell and coworkers (1994) concluded that this increased varus torque may contribute to the elbow pathology known as Little League elbow syndrome.

Sidearm Versus Overhead Throwing

The vast majority of sports medicine literature on baseball pitching has centered on overhand pitching techniques (Matsuo et al. 2000a, 2000b). The term overhand refers to pitching a baseball using an over-the-top or three-quarter motion. This technique of pitching is favored by most baseball pitchers regardless of skill level. Reasons for this as the preferred technique are the belief that risk for injury to the shoulder or elbow is minimal, along with the notion of maximal ball velocity (Fleisig et al. 1995). However, several pitchers employ an alternative method known as sidearm pitching.

To differentiate between overhand and sidearm pitching techniques, shoulder abduction angles in reference to trunk position during the arm cocking and arm acceleration phases are used to distinguish between the two. Overhand pitchers throw with shoulder abduction angles greater than 90° whereas a sidearm pitcher throws with less than 90° of shoulder abduction (Matsuo et al. 2000a, 2000b). When the contrasting techniques have been compared, several differences in biomechanics have been shown.

Observation of the kinematic relationships in the two throwing styles has shown that trunk angle or tilt is vastly different. With regard to trunk angle, trunk tilt compared to the vertical y-axis at ball release is the reference. Overhand throwers laterally tilt their trunk away from their throwing arm side whereas sidearm throwers tend to stay vertical or even bend their trunk toward their throwing side.

The most intriguing kinematic variable between the two techniques is elbow position at ball release. Due to lower shoulder abduction angles and ipsilateral trunk tilt, sidearm pitchers throw with a lower elbow position compared to overhand throwers. This lower elbow position leads to an increase in horizontal shoulder adduction, which accounts for a mechanical flaw known as "leading with the elbow" (Fleisig et al. 1995). This flaw leads to greater anterior shoulder and medial elbow forces (Fleisig et al. 1995). Various studies have shown that these factors may give rise to mechanical flaws in a sidearm pitcher's motion that can result in significant elbow or shoulder injury (Fleisig et al. 1995).

Windmill (Softball) Pitching

While much attention in the sports medicine literature has been directed toward overhand pitching in baseball, the mechanics of softball pitching have been minimally researched and often misunderstood. While there are numerous variations of the softball pitch, the most common technique is the windmill pitching motion. The windmill pitching motion is a complex set of movements involving both the upper and lower extremities working in unison to pitch the softball. The motion can be broken down into four distinct phases: windup, stride, delivery, and follow-through (Barrentine et al. 1998a).

Windup

The initial phase or the windup involves the pitcher's generating movement and momentum. The windup begins with the pitcher in the ready or set position. The pitcher then internally rotates the throwing shoulder and shifts the weight onto the ipsilateral leg. Next the pitcher extends the shoulder while also extending the elbow. The opposite leg will begin to undergo hip flexion in anticipation of the stride phase. The windup phase ends with the stride foot losing contact with the ground or the toe-off.

Stride

During the stride phase, the lead or stride foot loses contact with the ground while the throwing shoulder comes from an extended position to a forward flexed overhead position (the 12 o'clock position). This overhead motion is called the **top of the backswing** or TOB. At the TOB the humerus is externally rotated, firing the external rotators of the shoulder (infraspinatus, teres minor, posterior deltoid) (Maffet et al. 1994). The back foot pushes the body forward while the stride leg undergoes hip flexion and knee extension to propel the body toward the plate. The length of the pitcher's stride is between 60% and 70% of the athlete's height (Werner et al. 2006).

Delivery

The next phase of the motion is referred to as the delivery phase. This phase begins with the stride foot coming back into contact with the ground and the shoulder coming forward from the TOB. During this phase the biceps is activated along with the stabilizing muscles of the scapula and posterior shoulder. As the throwing shoulder comes forward, the hips rotate toward home plate and the shoulder releases the ball, propelling it toward home plate. As the lead foot makes contact with the ground, the weight of the pitcher is transferred from the back foot to the stride foot. The elbow remains extended until ball release.

Follow-Through

The final phase is referred to as the follow-through. The follow-through lasts from ball release until the throwing shoulder has completed its forward motion. Compared to baseball, the softball follow-through is much shorter. During this phase there is a full transfer of weight from the back foot to the lead foot. The throwing shoulder continues to move forward until full deceleration. Deceleration is achieved by activation of the biceps resulting in forearm and elbow flexion. Unlike what is seen in baseball, a softball pitcher's body usually goes in the opposite direction of the pitch due to the transference of weight from the back to lead foot. In the follow-through phase of the pitching motion, pitchers often go into a fielding position in case the ball is hit toward them.

Baseball Versus Football Throwing

Many talented athletes are both the quarterback on their school's football team and a pitcher on their school's baseball team. However, it is unknown whether participation in both activities is beneficial or detrimental to the athlete's performance and safety. In theory, a football can be used as an overload weighted implement for strengthening the arm of a baseball pitcher, because it has been documented that overload training can increase ball velocity once pitching with a regulation-weight baseball resumes (Brose & Hanson 1967, DeRenne & House 1993, Fleisig et al. 2009, 2011b, Litwhiler & Hamm 1973). To compare and contrast baseball pitching and football passing, Fleisig and colleagues (1996) studied 26 baseball pitchers and 26 football quarterbacks using motion analysis. The 26 high school and college pitchers threw from a mound to a strike zone ribbon located 60.5 feet (20 m) away; the 26 high school and college quarterbacks threw drop-back passes to a net located approximately 20 yards (18.2 m) away. The football passing motion was similar enough to the baseball pitching motion that the two activities could be analyzed and compared with respect to the six phases previously described for pitching. Although maximum external rotation occurred earlier for quarterbacks, maximum angular velocity of pelvis rotation, upper torso rotation, elbow extension, and shoulder internal rotation occurred earlier for pitchers and achieved greater magnitude. The quarterback had a shorter stride and stood more erect at ball release. During arm cocking, a quarterback demonstrated greater elbow flexion and greater shoulder horizontal adduction (55° for football and 49° for baseball), which produced greater shoulder anterior force and medial elbow force. To decelerate the arm, the pitcher generated greater flexion torque and compressive force at the elbow and compressive force, adduction torque, and posterior force at the shoulder.

A baseball pitcher's shoulder anterior force is greatest during throwing of a fastball. Football passing generates significantly less shoulder joint forces and torques compared with baseball pitching (Fleisig et al. 1996).

Relationship Between Baseball Pitching and Injury Risk

Baseball pitching and injury risk has been an area of research and interest for several years. What are the specific factors that can cause shoulder or elbow injury in the overhead throwing athlete? Several investigators have analyzed numerous risk factors. Fleisig and colleagues (2011a) reported that the most significant risk of serious shoulder or elbow injury (or of both) in youth baseball pitchers was pitching more than 100 innings in a year; this resulted in a 3.5 times greater likelihood of sustaining injury (when compared with pitching less than 100 innings). Also, pitchers who concomitantly played catcher seemed more likely to be injured. Furthermore, pitching when one is fatigued has been shown in several studies to result in a higher injury rate (Fleisig et al. 2009, Lyman et al. 2002). Davis and colleagues (2009) reported that youth baseball pitchers with better mechanics generated lower shoulder and elbow joint forces; therefore proper mechanics may help prevent injuries in youth baseball pitchers. Whether throwing a curveball or slider causes injury continues to be controversial; some authors believe it does cause injury (Lyman et al. 2002) and others (Fleisig et al. 2006, 2011a, 2011b, Nissen et al. 2009) that it does not. More research is needed to resolve this controversy.

TENNIS SERVING AND SWINGING MECHANICS

In addition to the throwing motion, discussing the mechanics of several other overhead sport movement patterns will provide an overview of the demands these activities place on the shoulder. This section covers the tennis serve and groundstrokes, along with overhead volleyball mechanics, the golf swing, and swimming strokes.

Tennis Serve

The tennis serve is the most complex stroke in competitive tennis (Girard et al. 2005). The complexity of the movement results from the combination of limb and joint movements required to summate and transfer forces from the ground up through the kinetic chain and out into the ball. Effective servers maximally use their entire kinetic chain via the synchronous use of selective muscle groups, segmental rotations, and coordinated lower extremity muscle (quadriceps, hamstrings, internal and external hip

rotators) activation. This lower body–core force production is then transferred up into the upper body and out through the racket into the ball. If any of the links in the chain are not synchronized effectively, the outcome of the serve will not be optimal (Kibler 2009).

The serve has been studied similarly to the throwing motion in baseball, although some significant differences exist between the serving motion and the throwing motion. These differences include planes of motion used, the nondominant arm tossing the tennis ball, the trajectory of forces produced and released, the tennis racket (which alters the lever arm), the technical components of the serve, and the variety of placements and the goals of the motion (spin, speed, angle, direction, and so on).

The components usually seen in the traditional throwing analysis (Fleisig et al. 1995, Jobe et al. 1983) have been altered in a proposed eight-stage tennis-specific serve model (figure 2.5; Kovacs & Ellenbecker 2011). The eight-stage model has three distinct phases: preparation, acceleration, and follow-through. Each stage is a direct result of muscle activation and technical adjustments made in the previous stage by the server. When one is evaluating a serve, the total body perspective is most important, not individual segments. However, knowledge of both the total body perspective and key insight on joint positions, muscle activations, and movement patterns in each stage will provide the clinician with the information necessary to better understand the overall demand this important stroke places on the human shoulder.

Over 25 years ago, the kinetic chain was first studied in nationally ranked tennis players (Elliott et al. 1986). During their early analysis, Elliott and colleagues (1986) found that players increased the maximum linear velocity from the knee to the racket. In an efficiently functioning kinetic chain, the legs and trunk segments are the engine for the development of force and the stable proximal base for distal mobility (Elliott et al. 1995, Kibler 1995, Zatarra & Bouisset

Three Phases   Eight Stages

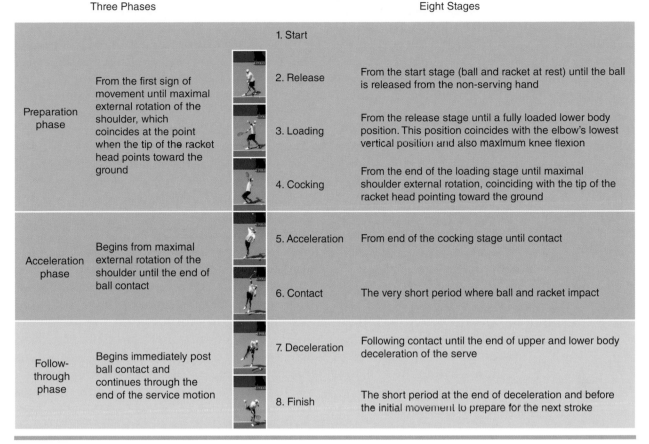

Figure 2.5   Eight-stage model of a high-performance tennis serve.

Adapted, by permission, from M. Kovacs and T.S. Ellenbecker, 2011, "An 8-stage model for evaluating the tennis serve: Implications for performance enhancement and injury prevention," *Sports Health* 3(6): 504-513. Photos courtesy of the USTA.

1988). This link develops 51% to 55% of the kinetic energy and force delivered to the hand (Kibler 1995). The link also creates the back leg to front leg angular momentum to drive the arm up and forward (Groppel 1984, Van Gheluwe & Hebbelinck 1986). The high cross-sectional area of the legs and trunk, the large mass, and the high moment of inertia create an anchor that allows for centripetal motion to occur (Cordo & Nasher 1982, Zattara & Bouisset 1988). In an analysis of the kinetic chain using mathematical modeling, a 20% reduction in kinetic energy from the trunk required a 34% increase in velocity or a 70% increase in mass to achieve the same kinetic energy to the hand (Kibler 1995). These data highlight the importance of developing effective lower body force and efficient energy transfer up through the kinetic chain.

The eight-stage model has three distinct phases: preparation, acceleration, and follow-through. The phases reflect the distinct dynamic functions of the serve: storing energy (preparation phase), releasing energy (acceleration phase), and deceleration (follow-through phase).

Preparation Phase

The start of a player's serve reflects style or individual tendency rather than substance. Muscular activation in the shoulder and scapular regions is very low during this phase because demand is low, similar to the situation in the windup phase of the throwing motion (Ryu et al. 1988). The goal of the start of the serve is to align the body to use the ground for force–power generation throughout the service motion.

The release stage occurs when the ball is released from the nondominant hand (left hand for a right-handed server). The location of the toss relative to the player affects shoulder abduction and subacromial humeral position. The toss should be out slightly lateral to the overhead position of the server, facilitating ball contact at approximately 100° of arm abduction (Fleisig et al. 2003). Improper toss location too close to the head (12 o'clock position) can increase arm abduction and cause subacromial impingement (Flatow et al. 1994). Trunk position and toss location are factors in shoulder pain during the acceleration and contact phases of the tennis serve (Ellenbecker 1995).

The loading stage positions the body segments to generate potential energy (figure 2.6). There are two broad types of lower body loading (foot position) options; these include the foot-up or pinpoint stance

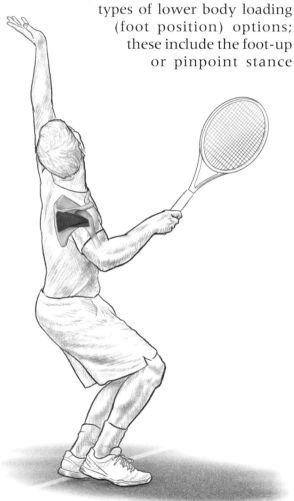

Figure 2.6   Loading stage of the tennis serve.

(figure 2.7a) or the foot-back (figure 2.7b) technique. Players using a foot-up or pinpoint technique develop greater vertical forces, which allows them to reach a greater height than the foot-back technique, while players using the foot-back technique generate greater horizontal forces (Elliott & Wood 1983). Ball velocities were shown not to be different between foot-up and foot-back technique (Elliott & Wood 1983). The back leg provides most of the upward and forward push, whereas the front leg provides a stable post to allow rotational momentum (Bahamonde & Knudson 2001).

A front knee flexion angle greater than 15° during the loading stage is recommended for effective front "leg drive" (Elliott et al. 2003). Elite servers with optimal front leg drive had lower anterior shoulder and medial elbow loads. The benefits of effective kinetic chain involvement include reducing injury potential in the high-performance tennis serve.

During the loading and cocking phases, the spine moves into hyperextension, ipsilateral lateral flexion, and ipsilateral rotation. This loads the spinal facets and is a potential factor in the development of spondylolysis in elite developing players (Alyas et al. 2007). Electromyographic studies demonstrate high trunk muscle activation in this stage, needed to protect the spine and optimally position and stabilize the body to allow and enhance the flow-transfer of energy through the kinetic chain (Chow et al. 2009).

The cocking phase position (figure 2.8 on page 40) depends on an efficient loading stage (stage 3). Increasing the efficiency of the dominant arm in driving the racket down and behind the torso lengthens the trajectory of the racket to the ball (Elliott 2002). This position allows for greater potential energy but does require optimal range of motion, positioning, and stabilization throughout the shoulder region.

Acceleration Phase

High internal rotator eccentric loads are applied during the late preparation phase (backswing), later transitioning into the acceleration phase (stage 5) before impact

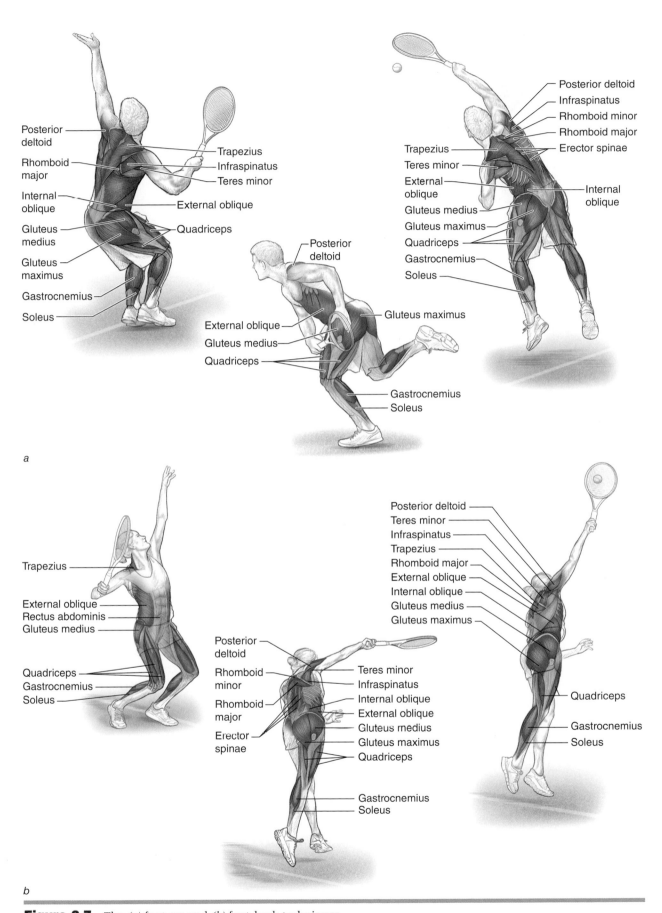

Figure 2.7 The (a) foot-up and (b) foot-back techniques.

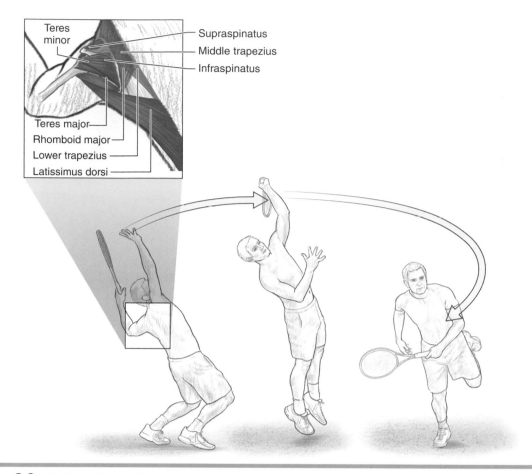

Teres minor
Supraspinatus
Middle trapezius
Infraspinatus
Teres major
Rhomboid major
Lower trapezius
Latissimus dorsi

Figure 2.8 Cocking phase of the tennis serve.

(Bahamonde 1997). Effective leg drive forces the racket in a downward motion away from the back. This energy is recovered to assist in generating racket velocity during the acceleration phase of the service motion (Elliott et al. 2003).

At the instant of maximum external rotation, the shoulder has been shown to be abducted 101 ± 13°, horizontally adducted 7° ± 13°, and externally rotated 172° ± 12°; the elbow flexed 104° ± 12°; and the wrist extended 66° ± 19° (Fleisig et al. 2003). This resulted in a near-parallel position between the racket and the trunk. The magnitude of external rotation is similar to that for elite baseball pitchers, 175° to 185° (Dillman et al. 1993, Fleisig et al. 1999). This degree of external rotation is a combination of glenohumeral, scapulothoracic, and trunk extension motions (Dillman et al. 1993).

Repeated external rotation in the tennis serve can lead to increased shoulder external rotation on the dominant arm at the expense of internal rotation (Ellenbecker 1992, Ellenbecker et al. 2002). These increases in external rotation do not match the magnitude of the increases reported in the dominant arm of professional baseball pitchers (Ellenbecker et al. 2002, Wilk et al. 2009a). Loss of both internal rotation and total rotation (see chapter 3) up to 10° in elite-level tennis players occurs at 90° in the abducted shoulder (Ellenbecker 1992, Ellenbecker et al. 2002, Kibler et al. 1996, Roetert et al. 2000). Stretches of the posterior shoulder (sleeper and cross-arm) (Kibler et al. 2003, Manske et al. 2010, McClure et al. 2007) counter internal rotation losses in developing and elite-level competitive tennis players (Ellenbecker & Cools 2010, Ellenbecker et al. 2010, Harryman et al. 1990, Kibler et al. 1996, Manske et al. 2010).

During the cocking stage, shoulder loads in the abducted, externally rotated position can lead to injury (Burkhart et al. 2003). Muscle activity (% maximal voluntary contraction [% MVC]) during the cocking stage is moderately high in the supraspinatus (53%), infraspinatus (41%), subscapularis (25%), biceps brachii (39%), and serratus anterior (70%) to provide stabilization (Ryu et al. 1988). The moderately high activity during this stage demonstrates the importance of both anterior and posterior rotator cuff and scapular stabilization for proper execution of the cocking stage.

Tennis serves depend on glenohumeral position during the cocking stage: 7° of horizontal adduction from the coronal plane places the glenohumeral joint anterior to the coronal plane (Fleisig et al. 2003). There is increased contact pressure between the supra- and infraspinatus and the posterior glenoid (internal impingement) in cadavers with the abducted, externally rotated shoulder (Mihata et al. 2010). This hyperabduction position is a risk factor in the throwing shoulder (Fleisig et al. 1995). Premature dropping of the tossing arm, coupled with early hip and trunk forward rotation, can lead to an exaggerated horizontal abduction or "arm lag," subjecting the shoulder to posterior impingement and loading the anterior capsular structures (Burkhart et al. 2003, Mihata et al. 2010).

The position of maximal external rotation in the cocking phase shows high abduction angles (83° [Elliott et al. 1986] and 101° [Fleisig et al. 2003]), which risks impingement (Wuelker et al. 1998). Lower external-to-internal rotation ratios on the dominant extremity in elite-level tennis players indicate selective development of the internal rotators relative to the external rotators (Ellenbecker 1991, 1992, Ellenbecker & Roetert 2003). Elite junior tennis players show normal external-to-internal rotation ratios (ratios of external to internal rotation between 66% and 75% [dominant] and 80% to 85% [nondominant arm]) at 90° abduction with isokinetic testing with the glenohumeral joint in 90° of abduction simulating the tennis serve position (Ellenbecker & Roetert 2003).

The acceleration stage is determined by the previous four stages. Elite servers have a quicker acceleration phase (stages 5 and 6) than beginner servers as a result of a more vigorous knee extension from stages 3 to 6 (Girard et al. 2005). Advanced servers move from maximum glenohumeral joint external rotation to ball contact in less than 1/100 of a second (Fleisig et al. 2003). Shoulder internal rotation velocities during the tennis serve in elite players have been reported as high as 1371°/sec in female players and 2420°/sec in male players (Fleisig et al. 2003).

High muscle activity (% maximum voluntary isometric contraction [% MVIC]) was found in the pectoralis major (115%), subscapularis (113%), latissimus dorsi (57%), and serratus anterior (74%) during internal rotation of the humerus, consistent with EMG recordings during the acceleration phase of throwing (Fleisig et al. 1995, Ryu et al. 1988). The pectoralis major, deltoid, trapezius, and triceps are active during the acceleration phase (Miyahita et al. 1980, Van Gheluwe & Hebbelinck 1986).

Power production during the acceleration stage (concentric action) depends on strength and neuromuscular coordination (Nagano & Gerritsen 2001). Vertical force production in the serve is approximately 1.68 to 2.12 times body weight (Elliott & Wood 1983, Girard et al. 2005).

At ball contact, the trunk has an average tilt of approximately 48° above horizontal, the arm is abducted 101°, and the elbow, wrist, and lead knee are slightly flexed in Olympic tennis players (Fleisig et al. 2003) (figure 2.9). Elite tennis players generate racket velocities of approximately 38 to 47 m/sec (85-105 miles/h [137-169 km/h]) (Chow 2003, Reid et al. 2008). The mean shoulder abduction just before contact is approximately 100° (Fleisig et al. 2003), which is similar to the 100° ± 10° angle that produces maximal ball velocity and minimal shoulder joint loading in baseball pitching (Matsuo et al. 2000a, 2000b, Reid et al. 2008). This suggests an optimum contact point of approximately 110° ± 15° for the tennis serve.

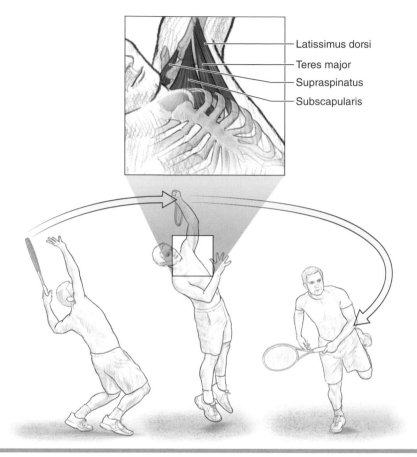

Figure 2.9 Ball contact during the tennis serve.

At ball contact, ball velocity is most determined by shoulder internal rotation and wrist flexion (Elliott et al. 1986, 1995). Elbow flexion (20° ± 4°), wrist extension (15° ± 8°), and front knee flexion (24° ± 14°) are minimal at contact (Fleisig et al. 2003). Trunk is tilted 48° ± 7° above horizontal in Olympic professional tennis players (Fleisig et al. 2003).

Follow-Through Phase

The follow-through phase (stages 7 and 8) is the most violent of the tennis serve, requiring extensive deceleration eccentric loads in both the upper and lower body (figure 2.10). Continued glenohumeral internal rotation and forearm pronation occur during the acceleration stage and continue after ball contact during deceleration. This coupled motion has been termed **long axis rotation** (Elliott et al. 1995, 2003).

The deceleration force activity between the trunk and the arm during the deceleration stage can be as high as 300 Nm (Ellenbecker et al. 2010). This force stabilizes the shoulder against the distraction forces of 0.5 to 0.75 times body weight (Ellenbecker et al. 2010). There is also moderately high activity in the posterior rotator cuff, serratus anterior, biceps brachii, deltoid, and latissimus dorsi musculature (Ryu et al. 1988). The posterior rotator cuff activation ranges between 30% and 35% as the humerus is decelerated following contact (Ryu et al. 1988) to offset the distraction forces and to maintain glenohumeral congruity. Serratus anterior MVIC (53%) indicates the continued need for scapular stabilization (Ryu et al. 1988).

The last stage of the service motion results in lower body landing, which generates eccentric forces. Larger horizontal braking

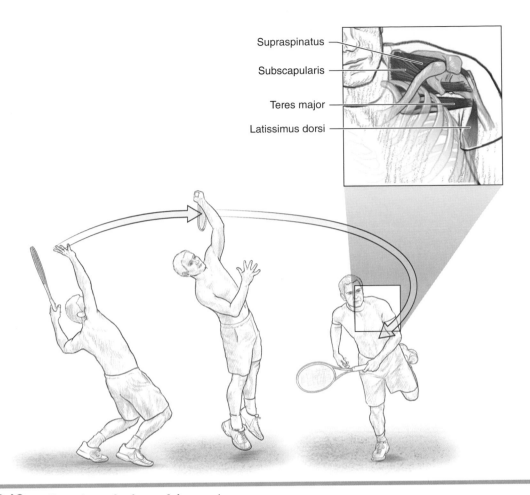

Supraspinatus
Subscapularis
Teres major
Latissimus dorsi

Figure 2.10   Follow-through phase of the tennis serve.

forces are developed with the front foot (at landing stage 8) using the foot-up technique (vs. the foot-back technique) since the center of mass is shifted forward, which may hinder serve and volley players (Bahamonde & Knudson 2001).

Tennis Groundstrokes

The forehand and backhand groundstrokes are excellent examples of swing mechanics in upper extremity sports. The forehand and backhand can both be broken down into three phases: preparation, acceleration, and follow-through. The EMG activity during the preparation phases of both the forehand and the backhand groundstroke is very low and does not deserve significant discussion (Ryu et al. 1988). The modern game of tennis typically consists of open stance positions in the lower extremity on the forehand, which accentuate the player's ability to use angular momentum for power generation (Roetert & Groppel 2001). Despite the lower extremity position in an open stance during the preparation phase of the forehand, it is imperative that the upper body be turned sideways, optimizing shoulder–hip separation angles to enable large trunk and lower extremity kinetic chain influence (Roetert & Kovacs 2011, Segal 2002) (figure 2.11a). This increased segmental rotation created by the open stance can be a liability when performed incorrectly. Premature opening of the pelvis and early rotation of the shoulders can lead to arm lag and hyperangulation at the shoulder joint, which can increase the risk of shoulder injury (Ellenbecker 2006, Roetert & Groppel 2001, Segal 2002).

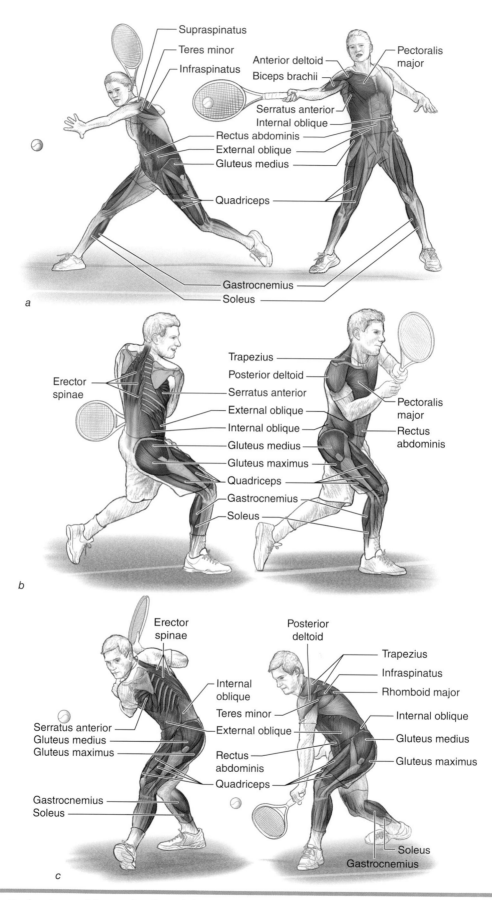

Figure 2.11 Backswing and forward swing of three types of tennis groundstrokes: *(a)* forehand, *(b)* two-handed backhand, and *(c)* one-handed backhand.

Acceleration during the forehand involves very high muscular activity from the subscapularis, biceps brachii, pectoralis major, and serratus anterior (MCIV of 102%, 86%, 85%, and 76%, respectively). Acceleration during the backhand groundstroke also involves high levels of muscular activity in the middle deltoid (118%), supraspinatus (73%), and infraspinatus (78%) (Ryu et al. 1988). Players use the two-handed backhand (figure 2.11*b*) more frequently than the one-handed backhand (figure 2.11*c*) in the modern game, but both types of backhand strokes are used by both recreational and elite-level players. The traditional closed stance or square stance is used by players for both the one- and two-handed backhands as pictured, with the front leg crossing over the midline of the body to allow for greater trunk and lower extremity rotation. Lower overall muscular activity is reported during the follow-through phases of the backhand compared with that during the acceleration phase. The serratus anterior activity remains very high in virtually all phases of the forehand and backhand groundstrokes, which has ramifications for rehabilitation as this muscle is frequently found to be deficient both in patients with instability (McMahon et al. 1996) and in patients with subacromial impingement (Cools et al. 2005, Ludewig & Cook 2000).

Relationship Between Tennis Strokes and Injury Risk

Research completed by the United States Tennis Association (USTA) Sport Science Committee (Kovacs et al. 2014) has provided key epidemiological information regarding the injury and training characteristics of elite junior tennis players. Prior studies by Reese and colleagues (1986) and others (Pluim et al. 2006) have reported shoulder injury rates of 8% to 24% in elite junior tennis players. In the USTA investigation by Kovacs and coworkers (2014), 861 elite-level players were studied between the ages of 10 and 17 years. Overall, 41% of all players reported at least one overuse injury that limited tennis play and competition in the past year. Elbow injuries composed 3% of those injuries reported among the elite junior players. Furthermore, of the 41% of players reporting a musculoskeletal injury, 33% of these players reported a second musculoskeletal injury during that time period. The repetitive overuse required to obtain high levels of skill, coupled with competition demands, has been reported to create muscular imbalances and range of motion alterations that may place the elite tennis player at a risk for injury. Further research to identify specific risk factors is needed in the sport of tennis.

VOLLEYBALL OVERHEAD MOTIONS

The sport of volleyball also has significant potential for shoulder injury due to the repetitive nature of the overhead spiking, serving, and blocking activities. Studies have shown that up to 8% to 20% of all injuries reported in volleyball are shoulder injuries (Briner & Kaemar 1997). Several types of overhead motions are used by volleyball players when training and competing. The spike or attack is the most explosive and is used to terminate a point, with speeds reported at up to 28 m/sec in elite players (Reeser et al. 2010). An elite-level volleyball player can execute up to 40,000 spikes in a single season. Additionally, two types of serves are used, the traditional float server and the more explosive jump serve. These overhead motions can be broken down for biomechanical study into five phases, similar to throwing or the tennis serve: windup, cocking, acceleration, deceleration, and follow-through (Rokito et al. 1998).

Reeser and colleagues (2010) performed a biomechanical study of the cross-body spike and straight-ahead spike in elite volleyball players. They found players to use approximately 160° to 163° of combined external rotation during the cocking phase of the spike, and ball contact to occur at 130° to 133° of abduction. This position of abduction at ball contact is moderately higher than values reported for baseball pitching (Fleisig et al. 1995) and the tennis serve (Elliott et al. 1986, Fleisig et al. 2003). At ball contact, the horizontal adduction angle averaged 29° to 33°, placing the shoulder in the scapular plane at values very similar to those reported in other overhead sports (Saha 1983). Similar values for shoulder external rotation (158°-164°), shoulder abduction at ball contact (129°-133°), and horizontal abduction (23°-30°) were reported by Reeser and coauthors (2010) for the jump serve and traditional float serve in elite volleyball players.

Shoulder internal rotation velocities in one study ranged between 2444°/sec and 2594°/sec during arm acceleration before ball contact (Reeser et al. 2010). Similar internal rotation velocities were reported for the jump serve, with significantly slower (1859°/sec) velocities present during the float serve. Muscular activity patterns of the rotator cuff are similar to observations in other reports in overhead athletes, with greatest subscapularis (65% MVIC), pectoralis major (59% MVIC), and latissimus (59% MVIC) activity occurring during the explosive internal rotation in the acceleration phase of the volleyball spike. Interestingly, the teres minor shows a peak in activity of 51% MVIC during acceleration to provide posterior stabilization to the accelerating humerus (Rokito et al. 1998). Activation levels of 34% to 37% MVIC are reported in the supraspinatus, infraspinatus, and teres minor during arm deceleration in the volleyball spike, highlighting the important need for eccentric stabilization to resist distraction forces at the glenohumeral joint and maintain glenohumeral joint integrity (Escamilla 2009, Rokito et al. 1998).

GOLF SWING MECHANICS

Similar to the situation with the other sports reviewed in this chapter, to isolate and identify the functions of the major muscles controlling the various body segments during the golf swing, dynamic EMG and high-speed motion analysis has been used and helps to provide a greater understanding of the demands of golf on the shoulder complex. For discussion and analysis purposes, the golf swing has been broken down into the following five phases (Pink et al. 1993) (figure 2.12):

- Take-away: from address to the ball to the end of the backswing
- Forward swing: from the end of the backswing until the club is horizontal
- Acceleration: from horizontal position of the club to ball contact
- Early follow-through: from ball contact to horizontal club position
- Late follow-through: from horizontal club position to the end of the swing

This section describes and compares the muscle activity patterns of the primary shoulder and scapular muscles (but note that there are also significant contributions from other body segments during a golf swing).

Take-Away

Before initiation of the backswing, proper setup and ball address must be achieved. This initial posture greatly influences the balance of forces throughout the golf swing and is therefore critical to the achievement of the proper swing plane. The take-away phase has been described as a "coiling" or "loading" of the body in order to enhance the velocity and kinetic energy of the club head (Pink et al. 1990). Electromyographic analysis reveals relatively low activity of the trunk musculature during this segment of the golf swing, as the trunk is simply preparing for the swing (Pink et al. 1990). Electromyographic analysis of the scapular muscles of the trailing arm reveals relatively high activity of the upper, middle, and lower portions of the trapezius during take-away in order to help the scapula retract and upwardly rotate (Kao et al. 1995). Similarly, the levator scapulae and rhomboid muscle of the trailing arm are active during this period to help with such

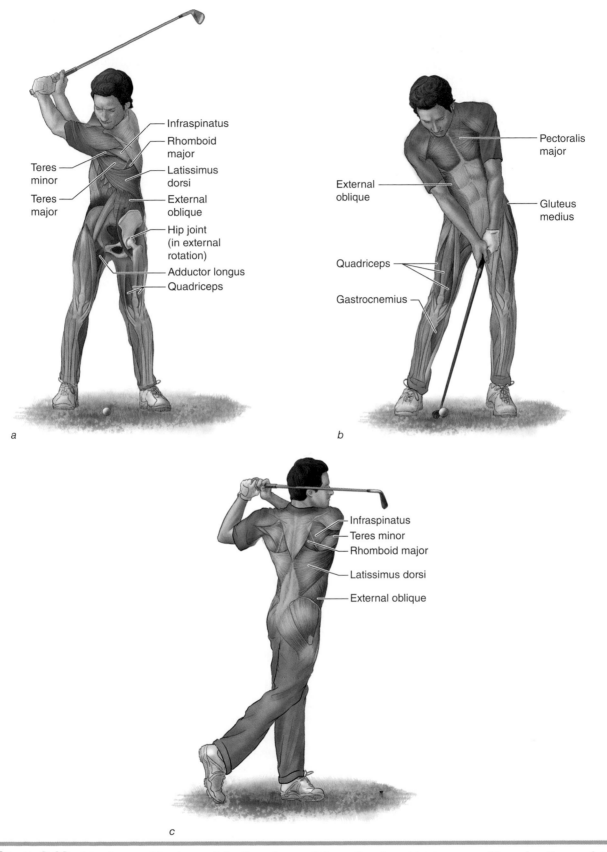

Figure 2.12 Muscles used in three of the five phases of the golf swing: *(a)* take-away, *(b)* acceleration, and *(c)* follow-through.

scapular movements (Kao et al. 1995). In the leading arm during take-away, the activity of the scapular stabilizing muscles is relatively low to allow for scapular protraction.

Electromyographic analysis of the rotator cuff muscles exhibits contributions from the supraspinatus and infraspinatus in the trailing arm as they act to approximate and stabilize the shoulder (Jobe et al. 1986, Pink et al. 1990). Of the rotator cuff muscles in the leading arm, only the subscapularis was shown to display marked activity during the take-away phase. It should be noted that the pectoralis major, latissimus dorsi, and the deltoid muscles of both arms are relatively inactive in the backswing of the golf club (Jobe et al. 1986, Pink et al. 1990).

Forward Swing

During forward swing, trunk rotation movement is initiated. Analysis of the trailing arm scapular muscles shows that the three portions of the trapezius have lower activation to allow for scapular protraction (Kao et al. 1995). However, the levator scapulae and rhomboid muscles display marked activity to control scapular protraction and rotation of the trailing arm. Analysis of the serratus anterior muscle in the trailing arm shows increased activity during forward swing to aid in scapular protraction and stabilization (Kao et al. 1995). Electromyographic studies of the lead arm demonstrate high activity of the trapezius, levator scapulae, rhomboids, and serratus anterior as they all contribute to scapular motion and stabilization as the arms move toward the ball (Kao et al. 1995).

Of the trailing shoulder muscles during forward swing, the subscapularis, pectoralis major, and latissimus begin firing at marked levels as the trailing arm increasingly accelerates into the internal rotation and adduction. The lead arm subscapularis and latissimus dorsi are both moderately active during the forward swing phase.

Acceleration

During the acceleration phase, the body segments work together in a coordinated

sequence in order to maximize club head speed at ball impact. The serratus anterior is the primary scapular stabilizer that is active in the trailing arm during acceleration (Kao et al. 1995). The serratus has high levels of involvement in order to allow for a strong scapular protraction and contribute to maximizing club head speed. Conversely, EMG analysis reveals strong contractions of the scapular muscles in the lead arm during acceleration (Kao et al. 1995). The trapezius, levator scapulae, and rhomboid muscles are firing to aid in scapular retraction, upward rotation, and elevation. The serratus anterior of the lead arm continues to display high levels of activation throughout. This important muscle is highly involved during the golf swing, similarly to what is seen during throwing and the tennis serve as discussed in earlier sections of this chapter.

Electromyographic investigations display high levels of subscapularis, pectoralis major, and latissimus dorsi activity to provide power to the trailing arm during acceleration (Jobe et al. 1986). These important muscles further increase in activity from forward swing to assist in rotation and forceful adduction of the arm during this phase. The latissimus dorsi contributes most of its power in the forward swing, while the pectoralis major supplies the most power during acceleration (Pink et al. 1990). Similarly, the subscapularis, pectoralis major, and latissimus dorsi of the lead arm fire at high rates during the acceleration phase (Jobe et al. 1986, Pink et al. 1990).

Early Follow-Through

After ball contact has been made, the follow-through phase is initiated. During early follow-through, nearly all the body segments work to decelerate their rotational contributions, often through eccentric muscle contractions (Jobe et al. 1986, Pink et al. 1993). The scapular muscles of both the trailing and lead arms display decreased activity throughout the follow-through phases, allowing for coordinated scapular protraction (Kao et al. 1995). Despite this decrease in scapular activity, the serratus anterior muscles of both arms show fairly consistent muscle firing patterns providing vital scapular stabilization throughout the follow-through phases (Kao et al. 1995).

In the trailing shoulder, marked activity of the subscapularis, pectoralis major, and latissimus dorsi muscles continues into the early follow-through phase (Jobe et al. 1986). For the lead shoulder, the subscapularis continues its high level of activity, while the pectoralis major and latissimus dorsi decrease their contributions (Jobe et al. 1986, Pink et al. 1990).

Late Follow-Through

Activity of the scapular muscles of both arms decreases to lower levels as the swing comes to an end (Kao et al. 1995). The subscapularis of the trailing shoulder is one of the only muscles that remains highly active during this phase (Jobe et al. 1986, Pink et al. 1990). Analysis of the lead arm reveals marked activity of the infraspinatus and the supraspinatus rotator cuff muscles used for glenohumeral stabilization (Pink et al. 1990).

One final discussion regarding the golf swing concerns a common mechanical fault that many golfers have, placing their glenohumeral joints at risk. During take-away, the lead arm is placed into increasing degrees of internal rotation and cross-body adduction. This position may predispose the golfer to impingement-type problems as the rotator cuff tendons and bursae are compressed within the shoulder (Mallon 1996). Additionally, at the end of the backswing, forces on the acromioclavicular joint of the lead arm are shown to be high, contributing to the incidence of pain often seen in the golfer's shoulder. The posterior rotator cuff and scapular muscles of the lead arm are also at risk for injury at the TOB as they are placed under a stretch load to achieve that position (Mallon 1996).

SWIMMING MECHANICS

The mechanics of swimming have significant implications for shoulder injury and for clinicians who evaluate and treat swimmers with shoulder pain. While it is beyond the scope of this chapter to completely review all the swimming mechanics relating to shoulder function, this section presents a brief review.

Shoulder injuries in swimmers are very common. McMaster and Troup (1993) report injury incidence ranging between 47% and 73% among all junior and collegiate elite-level swimmers, with a 50% incidence of shoulder injury among masters-level swimmers (Stocker et al. 1995). The highly repetitive stresses inherent in swim competition and training result in approximately 1 to 1.3 million arm revolutions in a competitive swimmer over the course of a year (Johnson et al. 1987, Richardson et al. 1980). Swim training consists of 5 to 7 days per week, with workouts ranging from 8000 to 20,000 yards (7315-18,288 m) per day. Thus, swimmers require an extensive amount of highly repetitive posterior shoulder preventive work as well as a highly endurance-oriented approach to their rehabilitation once injured (Davies et al. 2009).

Freestyle Stroke

The freestyle stroke is commonly divided into phases. Numerous classifications have been used to categorize the phases. One classification system is (1) above the water (early recovery and late recovery phases, ~35%) and (2) below the water (early pull-through and late pull-through phases, ~65%). The above-water phase is often described as the recovery phase and is further divided into three components: elbow lift, midrecovery, and hand entry. The arm motions in this phase consist of glenohumeral abduction and external rotation, as well as elbow flexion to extension (figure 2.13) (Pink et al. 1991).

The underwater phase is often referred to as the pull-through phase and is further subdivided into three components: hand entry, mid pull-through (which is the down-sweep and the in-sweep), and the end pull-through (which is the up-sweep phase) (figure 2.13). When the arm is doing most of the work in propelling the body forward using the resistance of the water, the glenohumeral joint

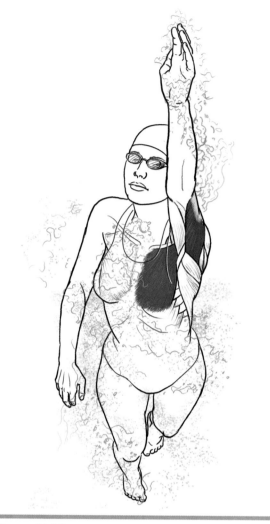

Figure 2.13 Underwater phase of the freestyle stroke.

is in the adducted, internally rotated, and extended position and the elbow progresses from flexion to extension.

Counsilman (1994) and Costill and associates (1992) have described the importance of head position and breathing patterns. An exaggerated head-down position will lead to deeper arm pull as well as body malalignments during the pull-through and recovery phases. An exaggerated head-up position will result in concomitant lowering of the hips in the plane of the water and in excessive drag and water resistance. The side of pain has been inconsistently correlated to the side of breathing in numerous studies (McMaster 1993), but no consensus exists in the literature.

Counsilman (1994) and Costill and colleagues (1992) have described body roll of 40° to 60° during the recovery phase, which minimizes the amount of horizontal abduction necessary for initiating the recovery phase and allows the overhead movement of the arm to occur with the external rotation necessary to avoid mechanical and vascular impingement. Excessive roll will lead to a crossover entry or crossover during the propulsive phase or both. Lack of body roll in the recovery phase will restrict the achievement of full external rotation, increase the degree of mechanical stress, and provide for an abnormal hand placement during entry.

Muscular Activity During Swimming

As seen in other sections of this chapter, much can be learned about the demands of a sport by examining the muscular recruitment and activation patterns using EMG. Two main studies have been done using both symptomatic and asymptomatic swimmers. Pink and colleagues (1991) performed an EMG study of the freestyle swimming stroke in swimmers who were not presently injured and were without any pain. Their findings show a unique role of each rotator cuff muscle during the freestyle stroke. The subscapularis was the only rotator cuff muscle that was active throughout the entire freestyle stroke cycle. The lowest level of EMG activity of the subscapularis during the stroke was 26% MVC. The serratus anterior, similarly to what occurs in throwing and the tennis serve, had findings similar to those for the subscapularis in that it had a rather constant level of activity (20% MVIC) or greater during all phases of the freestyle stroke.

Monad (1985) found that 15% to 20% MVC was the highest level at which sustained activity could be performed without fatigue. Interestingly, both the subscapularis and the serratus anterior continually fired above 20% MVC throughout the freestyle swim stroke. These two muscles appear to be susceptible to fatigue and have significant implications for rehabilitation.

Scovazzo and colleagues (1991) performed an EMG study of the painful shoulder during freestyle swimming. The following changes were noted when compared to the normal EMG activity in nonpainful swimmers. All three portions of the deltoid muscle showed decreased EMG activity as compared to that in uninjured swimmers. The infraspinatus demonstrated statistically more EMG activity whereas the subscapularis had significantly less EMG activity when compared to that in swimmers without shoulder injury. This alteration of muscular activation was likely a protective mechanism by the swimmer, with the increased EMG activity of the infraspinatus (external rotation) being used to try to stress-shield the subacromial area and prevent the powerful and usually overdeveloped internal rotator musculature from destabilizing the glenohumeral joint in the injured swimmer.

Additionally, the scapulothoracic muscles also all demonstrated significantly different EMG activity. The rhomboids and upper trapezius muscles had less EMG activity at hand entry whereas the rhomboids had significantly more activity at mid pull-through and the serratus anterior had significantly less overall activity during this important phase. This again is likely a compensatory protective pattern of the swimmer to try to minimize the pain in the shoulder.

In a comparison of the injured swimmer with the uninjured swimmer, the two largest and most powerful internal rotators of the glenohumeral joint (pectoralis major and latissimus dorsi, which are also the primary power muscles under the water for the pull-through phase of the freestyle stroke) demonstrated no significant differences (Scovazzo et al. 1991).

To summarize the findings of these EMG studies in both injured and uninjured swimmers, there were no significant differences in the EMG activity of the following muscles: pectoralis muscles, latissimus dorsi, teres minor, posterior deltoid, or supraspinatus. Typically one would think, since the supraspinatus is the muscle most commonly involved in the impingement syndrome, that it would have different EMG responses.

However, these studies did not demonstrate any significant changes in the EMG activity of the supraspinatus. There were significant changes in the following muscles between injured and uninjured swimmers: anterior deltoid, middle deltoid, infraspinatus, subscapularis, upper trapezius, rhomboids, and serratus anterior. The main three scapular stabilizers (rhomboids, trapezius, and serratus anterior) all demonstrated significant deficits in the swimmers with painful shoulders. These results have obvious implications for rehabilitation of the swimmer with a painful shoulder.

Relationship Between Swimming Strokes and Injury Risk

Counsilman (1994) and others (Bak 1996, Costill et al. 1992) have reported that 60% to 80% of all swim training occurs using the freestyle or crawl stroke. Given this high percentage, the main focus of the discussion in this chapter is on the mechanics of the freestyle stroke. Swimmer's shoulder has been characterized as an inflammatory condition caused by the mechanical impingement of soft tissue against the coracoacromial arch (Bak 1996, Davies et al. 2009, McMaster & Troup 1993). When this rotator cuff impingement occurs, it creates a "wringing-out" effect on the supraspinatus tendon (Penny & Smith 1980). This condition is most often caused by the repetitive overhead arm motion of the freestyle stroke. The pain associated with swimmer's shoulder may be caused by two commonly described sources of impingement in the shoulder. One type of impingement occurs during the pull-through phase of the freestyle stroke. The pull-through phase begins when the hand enters the water and terminates when the arm has completed pulling through the water and begins to exit the surface. At the beginning of pull-through, termed hand entry, if a swimmer's hand enters the water across the midline of the body, this will place the shoulder in a position of horizontal adduction, which mechanically impinges the long head of the biceps against the anterior part of the coracoacromial arch.

A second type of impingement may occur during the recovery phase of the freestyle stroke. The recovery phase is the time of the stroke cycle when the arm is exiting the water and lasts until the hand enters the water again. As a swimmer fatigues it becomes more difficult for the swimmer to lift the arm out of the water, and the muscles of the rotator cuff (which work to externally rotate and depress the head of the humerus against the glenoid) become less efficient (figure 2.14). When these muscles are not working properly, the supraspinatus muscle will be mechanically impinged between the greater tuberosity of the humerus and the middle and the posterior portions of the coracoacromial arch.

CONCLUSION

Based on the kinetics and kinematics of the throwing motion, tennis serve, volleyball spike, golf swing, and freestyle stroke, it is imperative for the overhead throwing athlete to perform specific physical conditioning before, during, and after the competitive season. Based on the kinetic chain concept, the conditioning program should include the entire body, from legs to the upper arm and hand. The exercises should be sport specific (e.g., baseball or tennis specific or both) and target the critical muscles necessary to perform proper throwing and upper extremity mechanics. This type of conditioning is beyond the scope of this book and chapter, but should be performed in addition to the shoulder-specific exercises and prevention patterns emphasized in the book. Additionally, the exercise program should change based on the time of year, according to the principles of periodization. For a thorough description of a year-round conditioning program, the reader is encouraged to examine several of these published programs (Ellenbecker & Cools 2010, Roetert & Ellenbecker 2007, Wilk 1996, 2000, Wilk et al. 2002, 2007, 2009a, 2011). The overhead throw, tennis serve, and many other overhead sport functions are highly dynamic activities (particularly overhead pitching) in which body segments move through tremendous arcs of motion and at astoundingly high speeds, thus producing large joint forces and torques at the shoulder joint. Frequently, shoulder injuries can develop because of these excessively high forces. A thorough understanding of the throwing mechanism and other upper extremity sport mechanics is necessary for clinicians to properly diagnose and establish appropriate and efficient treatment programs for the overhead athlete.

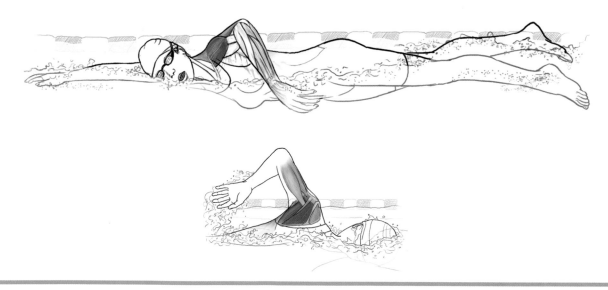

Figure 2.14   Recovery phase of the freestyle stroke.

II

EXAMINATION AND PATHOLOGY OF SHOULDER INJURIES

The most critical part in the process of treating a musculoskeletal injury is first evaluating the injured area or region to determine the injured structure or structures, as well as ultimately understanding the cause of the injury. Part II provides detailed information on the comprehensive evaluation of the shoulder complex, reviewing key musculoskeletal tests in detail to allow for not only the optimal performance of the test but also for interpretation of the findings and the injured patient's responses to the test. Part II of this book discusses common shoulder pathologies, as well as the tests used to identify and lead to the diagnosis of these injuries, to provide the reader with a complete resource for high-level evaluation of the shoulder complex. Performing the examination of the shoulder complex is a required precursor to the development of a treatment program to successfully treat the patient with a shoulder injury.

Clinical Examination of the Shoulder

One of the most important components of management of shoulder injuries is the successful performance and application of a comprehensive clinical examination. While several texts (Ellenbecker 2004a, Magee 1997, McFarland 2006) are dedicated solely to presenting and providing complete descriptions of the shoulder examination, this chapter presents an overview of key components of the shoulder examination to facilitate a complete understanding of clinical examination and thereby lead the clinician to accurately utilize the treatments of shoulder pathology provided later in this book. The chapter also includes several updated references to systematic reviews profiling the diagnostic accuracy of many traditional and recently recommended manual orthopedic tests.

SUBJECTIVE EVALUATION (HISTORY)

A detailed subjective examination is critically important; it has been documented and wit-nessed by nearly all clinicians when observing high-level orthopedic surgeons and other skilled medical professionals that many diagnoses could be made simply through the effective use of the subjective examination and simply listening to the patient. Two key areas pertinent to subjective examination methodology are the areas of localization of symptoms and rule-out questions, apart from gaining detailed insight into the injury mechanism from sport activities (Ellenbecker 2004a).

Localization and rule-out questions involve establishing that a shoulder injury without involvement from either systemic or referral causes is being treated. An example might be an athlete presenting with shoulder pain secondary to sliding headfirst into a base who is suffering a neck flexion and lateral flexion overpressure type of injury. The description of the injury, coupled with the patient's report of shoulder pain as linked only to neck lateral flexion, would alert the clinician that the shoulder pain presentation is likely not from local causes in the shoulder and that a more expanded clinical examination will be necessary. Detailed questions aimed at localizing the symptoms to the shoulder joint or surrounding structures are of key importance early in the subjective exam for shoulder injury.

Secondly, it is of vital importance that the clinician understand key injury mechanisms and sport biomechanics to be able to specifically question the patient about not only the activity resulting in injury but also the specific stage or timing in the activity that produced or is characteristic of the injury or pain-provoking symptom. For example, it would not be sufficient just to know or state that serving creates shoulder pain or injury in an elite-level tennis player. Rather, information is needed on the specific stage of the activity at which pain is brought on, for example during arm cocking or deceleration phases (Elliott et al. 1986, Fleisig et al. 2003). Additionally, detailed questioning about equipment such as racket type, string tension, and grip size for a tennis player, or changes in mechanics or specific characteristics of sport mechanics (i.e., breathing on only one side for a high-level developmental swimmer with unilateral shoulder pain), would also be of critical importance. While it is not possible for the clinician to have the highest-level knowledge of each sport's mechanics and specific characteristic musculoskeletal demands and subsequent adaptations, texts (e.g., Magee et al. 2011) profiling many of these elite sport-specific issues can assist the clinician. Additionally, in order to provide the highest level of care, it is important for each clinician to establish a network of sport biomechanics experts as a referral network for each sport that the clinician frequently encounters.

POSTURE EVALUATION

Evaluation of posture for the patient with shoulder dysfunction begins with shoulder heights evaluated in the standing position, as well as use of the hands-on-hips position to evaluate the prominence of the scapula

against the thoracic wall. Typically, the dominant shoulder is significantly lower than the nondominant shoulder in neutral, nonstressed standing postures, particularly in unilaterally dominant athletes like baseball and tennis players (Priest & Nagel 1976) (figure 3.1). Although the exact reason for this phenomenon is unclear, theories include increased mass in the dominant arm, leading the dominant shoulder to be lower secondary to the increased weight of the arm, and elongation of the periscapular musculature on the dominant or preferred side secondary to eccentric loading.

In the standing position, the clinician can observe the patient for symmetrical muscle development and, more specifically, focal areas of muscle atrophy. One of the positions recommended, in addition to a position with the arms at the sides in a comfortable standing posture, is the hands-on-hips position, which places the patient's shoulders in approximately 45° to 50° of abduction with slight internal rotation. The hands are placed on the iliac crests of the hips such that the thumbs are pointed posteriorly (figure 3.2). Placement of the hands on the hips allows

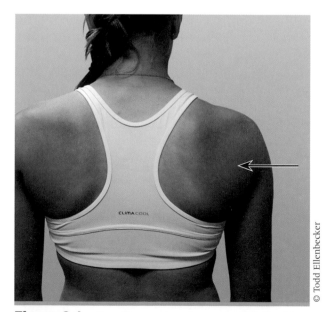

© Todd Ellenbecker

Figure 3.1 Standing posture in an overhead athlete showing the lower dominant shoulder and infraspinatus atrophy in the infraspinatus fossa.

the patient to relax the arms and often enables the clinician to observe focal pockets of atrophy along the scapular border, as well as more commonly over the infraspinous fossa of the scapula. Thorough visual inspection using this position can often identify excessive scalloping that may be present in patients with rotator cuff dysfunction, as well as in patients with severe atrophy who may have suprascapular nerve involvement (Safran 2004). Impingement of the suprascapular nerve can occur at the suprascapular notch and the spinoglenoid notch and also from paralabral cyst formation commonly found in patients with superior labral lesions (Piatt et al. 2002). Further diagnostic testing of the patient with extreme wasting of the infraspinatus muscle is warranted to rule out suprascapular nerve involvement.

SCAPULAR EVALUATION

Objective examination of the patient with a shoulder injury must include scapular testing and observation (Ellenbecker 1995). Tests

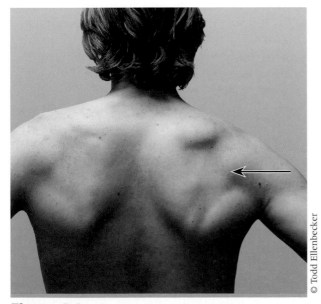

Figure 3.2 The hands-on-hips position shows the prominence of the inferior angle of the scapula and infraspinatus atrophy in the infraspinous fossa.

are indicated to diagnose scapular posterior displacement (often referred to as winging) in multiple positions (waist level and 90° of flexion or greater) with an axial load via the arms. A clinical method for testing scapular positioning can be performed using the Kibler scapular slide test in both neutral and 90° elevated positions (Kibler 1991). A tape measure is used to measure the distance from a thoracic spinous process to the inferior angle of the scapula. A difference of more than 1 to 1.5 cm is considered abnormal, and may indicate scapular muscular weakness and poor overall stabilization of the scapulothoracic joint (Kibler 1991).

Greater understanding of the importance that the scapulothoracic joint has in shoulder dysfunction has led to the development of a more advanced and detailed classification system of scapular dysfunction. It is important to note that several movements and translations occur in the scapulothoracic joint during arm elevation. These include scapular upward and downward rotation, internal rotation (IR) and external rotation (ER), and anterior and posterior sagittal plane tilting. In addition to these three rotational movements, two translations occur, superior and inferior translation, as well as protraction and retraction (Kibler 1991). It is important to note that with normal healthy arm elevation, scapular upward rotation, posterior tilting, and ER occur (Bourne et al. 2007). While scapular movement and biomechanics are very technical and complex, clinical evaluation of the scapulothoracic joint is an integral part of the complete evaluation of the patient with shoulder dysfunction. Kibler and colleagues (2002) have outlined three primary scapular dysfunctions. The classification system proposed by Kibler et al. (2002) can assist the clinician in evaluating the patient with more subtle forms of scapular malady. Subtle forms of scapular winging are frequently seen in patients and athletes presenting to the clinic with shoulder dysfunction (Ellenbecker 1995, 2004a, Kawasaki et al. 2012).

Kibler et al. (2002) have developed a classification system for subtle scapular dysfunction.

This classification system consists of three primary scapular conditions named for the portion of the scapula that is most pronounced or most prominently visible when viewed during the clinical examination. The scapular examination recommended by Kibler and colleagues (2002) includes visual inspection of the patient from a posterior view in resting stance; again in the hands-on-hips position (hands placed on the hips such that the thumbs are pointing backward on the iliac crests); and during active, repeated movements bilaterally in the sagittal, scapular, and frontal planes (Kibler et al. 2002). These three scapular dysfunctions are termed inferior angle, medial border, and superior (Kibler et al. 2002). The scapular classification of Kibler and colleagues (2002) ultimately contains three scapular dysfunctions that are also commonly referred to as type I (inferior angle), type II (medial border), and type III (superior) and represent common scapular patterns of dysfunction. A fourth classification (type IV) is normal scapulohumeral rhythm and represents the normal pattern or scapulohumeral rhythm without the presence of abnormal scapular movement or positioning in this system (Kibler et al. 2002).

In inferior angle scapular dysfunction (Kibler type I), the inferior border of the scapula is very prominent (figure 3.3a). This results from an anterior tipping of the scapula in the sagittal plane. It is most commonly seen in patients with rotator cuff impingement as the anterior tipping of the scapula causes the acromion to be positioned in a more offending position relative to an elevating humerus (Kibler et al. 2002). The medial border dysfunction (Kibler type II) results in the patient's entire medial border being posteriorly displaced from the thoracic wall (figure 3.3b). This occurs from IR of the scapula in the transverse plane and is most often witnessed in patients with glenohumeral joint instability. The IR of the scapula results in an altered position of the glenoid commonly referred to as **antetilting**, which allows for an opening up of the anterior half of the glenohumeral articula-

tion (Kibler 1991, 1998). The antetilting of the scapula has been shown by Saha (1983) to be a component of the subluxation–dislocation complex in patients with microtrauma-induced glenohumeral instability. Finally, superior scapular dysfunction (Kibler type III) involves early and excessive superior scapular elevation during arm elevation (figure 3.3c). This typically results from rotator cuff weakness and force couple imbalances (Kibler 1991, 1998).

Kibler tested his scapular classification system using videotaped evaluations of 26 individuals with and without scapular dysfunction (Kibler et al. 2002). Four evaluators, each blinded to the other evaluators' findings, observed individuals and categorized them as having one of the three Kibler scapular dysfunctions or normal scapulohumeral function. Intertester reliability measured using a kappa coefficient was slightly lower (kappa = 0.4) than intrarater reliability (kappa = 0.5). Kibler's results support the use of this classification system to categorize subtle scapular dysfunction via careful observation of the patient in static stance positions and during active goal-directed movement patterns.

Additional studies have been performed to test the effectiveness of visual observation of scapular movement. McClure and colleagues (2009) measured athletes during forward flexion and abduction using a 3- to 5-pound (1.4 to 2.3 kg) weight via visual observation of scapular mechanics. They graded the scapular pathology as either obvious, subtle, or normal. Multiple examiners viewed the subjects, with coefficients of agreement ranging from 75% to 80% between examiners with this method (kappa coefficients 0.48-0.61). Their findings support the visual observation of scapular pathology. Additional support for the clinical evaluation of the scapula is reported by Uhl and colleagues (2009b). They measured 56 subjects (35 with pathology) during arm elevation in the scapular and sagittal planes. They reported coefficients of agreement of 71% (kappa = 0.40) when grading the scapula as yes pathology (Kibler types I, II, or III) versus no pathology

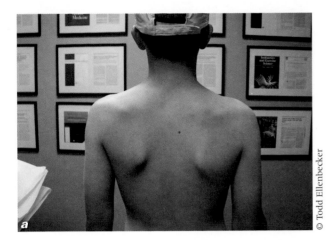

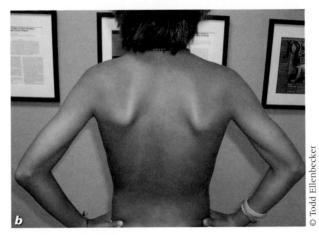

© Todd Ellenbecker

© Todd Ellenbecker

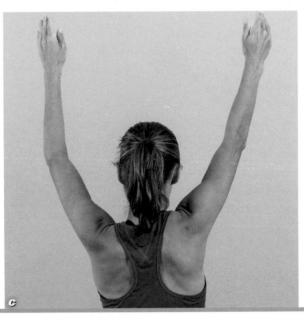

© Todd Ellenbecker

Figure 3.3 Scapular dysfunction: *(a)* inferior angle (Kibler type I), *(b)* medial border (Kibler type II), and *(c)* superior (Kibler type III).

(Kibler type IV), and coefficients of agreement of 61% (kappa = 0.44) when using the four-part Kibler classification (Kibler types I, II, III, and IV) (Uhl et al. 2009b).

Finally, Ellenbecker and colleagues (2012) have studied the Kibler scapular classification system in professional baseball players. They tested the interrater reliability of the Kibler system in professional pitchers and catchers and found low reliability (ranging between 0.157 and 0.264) coefficients with this clinical method of scapular evaluation. It is important to point out that these throwing athletes were uninjured and likely had

only subtle scapular pathology, which may have limited the accuracy and effectiveness of consistent scapular classification and observation. This study compared the Kibler four-part scapular classification system to the yes/no classification in professional baseball pitchers.

Several key issues are important to point out regarding the use of visual scapular evaluation methods. It is important to use multiple repetitions and multiple planes of movement to allow the evaluator to assess the effects of fatigue and several planes of elevation and their effect on the patient's ability to dynamically control and stabilize the scapula (Ellenbecker 2004a, Ellenbecker et al. 2012, Kibler et al. 2002). Additionally, the use of an external load may be necessary to further provoke and load the extremity to elicit scapular dysfunction especially in athletes with subtle presentations of shoulder pathology (Ellenbecker et al. 2012, McClure et al. 2009, Tate et al. 2009). Scapular disassociation away from the thorax often is most pronounced during the slow eccentric lowering of the extremities from overhead elevation rather than during the concentric phase of arm elevation, so the examiner should be sure to closely observe the scapula during all phases of movement. Finally, scapular dysfunction does not always present according to the previously outlined clear patterns of dysfunction, and multiple patterns or types of dysfunction can often occur simultaneously due to the complex movement patterns of the human scapula (Kibler 1998, 2002).

Additional clinical tests can be used during scapular evaluation in the patient with shoulder dysfunction. These include the scapular assistance test, scapular retraction test, and the flip sign. Each of these tests helps the clinician establish the important role that scapular stabilization and muscular control play in shoulder function and highlights the role or involvement of the scapula in shoulder pathology.

Scapular Assistance Test

Kibler (1998) has described the scapular assistance test (SAT). This test involves assistance of the scapula via application of one of the examiner's hands to the inferior medial aspect of the scapula and the second hand to the superior base of the scapula to provide an upward rotation assistance motion while the patient actively elevates the arm in either the scapular or sagittal plane (figure 3.4). A negation of symptoms or increased ease in arm elevation during the application of this pressure, as compared to the response of the patient doing the movement independently without the assistance of the examiner,

determines a positive or negative test. A positive SAT occurs when greater range of motion (ROM) or decreased pain (negation of impingement-type symptoms) occurs during the examiner's assistance of the scapula. Rabin and colleagues (2006) tested the interrater reliability of the SAT and found coefficient of agreements ranging between 77% and 91% (kappa range 0.53-0.62) for flexion and scapular plane movements, respectively. They concluded that the SAT is a clinical test acceptable for clinical use with moderate test–retest reliability. Additional research on the SAT by Kibler and colleagues (2009) showed an increase in the posterior tilt of the scapula by 7° during application of the clinician's stabilization and movement with a decrease in pain ratings of 56% (8

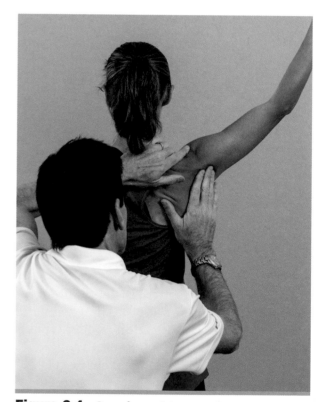

Figure 3.4   Scapular assistance test.

VIDEO 1 demonstrates the scapular assistance test.

mm visual analog scale [VAS]). This study demonstrates the favorable changes in scapular kinematics that can produce symptom reduction in patients with shoulder pain.

Additional research by Seitz and colleagues (2012) using the SAT also showed increases in scapular posterior tilt, upward rotation, and acromiohumeral distance in subjects with subacromial impingement as well as in normal controls. Their study did not identify differences in isometric rotator cuff strength with the SAT. Seitz and coworkers (2012) also examined the effects of the SAT in subjects with obvious scapular dyskinesis as well as in subjects with normal scapulohumeral rhythm. The SAT was equally effective at increasing posterior tilt, upward rotation, and acromiohumeral distance.

Scapular Retraction Test

Another test developed by Kibler is the scapular retraction test (SRT) (Kibler 1998, Uhl et al. 2009a). This test involves retraction of the scapula manually by the examiner during a movement that previously could not be performed secondary to weakness or loss of stability or a movement that was painful. Manual retraction of the scapula is performed using a cross-hand technique (figure 3.5) and is pictured for the movement of IR and ER at 90° of abduction, a common motion provoking pain in overhead athletes with posterior impingement and rotator cuff pathology (Ellenbecker 1995, 2004a, Mihata et al. 2010). Research by Kibler (Uhl et al. 2009a) profiling the kinematic and neuromuscular actions during the SRT showed an increase of 5° of scapular retraction during application of the clinician's pressure created by moving the scapula into retraction during this maneuver. Additionally, mean increases of 12° of posterior tilting and a reduction of scapular IR by 8° occurred during the performance of the SRT. Observed kinematic changes during the SRT place the glenohumeral joint in a biomechanically favorable position for function. Additional applications

of the SRT include stabilizing the scapula in a retracted position during manual muscle testing. Kibler and colleagues (2006) studied the SRT by measuring subject's ability to perform an **empty can test** (see more detail later in the chapter) both with and without scapular stabilization. They reported increases in muscular strength during the SRT with mean increases of 24% with scapular stabilization. The use of this maneuver demonstrates the important role proximal stabilization plays in shoulder function and can educate the patient on the need for and results of improved scapular control and stabilization.

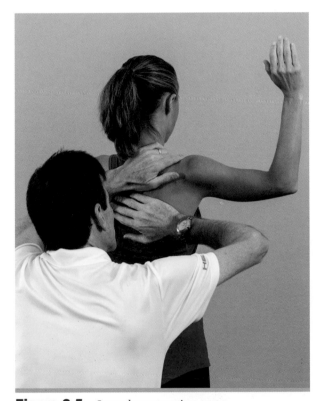

Figure 3.5   Scapular retraction test.

 VIDEO 2 demonstrates the scapular retraction test.

Flip Sign Test

One final scapular test or sign that can be used during evaluation of the shoulder is the flip sign. Kelley and associates (2008) originally described this test, which consists of resisted ER at the side applied by the examiner with close visual monitoring to the medial border of the scapula during the ER resistance (figure 3.6). A positive flip sign is present when the medial border of the scapular "flips" away from the thorax and becomes more prominent. This indicates a loss of scapular stability and would direct the clinician to further evaluate the scapula and integrate exercise progressions aimed at the serratus anterior and trapezius force couple to stabilize the scapula (Kelley et al. 2008). The test was originally described for patients with spinal accessory nerve lesions (Kelley et al. 2008) where excessive scapular dysfunction presents. One added clinical sign to observe is the apparent downward rotation of the scapula during the flip sign maneuver in patients with spinal accessory nerve lesions that result in massive trapezius weakness and subsequent loss of function.

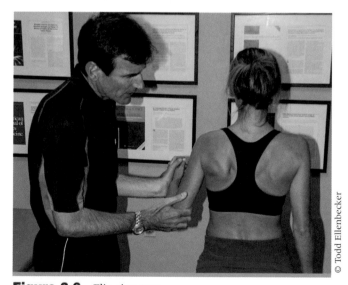

© Todd Ellenbecker

Figure 3.6 Flip sign test.

VIDEO 3 demonstrates the flip sign test.

EVALUATION OF GLENOHUMERAL JOINT RANGE OF MOTION

A detailed, isolated assessment of glenohumeral joint ROM is a key ingredient of a thorough evaluation of the patient with shoulder dysfunction. Measurement of several cardinal movements of the shoulder are important; however, glenohumeral joint IR, ER, and total ROM have significant clinical importance and are discussed at greater length and in more detail here.

Internal and External ROM Measurement

Selective loss of IR ROM on the dominant extremity has been consistently reported in patient populations as well as in overhead athletes such as elite tennis players (Chandler et al. 1990, Ellenbecker 1992, Ellenbecker et al. 2002), professional and youth baseball pitchers (Ellenbecker et al. 2002, Shanley et al. 2011, Wilk et al. 2011, 2012), and softball players (Shanley et al. 2011). A goniometric method using scapular stabilization by the examiner (figure 3.7) to minimize the scapulothoracic contribution or substitution is recommended by Ellenbecker and other authors to better isolate and represent glenohumeral rotational motion (Ellenbecker et al. 1993, Ellenbecker 2004a, Wilk et al. 2009). Wilk and colleagues (2009) studied three methods of glenohumeral joint IR ROM measurement. These included scapular stabilization using a C-shape type of grasp with the four lesser fingers on the scapula posteriorly and the thumb on the coracoid anteriorly as shown in figure 3.7. This method of stabilization produced an optimal amount of scapular stabilization and also proved reliable in both intrarater and interrater applications. The use of a consistent method for measurement of IR and ER ROM is of key importance and a critical part of the complete evaluation of both the overhead athlete and also the general orthopedic shoulder patient.

The loss of IR ROM is important to recognize and is clinically important for several reasons. The relationship between IR ROM loss (tightness in the posterior capsule of the shoulder) and increased anterior humeral head translation has been scientifically identified. The increase in anterior humeral shear initially reported by Harryman and colleagues in 1990 was manifested by a horizontal adduction cross-body maneuver similar to that seen during the follow-through of the throwing motion or tennis serve. Tightness of the posterior capsule has also been linked to increased superior migration of the humeral head during shoulder elevation (Matsen & Artnz 1990).

Research by Koffler and associates (2001), as well as Grossman and associates (2005), addressed the effects of posterior capsular tightness in a functional position of 90° of

abduction and 90° or more of ER in cadaveric specimens. These investigators found that humeral head kinematics were changed or altered either with imbrication of the inferior aspect of the posterior capsule or with imbrication of the entire posterior capsule. In the presence of posterior capsular tightness, the humeral head was found to shift in an anterior superior and posterior superior direction as compared to a normal shoulder with normal capsular relationships.

Muraki and colleagues (2010) tested the effect of posterior inferior capsular tightness on the contact area beneath the coracoacromial arch during the throwing motion. Their findings are somewhat consistent with the other studies showing that posterior inferior capsular tightness not only increased the subacromial contact of the rotator cuff but also increased the contact area or size of the area of contact compared to normal capsular conditions. This study also showed that the peak subacromial contact forces occurred during the follow-through phase of the simulated pitching motion. These studies point to the importance of identifying posterior shoulder tightness via IR ROM limitation both in patients with shoulder dysfunction and during preventive evaluations especially in overhead athletes.

Measurement of active and passive IR and ER at 90° of abduction—along with scapular plane elevation, forward flexion, and abduction—is performed during the examination of the patient with rotator cuff injury. Documentation of combined functional movement patterns such as the Apley scratch test for abduction and ER (Hoppenfeld 1976) and patterns such as IR with extension and adduction can also be important. However, specific, isolated testing of glenohumeral joint motion is necessary to identify important glenohumeral joint motion restrictions (Ellenbecker 2004a, Ellenbecker et al. 2002).

Additional ROM measures specifically recommended for the overhead athlete include horizontal (cross-arm) adduction. This measure also assesses the status of the posterior shoulder and includes not only the posterior capsule but also the posterior muscle–tendon

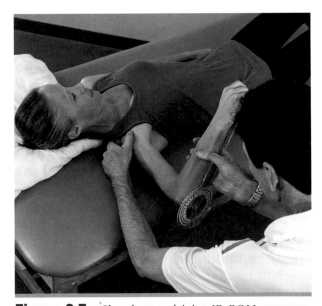

Figure 3.7 Glenohumeral joint IR ROM measurement test.

VIDEO 4 demonstrates the glenohumeral joint IR ROM measurement test.

part of a comprehensive evaluation of the patient with shoulder pathology. This includes both manual and instrumented testing of shoulder strength. The use of accurate, research-based methods is recommended to optimize the evaluation of shoulder strength.

Manual Muscle Testing

Since its initial development in the early 1900s during the study of muscle function in patients with poliomyelitis, manual muscle testing (MMT) has become a standard practice during the physical evaluation of patients with both neurological and orthopedic injuries (Daniels & Worthingham 1980). While it is beyond the scope of this book to completely review all aspects of MMT, this section covers several studies that have objectively identified positions for testing muscles in the shoulder complex, with particular emphasis on the rotator cuff (Kelly et al. 1996). The reader is referred to more detailed texts dedicated to MMT for comprehensive descriptions of and theory on the technique itself (Daniels & Worthingham 1980, Kendall & McCreary 1983).

Kelly and colleagues (1996) used EMG to determine the optimal position for testing the muscles of the rotator cuff in human subjects. Four criteria were used to establish which position was optimal for each rotator cuff muscle: maximal activation of the muscle, minimal contribution from shoulder synergists, minimal provocation of pain, and good test–retest reliability.

Supraspinatus

Kelly and colleagues (1996) found the optimal muscle testing position for the supraspinatus to be at 90° of elevation, with the patient in a seated position. The scapular plane position was used (in this research this represented 45° of horizontal adduction from the coronal plane) with ER of the humerus such that the forearm was placed in neutral and the thumb was pointing upward toward the ceiling. This was termed the **full can** testing position. Another frequently used test position to assess the strength of the supraspinatus muscle–tendon unit is the empty can test mentioned earlier in the chapter (figure 3.9). This test position has

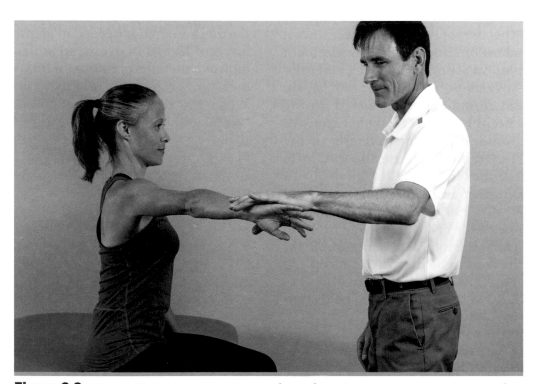

Figure 3.9 Supraspinatus (empty can) manual muscle test.

been advocated by Jobe and Bradley (1989) and has been found to produce high levels of supraspinatus muscular activation using indwelling EMG (Malanga et al. 1996).

VIDEO 5 demonstrates the supraspinatus (empty can) manual muscle test.

Infraspinatus

Kelly and colleagues (1996) reported that the optimal position to test for infraspinatus strength is with the patient in a seated position, with 0° of glenohumeral joint elevation and in 45° of IR from neutral as pictured in figure 3.10. An alternative position for testing the infraspinatus has been recommended

by Jenp and colleagues (1996). They recommend testing the infraspinatus in 90° of elevation in the sagittal plane, with the arm in half-maximal ER. Research published by Kurokawa and colleagues (2014) supported the recommendation by Kelly and colleagues (1996) using positron emission tomography. They found the infraspinatus most active during ER at 0° of abduction.

Teres Minor

Kelly and associates (1996) did not specifically report on the teres minor muscle; however, use of the Patte test to best isolate the teres minor has been recommended by both Walch and colleagues (1998) and Leroux and colleagues (1994). The position of the glenohumeral joint for the Patte test to isolate the teres minor has been reported as 90° of glenohumeral joint abduction in the scapular plane and 90° of ER (figure 3.11)

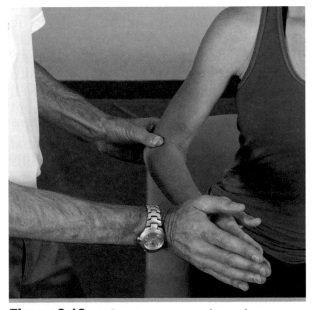

Figure 3.10 Infraspinatus manual muscle test.

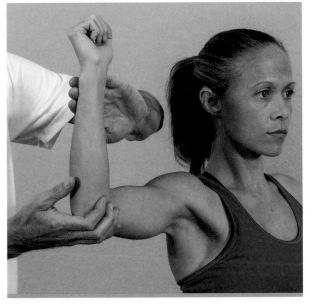

Figure 3.11 ER strength testing at 90 degrees abduction (teres minor).

VIDEO 6 demonstrates the infraspinatus manual muscle test.

VIDEO 7 demonstrates ER strength testing at 90 degrees abduction (teres minor).

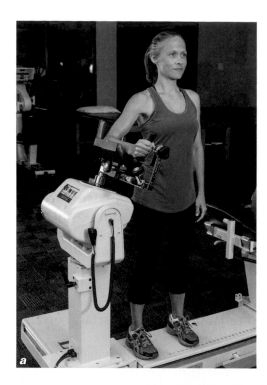

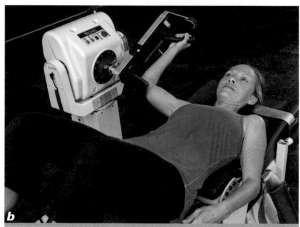

Figure 3.13 Isokinetic testing: *(a)* 30° of elevation in the scapular plane and *(b)* 90° of glenohumeral joint abduction.

In addition to the bilateral comparison of muscular strength and the use of normative data profiles in the literature, isokinetic testing allows the clinician to objectively measure agonist–antagonist muscular ratios. These are typically referred to as **unilateral strength ratios** (Ellenbecker & Davies 2000). These ratios provide valuable information on muscle balance. One critically important

variable to monitor in both evaluation and treatment of the shoulder is the ER/IR ratio (Davies 1992, Ellenbecker & Davies 2000). This ratio is typically 66% in normal healthy individuals, but in shoulder patients and in overhead athletes, this ratio can become grossly imbalanced and well below the 66% normal ratio (Ellenbecker & Mattalino 1999, Ellenbecker & Roetert 2003, Wilk et al. 1993). In the overhead athlete, this typically indicates significant development of the internal rotators without concomitant strength development of the external rotators (Ellenbecker & Davies 2000). In patient populations, low ER/IR ratios are most often due to selective weakness or atrophy of the external rotators (Warner et al. 1990). Davies (1992) and others (Ellenbecker & Davies 2000) have recommended biasing the ratio during shoulder rehabilitation of patients with rotator cuff injury and anterior instability to as much as 75% to enhance the ability of the posterior rotator cuff (external rotators) to provide stabilization.

Another ratio often used in shoulder rehabilitation and preventive screening is the eccentric ER to concentric IR ratio. This has been termed the "functional ratio" due to the key eccentric role of the external rotator musculature and concentric function of the internal rotators during the deceleration and acceleration phases of the throwing motion, respectively (Ellenbecker & Davies 2000). This ratio is thought to be functionally specific to actions of the throwing shoulder and can provide insight into the muscular strength of each muscle group in the specific mode of contraction used in the throwing motion.

Related Referral Joint Testing

Clinical testing of the joints proximal and distal to the shoulder allows the examiner to rule out referral symptoms and ensure that shoulder pain is from a local musculoskeletal origin. Overpressure of the cervical spine in the motions of flexion and extension and lateral flexion and rotation, as well as quadrant or Spurling test (Gould 1985) combining extension with ipsilateral lateral flexion and rotation, is commonly used to clear the cervical spine and rule out radicular symptoms (Gould 1985). Tong and colleagues (2002) tested the Spurling maneuver to determine the diagnostic accuracy of this examination maneuver. The Spurling test had a sensitivity of 30% and specificity of 93%. Caution therefore is in order when one is basing the clinical diagnosis solely on this examination maneuver. The test is not sensitive but is specific for cervical radiculopathy and can be used to help confirm a cervical radiculopathy.

Distally, screening the elbow joint is indicated due to the referral of symptoms distally as well as the common combination of injuries to the elbow and shoulder concomitantly in throwing athletes, and also elbow complications during sling use following many shoulder surgeries (Nirschl & Ashman 2004). Two recommended tests are the valgus stress test and the laterally based extensor provocation test (Ellenbecker & Mattalino 1997). The valgus stress test is used to evaluate the integrity of the ulnar collateral ligament (UCL). The position used for testing the anterior band of the UCL is characterized by 10° to 15° of elbow flexion and forearm supination. This elbow flexion position is used to unlock the olecranon from the olecranon fossa and decreases the stability provided by the osseous congruity of the joint. This places a greater relative stress on the medial ulnar collateral ligament (MUCL) (Morrey & An 1983). Reproduction of medial elbow pain, in addition to unilateral increases in ulnohumeral joint laxity, indicates a positive test. Grading the test is typically performed using the American Academy of Orthopaedic Surgeons (AAOS) guidelines of 0 mm to 5 mm, grade I; 5 mm to 10 mm, grade II; and greater than 10 mm, grade III (Ellenbecker et al. 1998). Laterally, provocation of the wrist and finger extensors through the use of an extensor provocation test (wrist extension manual muscle test

with the elbow placed in an extended position) to load the lateral epicondylar region is recommended (Nirschl & Ashman 2004).

FUNCTIONAL EVALUATION

There are limited tests in the literature for assessing the functional performance of the shoulder complex. For a complete description of upper extremity functional tests, the reader is referred to the work of Reiman and Manske (2009). Three tests that are recommended for orthopedic rehabilitation of shoulder disorders are discussed here.

Closed Kinetic Chain Upper Extremity Stability Test

The purpose of the closed kinetic chain (CKC) upper extremity stability test described by Goldbeck and Davies (2000) is to perform a power test of the shoulder complex by doing a modified crossover push-up type of maneuver. This test measures strength and endurance and closed chain kinetic stability of the upper extremities. It is performed by placing two pieces of athletic tape 3 feet (0.9 m) apart on the floor. The patient is instructed to assume a standard push-up position with hands just inside the two pieces of tape (see figure 3.14 for the setup for the test). The patient is then instructed to move the hands as rapidly as possible from one tape line to the other, touching each line alternatively in a windshield wiper-type fashion. Using a stopwatch, the number of touches are counted that can be performed in 15 seconds. This assesses the ability of the shoulder to function in a CKC environment without the deleterious movement pattern inherent in a traditional push-up, which places the shoulders behind the coronal plane of the body during the descent phase and stresses the anterior aspect of the shoulder.

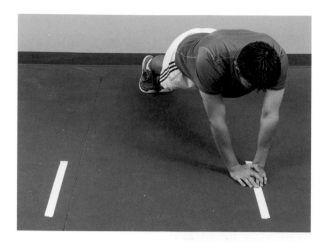
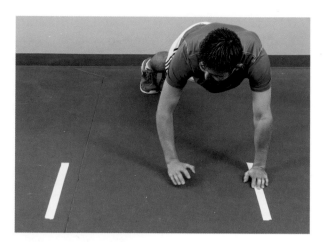
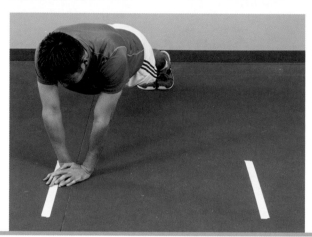

Figure 3.14 Setup and performance of the closed kinetic chain upper extremity test.

VIDEO 9 demonstrates the closed kinetic chain upper extremity test.

Functional Throwing Performance Index

If the patient is an overhead throwing athlete and has an injury to the dominant arm, an upper extremity-specific testing maneuver can be performed in a controlled environment. Davies and colleagues (1993) described the functional throwing performance index. This test was subjected to a test–retest reliability paradigm by Rankin and Roe (1996). The reliability of the index was 0.83. This test is characterized by a series of repetitive throws at a target; both accuracy and ability to functionally perform the throwing motion are scored.

Underkoffler Softball Throw

Finally, one additional test in the literature is the Underkoffler softball throw for distance. This procedure was initially reported by

Collins and Hedges (1978). This test includes the use of three maximal underhand throws, measured to the nearest 1/2 inch (1.3 cm) for distance. There are no reliability or validity data at this time for this assessment; however, this is an additional functional performance test for the upper extremity.

SPECIAL MANUAL ORTHOPEDIC SHOULDER TESTS

Discussion of several types of manual orthopedic tests is warranted, as their inclusion in the comprehensive examination sequence gives the clinician the ability to determine the underlying cause or causes of shoulder dysfunction. These tests include impingement, instability, rotator cuff, and labral tests.

Impingement Tests

Tests to identify glenohumeral impingement primarily involve the re-creation of subacromial shoulder pain using maneuvers that are known to reproduce and mimic functional positions in which significant subacromial compression is present. They include the following:

- Neer impingement test (forced forward flexion) (Neer & Welsch 1977) (figure 3.15)
- Hawkins impingement test (forced IR in the scapular plane) (Hawkins & Kennedy 1980) (figure 3.16)
- Coracoid impingement test (forced IR in the sagittal plane) (Davies & DeCarlo 1985) (figure 3.17)

- Cross-arm adduction impingement test (Magee 2009) (figure 3.18)
- Yocum impingement test (active combination of elevation with IR) (Yocum 1983) (figure 3.19)

The first four tests all involve passive movement of the glenohumeral joint. The Yocum impingement test assesses a patient's ability to control superior humeral head translation during active arm elevation in a compromised position.

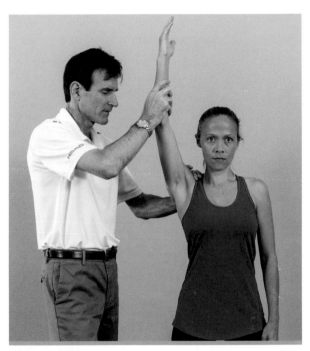

Figure 3.15 Neer forward flexion impingement test.

VIDEO 10 demonstrates the Neer forward flexion impingement test.

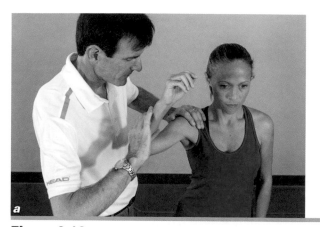

Figure 3.16   Hawkins impingement test: *(a)* start position and *(b)* end range of motion with forced internal rotation.

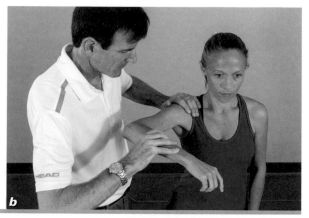

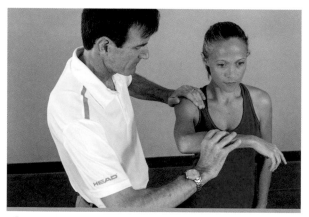

Figure 3.17   Coracoid impingement test.

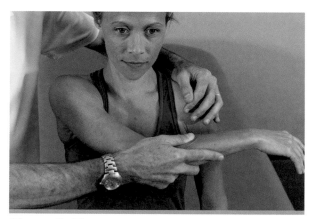

Figure 3.18   Cross-arm adduction impingement test.

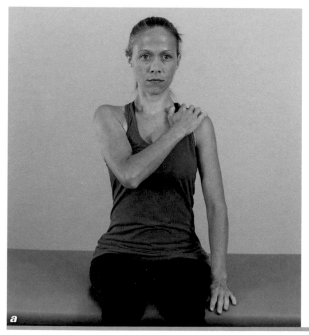

Figure 3.19   Yocum impingement test: *(a)* start and *(b)* finish.

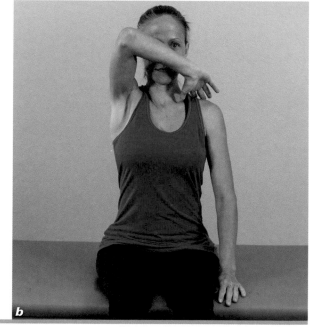

VIDEO 11 demonstrates the Hawkins impingement test.

VIDEO 12 demonstrates the coracoid impingement test.

VIDEO 13 demonstrates the cross-arm adduction impingement test.

VIDEO 14 demonstrates the Yocum impingement test.

Valadie and colleagues (2000) have provided objective evidence of the degree of encroachment and compression of the rotator cuff tendons against the coracoacromial arch during several impingement tests. These tests can be used effectively to reproduce a patient's symptoms of impingement and to give important insight into positions that should be avoided in future exercise progressions during treatment following evaluation. Use of exercises that simulate impingement positions is not recommended (Ellenbecker 1995, 2004a, 2004b).

The diagnostic accuracy of the impingement tests has been studied and profiled in several systematic reviews by Hegedus and colleagues (2008, 2012). They report the pooled specificity and sensitivity of the Neer impingement test to be 53% and 79%, respectively, and for the Hawkins impingement test to be 59% and 79%. These tests are important for the identification of rotator cuff impingement but must be used in combination with a complete examination to allow the clinician to discriminate between primary, secondary, and internal impingement for a more accurate and meaningful diagnosis (Moen et al. 2010). These additional forms of impingement are covered later in this book.

Before further discussion of the diagnostic accuracy of the clinical tests presented here, it is important to consider several terms and their definitions. These terms include specificity, sensitivity, and likelihood ratios. The specificity of a clinical test measures the ability of the test to be positive when the patient actually has the condition being tested for (Portney & Watkins 1993). The mnemonic acronym for specificity is **SPIN**, which stands for **S**pecificity **P**ositive rules the condition **IN**. Sensitivity estimates the ability of a clinical test to be negative when the patient does not have the given condition. The mnemonic acronym for sensitivity is **SNOUT**, which stands for **S**ensitivity **N**egative rules the condition **OUT**. While commonly used, specificity and sensitivity are less useful than likelihood ratios because they provide a less quantifiable estimate of the probability of a diagnosis (Michener et al. 2011). The best way to summarize likelihood ratio is to say that a likelihood ratio of +2.0 or greater reflects an important increase in the likelihood that the patient has the condition being tested for by the particular clinical test (Jaeschke et al. 1994). Similarly, a likelihood ratio of −0.50 or less reflects an important decrease in the likelihood that the patient does not have the condition being tested for via a negative response to that clinical test. The fact that no one impingement test has overwhelming metrics indicates the value of combining the results from multiple tests to assist or elevate the accuracy of impingement tests for the patient with suspected rotator cuff disease from compression or impingement origins. The reader is directed to systematic reviews and other publications for a complete description of the diagnostic accuracy of impingement tests as well as other tests discussed in this chapter (Ellenbecker 2004a, Hegedus et al. 2008, 2012).

Instability Tests

Another major type of clinical test that must be included during examination of the shoulder is instability testing. Two main types of instability tests are used and recommended—humeral head translation tests and provocation tests. This section discusses both types.

Humeral Head Translation Tests

Several authors believe that the most important tests used to identify shoulder joint instability are humeral head translation tests (Gerber & Ganz 1984, McFarland et al. 1996). These tests attempt to document the amount of movement of the humeral head relative to the glenoid through the use of carefully applied directional stresses to the proximal humerus. There are three main directions of humeral head translation testing: anterior, posterior, and inferior. Inferior humeral head translation testing is also referred to as **multidirectional instability** (MDI) (McFarland et al. 1996). It is important to know some reference values for the human glenohumeral joint when doing humeral head translation tests. Harryman and colleagues (1992) measured the amount of humeral head translation in vivo in healthy, uninjured subjects using a three-dimensional spatial tracking system. They found a mean of 7.8 mm of anterior translation and 7.9 mm of posterior translation when an anterior and posterior drawer test was used. Translation of the human shoulder in an inferior direction was evaluated with a MDI sulcus test (described in the next section). During in vivo testing of inferior humeral head translation, an average of 10 mm of inferior displacement was measured. Results from this detailed laboratory-based research study indicate that a ratio of approximately 1:1 of anterior-to-posterior humeral head translation can be expected in normal shoulders with manual humeral head translation tests. No definitive interpretation of bilateral symmetry in humeral head translation is available from this research. Important clinical recommendations for using humeral head translation tests include testing the uninjured shoulder first, using firm but not overly aggressive holds to promote patient relaxation, using fairly rapid accelerative movements with the humeral head, and comparing both the amount of translation and end feel during the translation test.

Multidirectional Instability Sulcus Test

One key test used to evaluate the stability of the shoulder is the MDI sulcus test (figure 3.20). This is the primary test used to identify the patient with MDI of the glenohumeral joint. Excessive translation in the inferior direction during this test most often indicates a forthcoming pattern of excessive translation in an anterior or posterior direction or in both anterior and posterior directions (McFarland et al. 1996). This test, when performed in the neutral adducted position, directly assesses the integrity of the superior glenohumeral ligament and the coracohumeral ligament (Pagnani & Warren 1994). These ligaments are the primary stabilizing structures against inferior humeral head translation in the adducted glenohumeral position (O'Brien et al. 1990). To perform this test, it is recommended that one examine the patient in the seated position with the arms in neutral adduction and resting gently in the patient's lap. The examiner grasps the distal aspect of the humerus using a firm but not overly aggressive grip with one hand while exerting several brief, relatively rapid downward pulls to the humerus in an inferior (vertical) direction. A visible "sulcus sign" (tethering of the skin between the lateral acromion and the humerus from the increase in inferior translation of the humeral head and the widening subacromial space) is usually present in patients with MDI (Hawkins & Mohtadi 1991).

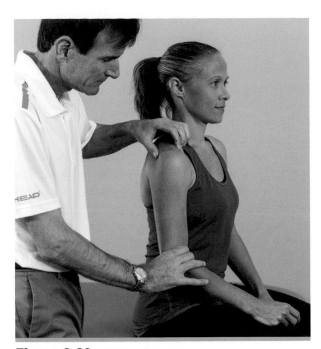

Figure 3.20 MDI sulcus test.

 VIDEO 15 demonstrates the MDI sulcus test.

Anterior and Posterior Translation (Drawer) Tests

Gerber and Ganz (1984) and McFarland and colleagues (1996) believed that testing for anterior and posterior shoulder laxity is best performed with the patient in the supine position because of greater inherent relaxation of the patient. This test allows the patient's extremity to be tested in multiple positions of glenohumeral joint abduction, thus selectively stressing specific portions of the glenohumeral joint anterior capsule and capsular ligaments. Seated humeral head translation tests are typically referred to as load and shift tests and involve testing of the glenohumeral joint in neutral (0° of glenohumeral joint abduction). Figure 3.21 shows the supine translation technique for assessing and grading the translation of the humeral head in anterior and posterior directions, respectively. It is important to note that the direction of translation must be along the line of the glenohumeral joint, with an anteromedial and posterolateral direction used because of the 30° version of the glenoid (Saha 1983). The examiner accomplishes this by ensuring that the patient's glenohumeral joint is placed in the scapular plane as seen in figure 3.21. Testing for anterior translation is performed in the range between 0° and 30° of abduction, between 30° and 60° of abduction, and at 90° of abduction to test the integrity of the superior, middle, and inferior glenohumeral ligaments, respectively (O'Brien et al. 1990, Pagnani et al. 1994). Posterior translation testing typically is performed at 90° of abduction because no distinct thickenings of the capsule are noted, with the exception of the posterior band of the inferior glenohumeral ligament complex (O'Brien et al. 1990).

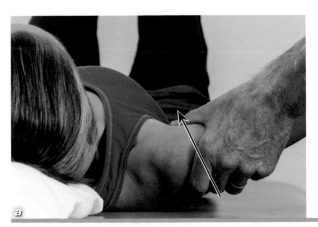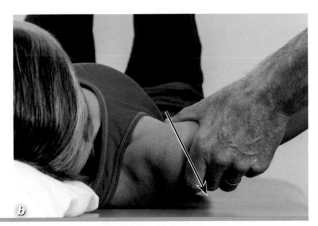

Figure 3.21 *(a)* Anterior and *(b)* posterior humeral head translation (drawer) tests.

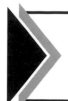

VIDEOS 16 AND 17 demonstrate the anterior and posterior humeral head translation (drawer) tests.

Grading (assessing the translation) for this test is performed using the classification of Altchek and Dines (1993). This classification system defines grade I translation as humeral translation within the glenoid without edge loading or translation of the humerus over the glenoid rim. Grade II represents translation of the humeral head up over the glenoid rim with spontaneous return on removal of the stress. The presence of grade II translation in an anterior or posterior direction without symptoms does not indicate instability but instead merely represents laxity of the glenohumeral joint. Unilateral increases in glenohumeral translation in the presence of shoulder pain and disability can ultimately lead to the diagnosis of glenohumeral joint instability (Ellenbecker 2004a, Hawkins et al. 1996). Grade III translation, which is not seen clinically in orthopedic and sports physical therapy, involves translation of the humeral head over the glenoid rim without relocation upon removal of stress. Ellenbecker and colleagues (2002) tested the intrarater reliability of humeral head translation tests and found improved reliability when using the main criterion of whether the humeral head traverses the glenoid rim. The use of end-feel classification and other estimators decreases intrarater and interrater reliability and interferes with the interpretation of findings from glenohumeral translation testing (Ellenbecker et al. 2002).

Subluxation–Relocation Test

The subluxation–relocation test may be one of the most important tests used to identify subtle anterior instability in the overhead throwing athlete or the individual with symptoms in overhead positions. The original apprehension test, which involves the combined movements of abduction and ER and monitoring the patient's "apprehension" response, is best suited to determining the presence of gross or occult instability of the glenohumeral joint. The subluxation–relocation test is a subtle form of provocation test that does not measure actual humeral head translation. Originally described by Jobe and Bradley (1989), the subluxation–relocation test is designed to identify subtle anterior instability of the glenohumeral joint. Credit for the development and application of this test is also given to Dr. Peter Fowler (Jobe & Bradley 1989). Fowler described the diagnostic quandary of **microinstability** (subtle anterior instability) versus rotator cuff injury or both in swimmers and advocated the use of this important test to assist in the diagnosis. The subluxation–relocation test is performed with the patient's shoulder held and stabilized in the patient's maximal end range of ER at 90° of abduction in the coronal plane. The examiner then provides a mild anterior subluxation force (see figure 3.22a), being sure to exert the subluxation force to the proximal humerus to create anterior translational stress or loading. The patient is then asked if this subluxation force reproduces her symptoms. Reproduction of patient symptoms of anterior or posterior shoulder pain with subluxation leads the examiner to reposition his hand on the anterior aspect of the patient's shoulder and perform a posteriorly laterally directed force, using a soft, cupped hand to minimize anterior shoulder pain from the hand–shoulder (e.g., examiner–patient) interface contact (see figure 3.22b). Failure to reproduce the patient's symptoms with end-range ER and 90° of abduction leads the examiner to reattempt the subluxation maneuver with 110° and 120° of abduction. This modification has been proposed by Hamner and colleagues (2000) to increase the potential for contact between the undersurface of the supraspinatus tendon and the posterior superior glenoid. In each position of abduction (90°, 110°, and 120° of abduction), the same sequence of initial subluxation and subsequent relocation is performed. Other

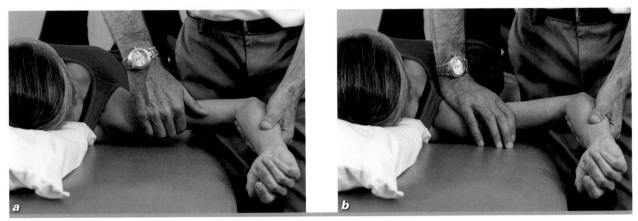

Figure 3.22   Subluxation–relocation test. *(a)* Subluxation in full external rotation and 90° of coronal plane abduction and *(b)* relocation.

VIDEO 18 demonstrates the subluxation–relocation test.

forms of this test include the anterior release test and relocation test (T'Jonck et al. 1996).

Reproduction of anterior or posterior shoulder pain with the subluxation portion of this test, with subsequent diminution or disappearance of anterior or posterior shoulder pain with the relocation maneuver, constitutes a positive test. Production of apprehension with any position of abduction during the anteriorly directed subluxation force phase of testing would indicate occult anterior instability. A positive test would primarily indicate subtle anterior instability and secondary glenohumeral joint impingement (anterior pain) or posterior or internal impingement in the presence of posterior pain with this maneuver. This test forms one of the key clinical indicators for identifying posterior impingement in the throwing athlete coupled with patient history of deep posteriorly directed pain in the position of 90° or more of ER in 90° of abduction (arm-cocking position). A posterior type II superior labrum anterior to posterior (SLAP) lesion has also been implicated in patients with a positive subluxation–relocation test (Morgan et al. 1998).

Beighton Hypermobility Index

Lastly, in addition to the previously mentioned translation and provocation tests used for instability testing of the patient with shoulder dysfunction, a series of tests to assess the overall mobility or presence of generalized hypermobility is valuable during clinical evaluation of the shoulder in the overhead athlete (Ellenbecker 2004a). The Beighton hypermobility scale or index was introduced by Carter and Wilkinson (1964) and modified by Beighton and Horan (1969). This scale is based on five tests, used to assess generalized hypermobility. Four of these are performed bilaterally, for a total of nine individual tests. The bilateral tests are passive hyperextension of the fifth metacarpophalangeal joint, passive thumb opposition to the forearm, elbow extension, and knee hyperextension. The fifth test, trunk flexion, is the one that is not performed bilaterally.

Several authors have documented the psychometric properties of the Beighton scale, with reliability estimates ranging from 0.74 to 0.84 (Juul-Kristensen et al. 2007). Several cutoff criteria have been used to determine how many of the individual tests must be positive to rate an individual as hypermobile, with no overwhelming consensus (Cameron et al. 2010). Some studies have used two of the nine measures as positive to grade in 1906 was the first to describe the presence of a detachment of the anterior labrum in patients with recurrent anterior instability. Bankart (1923, 1938) initially described a method for surgically repairing this lesion that now bears his name. A Bankart lesion, which is found in as many as 85% of dislocations (Gill et al. 1997), is described as a labral detachment that occurs at between 2 o'clock and 6 o'clock on a right shoulder and between the 6 and 10 o'clock positions on a left shoulder. Detachment of the anterior inferior glenoid labrum results in increases in anterior and inferior humeral head translation—a pattern commonly seen in patients with glenohumeral joint instability (Speer et al. 1994).

In addition to labral detachment in the anterior inferior aspect of the glenohumeral joint, similar labral detachment can occur in the superior aspect of the labrum. Superior labrum anterior posterior (SLAP) lesions are defined as detachments of the superior labrum anterior posterior from the superior glenoid. (See also chapter 6.) Snyder and colleagues (1990) classified superior labral injuries into four main types; additional classifications have been created as identification and study of the superior labrum have evolved. They reported a type I labral tear as fraying, with types II through IV tears involving actual detachment of the labrum away from the glenoid with or without involvement of the actual biceps tendon (Snyder et al. 1990). One of the consequences of a superior labral injury is the involvement of the biceps long head tendon and the biceps anchor in the superior aspect of the glenoid. This compromise of the integrity of the superior labrum and loss of the biceps anchor lead to significant losses in the static stability of the human shoulder (Cheng & Karzel 1997). Cheng and Karzel (1997) demonstrated the important role the superior labrum and biceps anchor play in glenohumeral joint stability by experimentally creating a SLAP lesion at between 10 and 2 o'clock positions. They found an 11% to 19% decrease in the ability of the glenohumeral joint to withstand rotational force, as well as a 100%

to 120% increase in strain on the anterior band of the inferior glenohumeral ligament. This demonstrates a significant increase in the load on the capsular ligaments in the presence of superior labral injury.

One final area of discussion preceding a description of the clinical tests used to evaluate glenoid labral injury is the proposed mechanism of injury for superior labral injury. This is particularly relevant as it helps the clinician to understand the positions used and maneuvers recommended to test for superior labral injury. Andrews and Gillogly (1985) first described labral injuries in throwers and postulated tensile failure at the biceps insertion as the primary mechanism of failure. The theory they originally proposed was based on the important role that the biceps plays in decelerating the extending elbow during the follow-through phase of pitching, coupled with the large distraction forces present during this violent phase of the throwing motion. Recent hypotheses have been developed based on the finding by Burkhart and Morgan (1998) of a more commonly located posterior type II SLAP lesion in the throwing or overhead athlete. This posteriorly based lesion can best be explained by the "peel-back mechanism" as described by Burkhart and Morgan (1998). The torsional force created when the abducted arm is brought into maximal ER is thought to "peel back" the biceps and posterior labrum. Several of the tests discussed in this chapter that are used to identify the patient with a superior labral injury use a position of abduction and ER similar to that for the peel-back mechanism as described by Burkhart and Morgan (1998). Kuhn and colleagues (2000) compared the amount of force required between two commonly reported mechanisms that are thought to cause SLAP lesions. These commonly reported mechanisms are the distraction force and peel back mechanisms, and they were performed on cadaveric specimens. They found significantly lower load to failure for the peel-back pathomechanical model than is seen with distraction, indicating the vulnerability of the superior labrum and of subsequent labral repair to this type of loading.

Tests given to assess the glenoid labrum can be general or location specific. Both are discussed in this section and presented for clinical use. The diagnostic accuracy has been reported in an extensive number of studies in the literature (Hegedus et al. 2012, Stetson et al. 2002).

General Labral Tests

Many general labral tests, such as the clunk test (figure 3.26), circumduction test (figure 3.27), and compression rotation test (figure 3.28), use a long axis compression exerted through the humerus to scour the glenoid and to attempt to trap the torn or detached labral fragment between the humeral head and the glenoid, much like a mortar and pestle type of mechanism (Andrews & Gillogly 1985, Ellenbecker 2004a, Liu et al. 1996, Stetson et al. 2002). The crank test is another test using a compression rotation type of movement mechanism to trap the labrum (Liu et al. 1996). The circumduction and clunk tests literally scour the perimeter of the glenoid in an attempt to trap the labral tear, with the compression and rotation

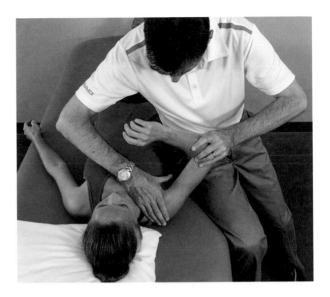

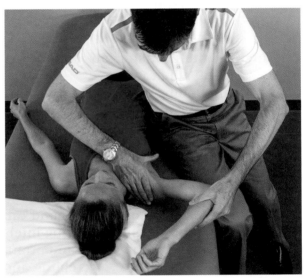

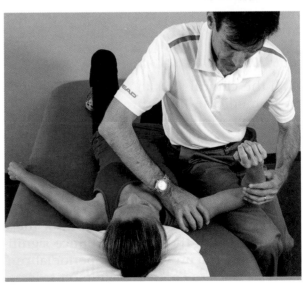

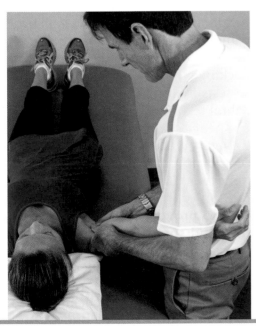

Figure 3.26 Clunk test.

Figure 3.27 Circumduction test.

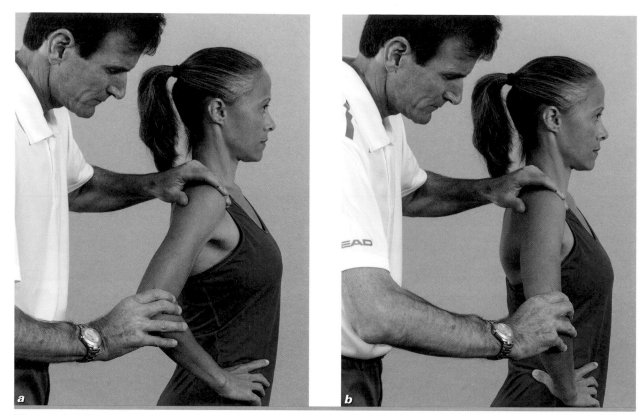

Figure 3.32 Anterior slide test: *(a)* start position and *(b)* end position.

VIDEO 21 demonstrates the anterior slide test.

Diagnostic Accuracy of Labral Tests

Diagnostic data from many of these labral tests show a large amount of variability in the research literature. Of particular importance is the difficulty involved when independent researchers report psychometric indices comparable to those reported in the literature by the originator of each test. One important variable in the interpretation of these tests for clinical application is the ability of virtually any examiner to reproduce the exceptional diagnostic accuracy reported in these tests.

Several groups (Cook et al. 2012, Hegedus et al. 2012, Michener et al. 2011, Pandya et al. 2008) have provided recent reviews of the diagnostic accuracy of clinical labral tests. Specificities and sensitivities for the O'Brien test range between 47% to 99% and 11% to 98%, respectively, in the review by Hegedus and colleagues (2012). Similar reports for the compression rotation test showed 24% to 26% and 76% to 98% in their review of the literature (Hegedus et al. 2012). Each of these studies ultimately compared the effectiveness of the clinical examination maneuver versus findings obtained at time of arthroscopic surgery or with magnetic resonance imaging (MRI) and identifies the difficulty in ultimately using a manual orthopedic test to accurately diagnose glenoid labral tears. Noncontrast MRI was reported in previous studies to have shown sensitivities ranging from 42% to 98% and specificity of 71% for the diagnosis of SLAP lesions (Ruess et al. 2006). Improved diagnostic accuracy has been reported with the use of contrast MRI or an MRI arthrogram, with sensitivities ranging between 67% and 92% and specificities of 42% to 91% (Jee et al. 2001). Further research will assist the clinician in the utilization of clusters of labral tests to obtain the most efficient and effective evaluation of the glenoid labrum.

CONCLUSION

This chapter presents the key components required in a comprehensive shoulder examination. It will prepare the reader for the treatment sections later in this book. The evaluation of mobility status, strength, and scapular dysfunction, coupled with skilled application of manual orthopedic shoulder tests, will enable the clinician to design high-level evidence-based rehabilitation programs to specifically treat the patient with shoulder dysfunction.

Injury Pathology of the Shoulder

Following the detailed initial evaluation of the patient with shoulder pathology, clinicians can develop a plan of care and rehabilitation goals based on the objective findings. These goals typically involve restoration of ROM and normalization of capsular tension; improvement of muscular strength, endurance, and ultimately muscle balance of the force couples surrounding the shoulder complex; and decreasing pain and patient symptoms to allow for a full return to function.

The goals of shoulder rehabilitation can be objectively measured and quantified through the use of goniometric ROM measurement, muscular strength testing (either manual or instrumented), pain provocation, and evaluation of hyper- or hypomobility (or both) with the manual orthopedic shoulder special tests (chapter 3), as well as shoulder-specific functional rating scales. These rating scales include the Simple Shoulder Test (SST) (Matsen et al. 1994), Modified American Shoulder Elbow Surgeons Rating Scale (ASES) (Beaton & Richards 1998), and Single Assessment Numeric Evaluation

(SANE) (Williams et al. 1999). Specific to overhead athletes is the Kerlan Jobe Orthopaedic Clinic (KJOC) Shoulder and Elbow Score (Kraeutler et al. 2013). These combined goals and the subsequent objective measures that accompany these goals allow for the development of evidence-based rehabilitation progressions that are discussed throughout the remaining chapters of this book. Before undertaking that discussion, however, a thorough consideration of shoulder pathology will provide reference information for the reader regarding the most common diagnoses seen in orthopedic and sports medicine settings.

ROTATOR CUFF INJURY

For many clinicians, the main understanding of the mechanism underlying rotator cuff injury is the impingement progression outlined by Neer (1972, 1983). Although this concept has greatly influenced treatment philosophies and surgical management of patients with rotator cuff injury, several other important mechanisms of rotator cuff injury have been proposed and tested. Understanding how each of these injury mechanisms affects the rotator cuff can lead to a more complete and global understanding of rotator cuff injury and can facilitate the development of evidence-based strategies to treat this important injury. This section discusses several key pathophysiological factors that lead to rotator cuff disease. These include primary and secondary impingement, tensile overload, macrotraumatic tendon failure, and posterior or undersurface impingement. Later chapters follow up by discussing treatment progressions emphasizing rotator cuff and scapular strengthening, as well as specific strategies to normalize ROM to return the patient to full function.

Primary Impingement

Primary compressive disease or impingement is a direct result of compression of the rotator cuff tendons between the humeral head and the overlying anterior third of the acromion, coracoacromial ligament, coracoid, or acromioclavicular joint (Neer 1972, 1983). The physiological space between the inferior acromion and the superior surface of the rotator cuff tendons is termed the **subacromial space**. It has been measured with the use of anteroposterior radiographs and was found to be 7 mm to 13 mm in patients with shoulder pain (Golding 1962) and 6 mm to 14 mm in those with normal shoulders (Cotton & Rideout 1964).

Biomechanical analysis of the shoulder has produced theoretical estimates of the compressive forces against the acromion with elevation of the shoulder. Poppen and Walker (1978) calculated this force at 0.42 times body weight. Peak forces against the acromion were measured at between 85° and 136° of elevation (Wuelker et al. 1994). The positions of the shoulder in forward flexion, horizontal adduction, and IR during the acceleration and follow-through phases of the throwing motion are likely to produce subacromial impingement due to abrasion of the supraspinatus, infraspinatus, or biceps tendon (Fleisig et al. 1995). These data

provide a scientific rationale for the concept of impingement or compressive disease as a cause of rotator cuff pathology.

Neer (1972, 1983) outlined three stages of primary impingement as it relates to rotator cuff pathology. Stage I, **edema and hemorrhage**, results from mechanical irritation of the tendon by the impingement incurred with overhead activity. This is characteristically observed in younger patients who are athletic and is described as a reversible condition with conservative physical therapy. The primary symptoms and physical signs of this stage of impingement or compressive disease are similar to those of the other two stages and consist of a positive impingement sign, a painful arc of movement, and varying degrees of muscular weakness. The second stage of compressive disease outlined by Neer is termed **fibrosis and tendinitis**. This occurs from repeated episodes of mechanical inflammation and may include thickening or fibrosis of the subacromial bursae. The typical age range for this stage of injury is 25 to 40 years. Neer's stage III impingement lesion, termed **bone spurs and tendon rupture**, is the result of continued mechanical compression of the rotator cuff tendons. Full-thickness tears of the rotator cuff, partial-thickness tears of the rotator cuff, biceps tendon lesions, and bony alterations of the acromion and the acromioclavicular joint may be associated with this stage. In addition to bony alterations that are acquired with repetitive stress to the shoulder, the native shape of the acromion is of relevance.

The specific shape of the overlying acromion process, termed **acromial architecture**, has been studied in relation to full-thickness tears of the rotator cuff. Bigliani and colleagues (1991) described three types of acromions: type I (flat), type II (curved), and type III (hooked). A type III or hooked acromion was found in 70% of cadaveric shoulders with a full-thickness rotator cuff tear, and type I acromions were associated with only 3% (Bigliani et al. 1991). In a series of 200 clinically evaluated patients, 80% with a positive arthrogram had a type III acromion (Zuckerman et al. 1992).

Secondary Impingement

Impingement or compressive symptoms may result from underlying instability of the glenohumeral joint (Andrews & Alexander 1995, Jobe et al. 1989). Attenuation of static stabilizers of the glenohumeral joint such as the capsular ligaments and the labrum, due to excessive demands incurred with throwing or overhead activities, can lead to anterior instability of the glenohumeral joint. Because of increased humeral head translation, the biceps tendon and the rotator cuff can become impinged as a result of the ensuing instability (Andrews & Alexander 1995, Jobe et al. 1989). A progressive loss of glenohumeral joint stability is created when the dynamic stabilizing functions of the rotator cuff are diminished through fatigue and tendon injury (Andrews & Alexander 1995). The effects of secondary impingement can lead to rotator cuff tears as instability and impingement continue (Andrews & Alexander 1995, Jobe et al. 1989).

Tensile Overload

Another etiologic factor in rotator cuff pathology is **repetitive intrinsic tension overload**. The heavy, repetitive eccentric forces incurred by the posterior rotator cuff musculature during the deceleration and follow-through phases of overhead sport activities can lead to overload failure of the tendon (Andrews & Alexander 1995, Nirschl 1988). The pathologic changes referred to by Nirschl as **angiofibroblastic hyperplasia** occur in the early stages of tendon injury and can progress to rotator cuff tears caused by continued tensile overload (Andrews & Alexander 1995, Nirschl 1988). The term angiofibroblastic hyperplasia refers to the pathologic response found in tendon injury from repetitive stresses leading to tendon degeneration, not primarily tendon inflammation as was previously considered.

Research conducted by Kraushaar and Nirschl (1990) in a histologic study of the extensor carpi radialis brevis, the primary tendon involved in lateral humeral epicon-dylitis, has identified specific characteristics inherent in the injured tendon. Based on their study, these investigators recommended that the term **tendinosis** rather than **tendinitis** be used to more accurately refer to tendon injury. Histopathologic study reveals that tendons taken from areas of chronic overuse in the human body do not contain large numbers of macrophages, lymphocytes, or neutrophils. Based on the histopathologic findings, tendinosis appears to be a degenerative process that is characterized by the presence of dense populations of fibroblasts, vascular hyperplasia, and disorganized collagen (Kraushaar & Nirschl 1990). Kraushaar and Nirschl (1990) point out that it is unknown why tendinosis is painful, given the absence of acute inflammatory cells, nor is it known why the collagen fails to mature.

Tensile stresses incurred by the rotator cuff during the arm deceleration phase of the throwing motion to resist joint distraction, horizontal adduction, and IR were reported to be as high as 1090 N in a biomechanical study of highly skilled pitchers (Fleisig et al. 1995). The presence of acquired or congenital capsular laxity, as well as labral insufficiency, can greatly increase tensile stresses to the rotator cuff muscle–tendon units (Andrews & Alexander 1995, Jobe et al. 1989).

Macrotraumatic Tendon Failure

Unlike the previously mentioned rotator cuff classifications, cases involving macrotraumatic tendon failure usually entail a previous or single traumatic event in the clinical history (Andrews & Alexander 1995). Forces encountered during the traumatic event are greater than the normal tendon can tolerate. Full-thickness tears of the rotator cuff with bony avulsions of the greater tuberosity can result from single traumatic episodes. According to Cofield (1985), normal tendons do not tear, as 30% or more of the tendon must be damaged to produce a substantial reduction in strength. Although a single traumatic event that resulted in tendon failure is often reported by the patient in the subjective examination, repeated microtraumatic insults and degeneration over time may have created a substantially weakened tendon that ultimately failed under the heavy load involved in the specific event described by the patient. Historically, full-thickness rotator cuff tears required surgical treatment and subsequent rehabilitation to achieve a positive functional outcome (Neer 1972); however, research by Kuhn and colleagues (2013) has shown that a structured rehabilitation program in patients with full-thickness rotator cuff tears can provide improved function and symptomatic relief in up to 75% of patients at two-year follow-up. Only 25% of patients required surgery during the two-year follow-up period in this study. Based on the results of this study, rehabilitation can be an appropriate first step even in patients with full-thickness rotator cuff tears. Surgery still may be indicated if patients do not show improved function or symptomatic relief (Kuhn et al. 2013).

Posterior or Undersurface Impingement

One additional cause for the undersurface tear of the rotator cuff in the young athletic shoulder is termed **posterior**, **inside**, or **undersurface impingement** (Jobe & Pink 1994, Walch et al. 1992). This phenomenon was originally observed by Walch and colleagues (1992) during shoulder arthroscopy with the shoulder placed in the 90/90 position. Placement of the shoulder in a position of 90° of abduction and 90° of ER causes the supraspinatus and infraspinatus tendons to rotate posteriorly. This more posterior orientation of the tendons aligns them such that the undersurfaces of the tendons rub on the posterior superior glenoid lip and become pinched or compressed between the humeral head and the posterior superior glenoid rim (figure 4.1) (Jobe & Pink 1994). Individuals having posterior shoulder pain brought on by positioning of the arm in 90°

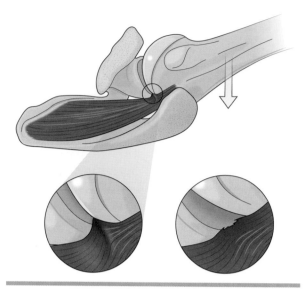

Figure 4.1 Posterior or undersurface impingement. Based on Walch et al. 1992.

of abduction and 90° or more of ER, typically from overhead positions in sport or industrial situations, may be considered potential candidates for undersurface impingement.

The presence of anterior translation of the humeral head with maximal ER and 90° of abduction that has been confirmed arthroscopically during the subluxation relocation test can produce mechanical rubbing and fraying on the undersurface of the rotator cuff tendons. Additional harm can be caused by the posterior deltoid if the rotator cuff is not functioning properly. The posterior deltoid's angle of pull pushes the humeral head against the glenoid, accentuating the skeletal, tendinous, and labral lesions (Jobe & Pink 1994). Walch and associates (1992) arthroscopically evaluated 17 throwing athletes with shoulder pain during throwing and found undersurface impingement that resulted in eight partial-thickness rotator cuff tears and 12 lesions in the posterior superior labrum. Impingement of the undersurface of the rotator cuff on the posterior superior glenoid labrum may be a cause of painful structural disease in the overhead athlete.

Additional research confirming the concept of posterior or undersurface impingement in the overhead athlete has been published (Halbrecht et al. 1999, Paley et al. 2000). Halbrecht and associates (1999) have confirmed, using MRI performed in the position of 90° of abduction and 90° of ER, contact of the undersurface of the supraspinatus tendon against the posterior superior glenoid in baseball pitchers with the arm placed in 90° of ER and 90° of abduction. Ten collegiate baseball pitchers were examined, and in all 10 pitchers, physical contact was encountered in this position. Paley and associates (2000) published a series on arthroscopic evaluation of the dominant shoulder of 41 professional throwing athletes. With the arthroscope inserted in the glenohumeral joint, they found that 41 of 41 dominant shoulders evaluated had posterior undersurface impingement between the rotator cuff and posterior superior glenoid. In these professional throwing athletes, 93% had undersurface fraying of the rotator cuff tendons, and 88% showed fraying of the posterior superior glenoid.

Mihata and colleagues (2010) studied the effect of glenohumeral horizontal abduction during the cocking phase of throwing and its effect on posterior impingement in the abducted shoulder. Their findings confirmed that the articular portion of the supraspinatus and infraspinatus tendons underwent greater contact pressure against the posterior superior glenoid, with 30° and 45° of horizontal abduction as compared to the scapular plane and only 15° of horizontal abduction. This has significant clinical ramifications, as throwing athletes with shoulder injury may possess mechanics that place the shoulder in greater amounts of horizontal abduction (arm-lag or hyperangulation positions) (figure 4.2). Close evaluation of the amount of horizontal abduction in the 90° abducted shoulder is a critical aspect of the complete evaluation and rehabilitation of the injured throwing athlete with posterior or undersurface impingement in order to minimize the contact pressures occurring at the articular surface of the rotator cuff.

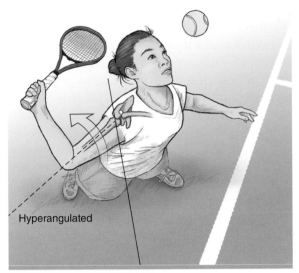

Hyperangulated

Figure 4.2 Hyperangulation in an elite tennis player showing excessive hyperangulation of the glenohumeral joint.

SHOULDER INSTABILITY

Many classification schemes and terms can be used in connection with glenohumeral joint instability. Examples of these include acute versus chronic, first-time versus recurrent, traumatic versus atraumatic, voluntary versus involuntary, subluxation versus dislocation, and unidirectional versus multidirectional (Hawkins & Mohtadi 1991). Each of these can be addressed, many by subjective questioning of the patient, as well as during objective testing. It is important that instability of the glenohumeral joint be thought of as a spectrum of disease or pathology (Hawkins & Mohtadi 1991).

Matsen and colleagues (1991) have used two acronyms, TUBS and AMBRI, to classify and descriptively define the continuum of shoulder instability. These two instability acronyms represent the ends of the instability spectrum. TUBS represents a patient with **T**raumatic **U**nidirectional Instability with a **B**ankart lesion that usually requires **S**urgery to correct or address the instability. The classic example of a

TUBS patient is the football quarterback who is tackled with the shoulder in a position of abduction and ER while preparing to throw. The forceful movements into greater degrees of ER, horizontal abduction, and abduction in this example often lead to the classic anterior unidirectional dislocation of the shoulder that requires surgery to repair the Bankart lesion (detachment of the anterior inferior labrum from the glenoid) to restore glenohumeral joint stability. The TUBS patient is also commonly referred to as the "torn loose" patient, based on the traumatic incident that produced the unidirectional dislocation.

The AMBRI type of instability occurs from an **A**traumatic onset and is most often **M**ultidirectional, occurring in patients with **B**ilateral glenohumeral joint laxity and generalized joint laxity. These patients typically respond best to **R**ehabilitation and, if surgery is required, an **I**nferior capsular shift is most often performed. The AMBRI patient is also commonly referred to as the "born loose" patient as opposed to the "torn loose" example mentioned in the preceding paragraph. A classic example of an AMBRI-type patient is a young female volleyball player with anterior shoulder pain and inability to perform overhead movements due to repetitive training.

Directions of Glenohumeral Joint Instability

As a follow-up to the discussion in the preceding chapter regarding the specific tests to identify glenohumeral joint instability, it is imperative that the actual directions of glenohumeral joint instability be discussed and clearly defined. Three typical directions of instability are discussed in the literature (Hawkins & Mohtadi 1991, Jobe & Bradley 1989). These are anterior, posterior, and multidirectional. These directions of instability are named according to the direction of the movement of the humeral head relative to the glenoid.

Anterior

Anterior glenohumeral joint instability results when the humeral head traverses excessively in an anterior direction relative to the glenoid, producing symptoms of pain, apprehension, or loss of function. Dislocations of the shoulder account for approximately 45% of the dislocations in the human body (Kazar & Relovszky 1969), and of those, 85% are anterior glenohumeral joint dislocations (Cave et al. 1974). Subcoracoid dislocation is the most common type of anterior glenohumeral joint dislocation (Matsen et al. 1998). The usual mechanism producing a subcoracoid dislocation is a combination of glenohumeral joint abduction, extension, and ER forces that produces a challenge to the anterior capsule and capsular ligaments, the glenoid rim, and the rotator cuff mechanism (Matsen et al. 1998).

Posterior

Posterior glenohumeral joint instability occurs when the humeral head traverses excessively in a posterior direction relative to the glenoid, producing symptoms. The most common posterior glenohumeral joint dislocation is the subacromial dislocation. Posterior dislocations are frequently locked (Hawkins et al. 1987). Posterior dislocations are reported to occur only 2% of the time; however, they are also the most frequently missed diagnosis with respect to shoulder instability (Matsen et al. 1998).

Multidirectional

In 1962, Carter Rowe was the first to report that atraumatic instability could occur in more than one direction. Neer and Foster (1980) called the combined type of instability **multidirectional**. Multidirectional instability consists of primarily an inferior instability with excessive inferior movement of the humeral head relative to the glenoid, with concomitant anterior or posterior (or both anterior and posterior) excessive symptomatic mobility as well. The multidirectional instability or MDI sulcus test is a key test used to identify patients with multidirectional instability (McFarland et al. 1996).

Additional Terminology

It is important to note the difference between instability and laxity. **Laxity** can be defined as translation of the humeral head relative to the glenoid when stress is applied (Matsen et al. 1992). In defining laxity, reference should be made to both humeral position and the direction of the force applied (Borsa et al. 1999). Instability can be defined as **excessive symptomatic translation** of the humeral head relative to the glenoid when stress is applied. According to Matsen and colleagues (1992), this excessive or "unwanted" translation compromises shoulder function and produces clinical symptoms. It is important when evaluating the patient with glenohumeral joint pathology that these terms be used in the proper context, as individuals possess varying amounts of glenohumeral joint laxity but only those with clinical symptoms and functional limitations can be characterized as having instability.

LABRAL LESIONS AND TEARS

The inherently complicated nature of injuries involving the superior aspect of the glenoid labrum can present a substantial clinical challenge. Successful return to unrestricted function requires integrating the appropriate diagnosis, surgical management, and rehabilitation in a coordinated effort. Injuries to the anterior inferior labrum can produce marked instability that requires high-level evaluation and treatment to attempt to improve function. This section reviews the most common labral injury mechanisms, providing a foundation for a greater understanding of treatment.

SLAP Lesions

In 1985, Andrews and colleagues originally described the detachment of the superior labrum in a subset of throwing athletes. Later Snyder and colleagues (1995) introduced the term **SLAP lesion**, indicating an injury located within the superior labrum extending anterior to posterior. They originally classified these lesions into four distinct categories based on the type of lesion present, emphasizing that this lesion may disrupt the origin of the long head of the biceps brachii (Snyder et al. 1995). Subsequent authors have added additional classification categories and specific subtypes, further expanding on the four originally described categories (Gartsman & Hammerman 2000, Maffet et al. 1995, Morgan et al. 1998). Based on these subtle differences in labral pathology, an appropriate treatment plan may be developed to adequately address the specific pathology present.

Pathomechanics

Several injury mechanisms are speculated to be responsible for creating SLAP lesions. These mechanisms range from single traumatic events to repetitive microtraumatic injuries. Traumatic events, such as falling on an outstretched arm or bracing oneself during a motor vehicle accident, may result in SLAP lesions due to compression of the superior joint surfaces superimposed on subluxation of the humeral head. Snyder and colleagues (1995) referred to this as a **pinching mechanism** of injury. Other traumatic injury mechanisms include direct blows, falling onto the point of the shoulder, and forceful traction injuries of the upper extremity.

Repetitive overhead activity, such as throwing a baseball, is another common mechanism of injury frequently responsible for producing SLAP injuries (Andrews et al. 1985, Burkhart & Morgan 1998, Kuhn et al. 2003, Morgan et al. 1998). Andrews and colleagues (1985) first hypothesized that SLAP pathology in overhead throwing athletes was the result of the high eccentric activity of the biceps brachii during the arm deceleration and follow-through phases of the overhead throw. The authors applied electrical stimulation to the biceps during arthroscopic evaluation and noted that the biceps contraction raised the labrum off of the glenoid rim, simulating the hypothesized mechanism (Andrews et al. 1985).

Burkhart and Morgan (1998) and Morgan and colleagues (1998) have hypothesized a "peel-back" mechanism that produces a SLAP lesion in the overhead athlete. They suggest that when the shoulder is placed in a position of abduction and maximal ER, the rotation produces a twist at the base of the biceps, transmitting torsional force to the anchor (figure 4.3). Pradham and colleagues (2001) measured superior labral strain in a cadaveric model during each phase of the throwing motion. They noted that increased superior labral strain occurred during the late cocking phase of throwing. Furthermore, Jobe (1995) and Walch and colleagues (1992) have also demon-

strated that when the arm is in a maximally externally rotated position there is contact between the posterior superior labral lesions and the rotator cuff.

A study by Shepard and colleagues (2004) simulated each of these mechanisms using cadaveric models. Nine pairs of cadaveric shoulders were loaded to biceps anchor complex failure in a position of either simulated in-line loading (similar to the deceleration phase of throwing) or simulated peel-back mechanism (similar to the cocking phase of overhead throwing). Results showed that seven of eight of the in-line loading group failed in the midsubstance of the biceps tendon, with one of eight fracturing at the supraglenoid tubercle. However, all eight of the simulated peel-back group failures resulted in a type II SLAP lesion. The ultimate strength of the biceps anchor was significantly different when the two loading techniques were compared (Kuhn et al. 2003, Shepard et al. 2004). The biceps anchor demonstrated significantly higher ultimate strength with the in-line loading (508 N) compared to the peel-back loading mechanism (202 N).

In theory, SLAP lesions most likely occur in overhead athletes from a combination of these two forces. The eccentric biceps activity during deceleration may serve to weaken the biceps–labrum complex, while the torsional peel-back force may result in the posterosuperior detachment of the labral anchor. The type II superior labral lesion is the most commonly encountered superior labral lesion and the one most often seen in rehabilitation of the overhead athlete.

Several authors have also reported a strong correlation between SLAP lesions and glenohumeral instability (Burkhart & Morgan 1998, Kim et al. 2001, O'Brien et al. 1998, Reinold et al. 2004, Resch et al. 1993, Wilk et al. 2001). Normal biceps function and glenohumeral stability are dependent on a stable superior labrum and biceps anchor. Pagnani and colleagues (1995a, 1995b) found that a complete lesion of the superior portion of the labrum large enough to destabilize the insertion of the biceps was

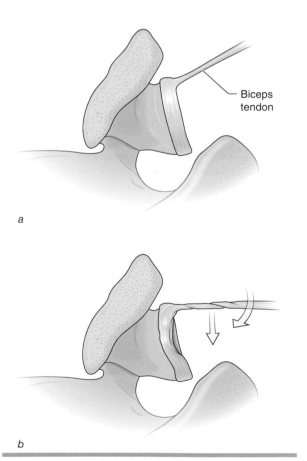

a

Biceps tendon

b

Figure 4.3 Peel-back mechanism that produces a SLAP lesion: *(a)* neutral position and *(b)* abduction external rotation position.

associated with significant increases in anterior posterior and superior inferior glenohumeral translation. Furthermore, Pagnani and colleagues (1995a, 1995b) reported that the presence of a simulated SLAP lesion in seven cadaveric shoulders resulted in a 6 mm increase in anterior glenohumeral translation. These studies are in agreement with the results of Glousman and colleagues (1988), who showed increased EMG activity of the biceps brachii in baseball pitchers with anterior instability. Furthermore, Kim and colleagues (2001) reported that maximal biceps activity occurred when the shoulder was abducted to 90° and externally rotated to 120° in patients with anterior instability. Because this position is remarkably similar to the cocking position of the overhand throwing motion, the finding of instability may cause or facilitate the progression of internal impingement (impingement of the infraspinatus on the posterosuperior glenoid rim) in the overhead athlete.

Classifications

The prevalence of SLAP lesions is disputed in the published literature. Some authors have reported encountering SLAP lesions in as many as 26% of shoulders undergoing arthroscopy (Handelberg et al. 1998, Kim et al. 2003, Maffet et al. 1995, Shepard et al. 2004, Snyder et al. 1995, Stetson & Templin 2002, Walch et al. 1992). These percentages

rise dramatically in reports specific to overhead throwing athletes. Andrews and colleagues (1985) noted that 83% of 73 throwers exhibited labral lesions when evaluated arthroscopically. Following a retrospective review of 700 shoulder arthroscopies, Snyder and colleagues (1995) identified four types of superior labrum lesions involving the biceps anchor (figure 4.4). Type I SLAP lesions were described as being indicative of isolated fraying of the superior labrum with a firm attachment of the labrum to the glenoid. These lesions are typically degenerative. Type II SLAP lesions are characterized by a detachment of the superior labrum and the origin of the tendon of the long head of the biceps brachii from the glenoid, resulting in instability of the biceps–labral anchor. A bucket-handle tear of the labrum with an intact biceps insertion is the characteristic presentation of a type III SLAP lesion. Type IV SLAP lesions have a bucket-handle tear of the labrum that extends into the biceps tendon. In this lesion, instability of the biceps–labrum anchor is also present, similar to what is seen in the type II SLAP lesion.

Maffet and colleagues (1995) noted that 38% of the SLAP lesions identified in their retrospective review of 712 arthroscopies were not classifiable using the I through IV terminology previously defined by Snyder and colleagues (1995). They suggested expanding the classification scale for SLAP

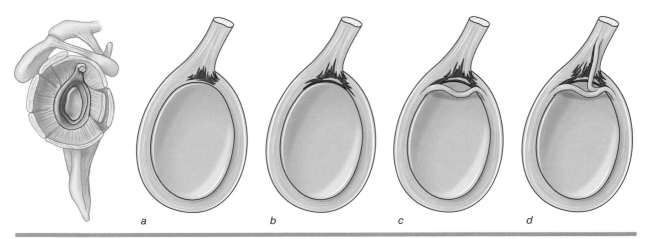

Figure 4.4   SLAP lesions *(a)* I, *(b)* II, *(c)* III, and *(d)* IV.

98

lesions to a total of seven categories, adding descriptions for types V through VII (Maffet et al. 1995). Type V SLAP lesions are characterized by the presence of a Bankart lesion of the anterior capsule that extends into the anterior superior labrum. Disruption of the biceps tendon anchor with an anterior or posterior superior labral flap tear is indicative of a type VI SLAP lesion. Type VII SLAP lesions are described as the extension of a SLAP lesion anteriorly to involve the area inferior to the middle glenohumeral ligament. These three types typically involve a concomitant pathology in conjunction with a SLAP lesion. Thus, the surgical treatment and rehabilitation will vary based on these concomitant pathologies. A detailed description of these variations is beyond the scope of this book.

Three distinct subcategories of type II SLAP lesions have been further identified by Morgan and colleagues (1998). They reported that in a series of 102 patients undergoing arthroscopic evaluation, 37% presented with an anterosuperior lesion, 31% presented with a posterosuperior lesion, and 31% exhibited a combined anterior and superior lesion (Morgan et al. 1998). These findings are consistent with clinical observations. Experience suggests that the majority of overhead athletes present with posterosuperior lesions, while individuals who have traumatic SLAP lesions typically present with anterosuperior lesions (Morgan et al. 1998). These variations may become important when one is selecting which special tests to perform based on the patient's history and mechanism of injury.

Finally, Powell and colleagues (2012) reported three additional types of SLAP lesions seen at the glenohumeral joint. A type VIII lesion is a SLAP lesion that extends posteriorly along the glenoid from the 12 o'clock position posteriorly and inferiorly to the 6 o'clock position. A type IX SLAP lesion is described as a panlabral lesion that extends the entire circumference of the glenoid labrum (figure 4.5). Lastly, a type X SLAP lesion is a glenoid labrum lesion that includes a SLAP lesion with

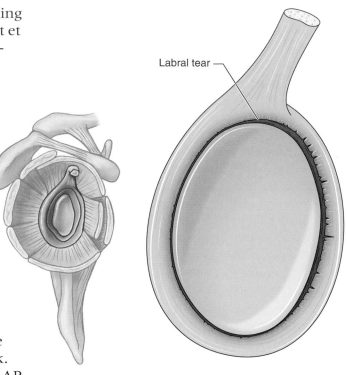

Figure 4.5 Type IX (panlabral) SLAP lesion.

a posterior inferior labrum detachment (i.e., posterior Bankart).

Bankart Lesion

In addition to tearing of the labrum that can occur at virtually any portion along the circular course of the labrum, detachments of the labrum from the glenoid rim occur and markedly affect glenohumeral joint stability. In addition to the SLAP lesion previously described, the other common labral detachment that is clinically encountered is the Bankart lesion. Perthes (1906) was the first to report the presence of a detachment of the anterior labrum in patients with recurrent anterior instability. Bankart (1923, 1938) initially described a method for surgically repairing this lesion that now bears his name.

A Bankart lesion, which is found in as many as 85% of dislocations (Gill et al. 1997), is described as a labral detachment that occurs at between 2 o'clock and 6 o'clock on a right shoulder and between the 6 and 10 o'clock positions on a left shoulder (figure 4.6). This anterior inferior detachment decreases glenohumeral joint stability by interrupting the continuity of the glenoid labrum and compromising the glenohumeral capsular ligaments (Speer et al. 1994). The anterior inferior aspect of the labrum serves as the attachment site for the inferior glenohumeral capsular ligament, and with labral detachment, compromises the function of the ligament's key role in providing anterior and inferior stability to the abducted shoulder (O'Brien et al. 1990). Detachment of the anterior inferior glenoid labrum creates increases in anterior and inferior humeral head translation—a pattern commonly seen in patients with glenohumeral joint instability (Speer et al. 1994).

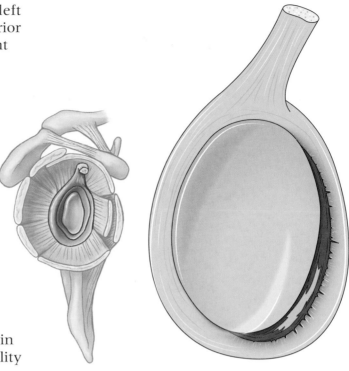

Figure 4.6 Bankart lesion.

CONCLUSION

This chapter has provided an overview of the primary pathologies encountered in the shoulder. These mainly include impingement, instability, and labral pathology. The information in this chapter will help to highlight the importance of the treatment progressions and techniques detailed throughout the remainder of this book. It is imperative that clinicians have a sound understanding of both the pathologies and the underlying causes and mechanisms behind them to aid in both evaluation and treatment of the patient with shoulder dysfunction.

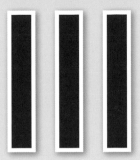

REHABILITATION OF SHOULDER INJURIES

Rehabilitation of patients both without surgery and following surgical procedures to address shoulder pathology requires a comprehensive approach to the management of shoulder range of motion status as well as the return of optimal levels of dynamic stabilization to the shoulder. The inherent mobility of the shoulder, coupled with its unique dependence on the dynamic stabilizers, requires the application of high-level resistive exercise progressions using multiple modes of therapeutic exercise. These progressions, based on musculoskeletal research, provide the clinician with a step-by-step progressive approach to improve strength and local muscular endurance in order to improve joint stabilization and ultimately optimize shoulder function. Part III contains a complete overview of both nonoperative and postsurgical rehabilitation guidelines to help clinicians apply evidence-based rehabilitation to patients with shoulder injury.

two adjacent joint surfaces. Osteokinematics is the study of bone movements in space. MacConaill (1949) explained that during any movement, a roll and a glide occur at the joint surfaces. Kaltenborn (1980) defined roll and glide as a rolling and gliding between two incongruent surfaces. The glenohumeral joint is a convex humerus articulating with a concave glenoid fossa. Thus the convex joint surface is moving in an opposite direction to the axis of movement. Using the convex-on-concave concept, during elevation of the shoulder a superior roll and inferior glide allows for glenohumeral elevation.

Joint mobilization of an extremity consists of two passive movements: (1) a passive and slight traction or separation force and (2) the translation or glide. The traction force is provided to avoid harmful compression of the articular surfaces. Kaltenborn (1980) states that compression should be strictly avoided in the treatment of a joint pathology. Often before a translation or glide is performed, a slight traction (or distraction) force is applied to take up the slack of the joint capsule.

The assessment of joint mobility is essential to determining the amount of joint motion, but also to determine if the restriction is due to the capsule or due to other structures (such as muscle or bone). As discussed later in this chapter, this assessment is critically important to guide the clinician in determining whether a joint mobilization should be used or a static stretching or contract–relax technique is more appropriately used to

address muscle–tendon unit tightness. The assessment and physical interpretation by the clinician of joint mobility is referred to as **joint play**. A scale recommended by Kaltenborn (1980) to grade joint play provides seven levels of mobility. Figure 5.1 illustrates hypomobility, normal mobility, and hypermobility.

Other terms that need to be defined preceding a discussion of specific mobilization techniques include **loose-packed** and **close-packed** position of the joint. Maximum loose-packed position of the joint or resting position is defined as a position in which the joint capsule is most relaxed and exhibits the greatest amount of joint play. In the past, this position has been used for prolonged immobilization of the joint in a cast or a splint or brace in order to avoid damaging the joint. For example, years ago when the knee joint was immobilized, it would be splinted or casted at 30° of knee flexion (i.e., loose-packed position of the knee joint). Loose-packed position of the glenohumeral joint is shoulder scapular plane abduction of approximately 55° and horizontal adduction of approximately 30°, and the humerus continues in the same direction as a vertical plane through the scapula (Kaltenborn 1980). Close-packed position of a joint is present when the joint capsule and ligaments are tight or maximally tensed and there is maximal contact between the articular surfaces. Thus it is difficult to separate the articular surfaces. Close-packed

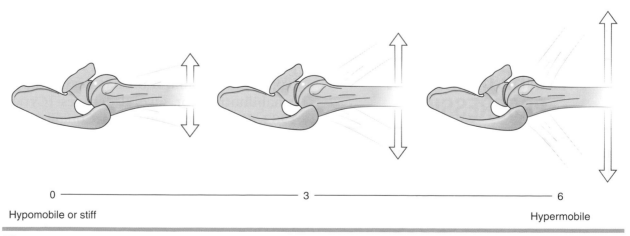

0 — Hypomobile or stiff — 3 — 6 — Hypermobile

Figure 5.1 Mobility spectrum of the human shoulder.

position of the glenohumeral joint is maximal abduction and ER.

Capsular patterns occur due to injury or a lesion of the capsule or synovium. The use of the term capsular patterns also suggests that the entire capsule is involved. Cyriax (1982) described capsular patterns for every joint in the human body. At the glenohumeral joint, the capsular pattern as initially described by Cyriax (1982) is characterized by the greatest or most limitation in ER, followed by abduction, and finally IR. Capsular patterns are important to recognize and perhaps more importantly serve as a guideline for treatment. The assessment of end feels is similar. **End feel** is characterized as the sensation or feel when the examiner tests passive movement of the joint as the joint is taken to the extreme of the possible ROM. According to Cyriax (1982), end feels can significantly add to the clinician's ability to diagnose a range of motion limitation and should be included in the evaluation of joint motion. He held that joints can exhibit a normal or physiological end feel or a pathological end feel. Each joint in the human body exhibits a different physiological end feel based on the anatomy of the joint and the direction of the movement tested. For example, a physiological end feel for elbow extension is a hard end feel (bone to bone), whereas the physiological end feel for elbow flexion is tissue approximation or soft end feel. At the glenohumeral joint, Cyriax described the normal physiological end feel as a capsular end feel. The following are the six physiological and pathological end feels as described by Cyriax (1982).

- Bone to bone: an abrupt halt to movement, when two bones meet

- Spasm: vibrant twang, muscle guarding possible (pathological)

- Capsular: "hardish" arrest of movement, feel of leather being stretched

- Springy block: intra-articular displacement present, a rebound is felt (pathological)

- Tissue approximation: soft feel when tissues from both sides of joint meet

- Empty feel: when end range cannot be reached due to pain, apprehensiveness

As already mentioned, Cyriax (1982) described the end feel of the glenohumeral joint as a capsular end feel. This is due to the capsular ligaments being stretched at end range. The end feel of the glenohumeral joint is different depending on the direction of movement. Thus, glenohumeral joint ER exhibits a capsular end feel, whereas IR often exhibits a hard or bony end feel. Glenohumeral joint flexion exhibits a different end feel that was not described by Cyriax, referred to here as a soft capsular end feel. Additionally, the horizontal adduction end feel is capsular.

The last term to define and discuss is the treatment plane. The **treatment plane** is an important factor to consider when using joint mobilization techniques. The treatment plane passes through the joint and lies at a right angle to a line running from the axis of rotation of the articular surface. Recognition of the treatment plane is important when one is performing joint mobilizations because the gliding bone must be parallel to the treatment plane. If the examiner does not glide parallel to the treatment plane, the mobilizing bone will strike against the stationary proximal joint surface and restrict the glide. A hard or bony end feel will also result. A specific example of this concept lies in the proper joint position during the posterior glide of the humerus. Inexperienced therapists often perform a posterior glide with the shoulder in the coronal plane and use a straight posterior glide of the humeral head relative to the glenoid. This imparts compressive force of the humeral head against the posterior glenoid due to the anatomical orientation of the glenohumeral joint. Instead, it is highly recommended that the therapist use a position of mobilization that places the humerus anterior to the scapular plane and use a posterior lateral glide direction to optimize the proper plane of mobilization. Figure 5.2 shows the improper and proper positions and glide orientation-direction for the posterior glide mobilization of the glenohumeral joint.

Joint mobilizations can be classified as one of five types: **straight plane glides** (distraction, anterior, posterior lateral, inferior, and lateral), **multiplane glides** (anteroinferior

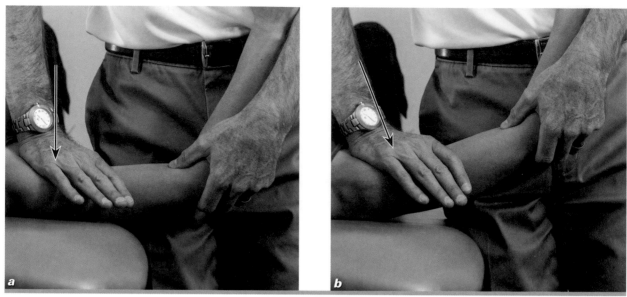

Figure 5.2 *(a)* Improper and *(b)* proper posterior glide glenohumeral joint positioning and direction of mobilization application.

glide, posterior inferior glide), **combined plane glides** (ER humeral head spin with anteroinferior glide, IR humeral head spin with posterior inferior glide, anteroinferior glide with abduction and ER, and posterior lateral glide with abduction and IR), **glides with passive movement** (inferior glide with abduction, inferior glide with flexion, anterior glide with ER, posterior lateral glide with IR), and **mobilization with movement** (as originally described by Mulligan 2016).

Application of Total Rotation ROM Concept

In addition to the use of joint mobilization in the patient with shoulder dysfunction, specific static stretching techniques are used to improve joint ROM. It is important to note again the importance of assessing the underlying mobility status of the patient, as many patients with shoulder dysfunction actually possess hypermobile shoulder profiles and do not need extensive joint mobilization or stretching as part of their rehabilitation. Use of examination procedures to assess anterior and posterior humeral head translation, as discussed earlier in this book (chapter 3), and to determine the accessory mobility of the

glenohumeral joint is of critical importance in guiding this portion of the treatment. For example, many patients with secondary rotator cuff impingement and tensile overload injury due to underlying shoulder instability should not undergo accessory mobilization techniques to increase mobility, as this would only compound their existing capsular laxity. However, patients with primary impingement often present with underlying capsular hypomobility and are prime candidates for specific mobilization techniques performed to improve glenohumeral joint arthrokinematics.

One specific area that has received a great deal of attention in the scientific literature is the presence of IR ROM limitation, particularly in the overhead athlete with rotator cuff dysfunction (Burkhart et al. 2003a, 2003b, Ellenbecker et al. 2002). To determine the optimal course of treatment for the patient with limited IR ROM, the clinical exam must identify the tissue involved. The limitation in shoulder IR ROM may be due to acute or chronic shortening of the posterior muscle–tendon units, humeral retrotorsion (often also called retroversion), or restrictions in the posterior capsule (Manske et al. 2013). When the tissue involved has been identified, the treatment can more effectively target the source of the limitation.

To determine tightness of the posterior glenohumeral joint capsule, an accessory mobility technique is recommended to assess the mobility of the humeral head relative to the glenoid. This technique most often is referred to as the posterior load and shift or the posterior drawer test (Gerber & Ganz 1984, McFarland et al. 1996). Figure 3.21 in chapter 3 shows the recommended technique for this examination maneuver, whereby the glenohumeral joint is abducted 90° in the scapular plane (note the position of the humerus 30° anterior to the coronal plane). The examiner is careful to use a posteriorly and laterally directed force along the line of the glenohumeral joint. The examiner then feels for translation of the humeral head along the glenoid face. One should not apply posterior glide accessory techniques to increase IR ROM in patients who present with a limitation in IR ROM and have grade II translation (translation over the rim of the glenoid) (Altchek & Dines 1993) because of the hypermobility of the posterior capsule made evident during this important passive clinical test.

Incorrect use of this posterior glide assessment technique may lead to the false identification of posterior capsular tightness. A common error in this examination technique is use of the coronal plane for testing, as well as use of a straight posterior-directed force by the examiner's hand rather than the recommended posterior lateral force. The straight posterior force compresses the humeral head into the glenoid because of the anteverted position of the glenoid, and this would lead to the inaccurate assumption on the part of the examining clinician that limited posterior capsular mobility is present.

The second important test used to determine the presence of IR ROM limitation is the assessment of physiological ROM. Several authors recommend measurement of glenohumeral IR with the joint in 90° of abduction in the coronal plane (Awan et al. 2002, Boon & Smith 2000, Ellenbecker et al. 1996). Care must be taken to stabilize the scapula, with

measurement taking place with the patient in the supine position so that the patient's body weight can minimize scapular motion. In addition, a posteriorly directed stabilization force is used by the examiner on the anterior aspect of the coracoid and shoulder during IR ROM measurement (figure 3.7 in chapter 3). Internal rotation ROM is compared bilaterally, with careful interpretation of isolated glenohumeral motion.

A rather consistent finding during examination of the overhead athlete is increased dominant arm ER, as well as reduced dominant arm glenohumeral joint IR (Brown et al. 1988, Ellenbecker 1992, 1995, Ellenbecker et al. 1996). Ellenbecker and colleagues (1996) noted that this consistent relationship could occur only in the condition in which glenohumeral joint rotation is measured with the scapula stabilized. Several mechanisms have been proposed to attempt to explain this glenohumeral ROM relationship of increased ER and limited IR (Crockett et al. 2002, Ellenbecker 1995, Meister et al. 2005). Tightness of the posterior capsule, tightness of the muscle–tendon unit of the posterior rotator cuff, and humeral retroversion all have been characterized as factors that limit internal glenohumeral joint rotation. Crockett and colleagues (2002) and others (Chant et al. 2007, Osbahr et al. 2002, Reagan et al. 2002) have shown unilateral increases in humeral retroversion in throwing athletes, which would explain the increase in ER noted with accompanying IR loss.

Reinold and colleagues (2007) demonstrated the acute effects of pitching on glenohumeral ROM. Sixty-seven professional baseball pitchers were measured for glenohumeral joint rotational ROM with the use of scapular stabilization before and immediately after 50 to 60 pitches at full intensity. Results showed a loss of 9.5° of IR and 10.7° of TROM during this short-term response to overhead throwing. This study shows significant decreases in IR and TROM of the dominant glenohumeral joint in professional pitchers following an acute episode of throwing. Reinold and colleagues (2007) suggest that muscle–tendinous adaptations from eccentric loading likely are implicated in this ROM adaptation following throwing (known as thixotropy). This musculotendinous adaptation may occur in addition to the osseous and capsular mechanisms previously reported (Reinold et al. 2007).

Careful glenohumeral rotational measurement using the total rotation concept (summing the ER and IR measures) guides the progression of either physiological ROM or light stretching used in rehabilitation or the inclusion of specific mobilization techniques used to address capsular deficiencies. The TROM concept can be used as illustrated in figure 5.3 to guide the clinician during rehabilitation, specifically in the area of application of stretching and mobilization, to best determine what glenohumeral joint requires additional mobility and which extremity should not have additional mobility because of the obvious harm induced by increases in capsular mobility and increases in humeral

head translation during aggressive upper extremity exertion.

Wilk and coworkers (2002) proposed the TROM concept, according to which the amounts of ER and IR at 90° of abduction are added together and a TROM arc is determined. The authors reported that the TROM in the throwing shoulders of professional baseball pitchers is within 5° of that of the nonthrowing shoulder (Wilk et al. 2011a). Furthermore, it is suggested that a TROM arc outside the 5° range may be a contributing factor to shoulder injuries.

In the study by Wilk and associates (2012), pitchers whose TROM comparison was outside the 5° acceptable difference range exhibited a 2.5 times greater risk of sustaining a shoulder injury. Furthermore, 29 of the 37 injuries (78%) were sustained in throwers whose TROM was greater than 176°. Stretching to increase IR passive range of motion (PROM), thereby treating

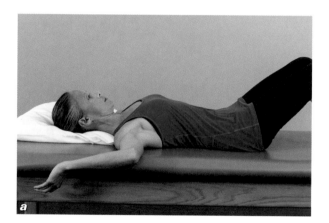
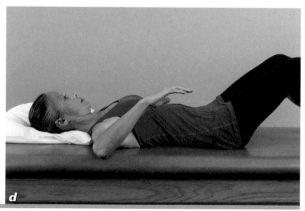
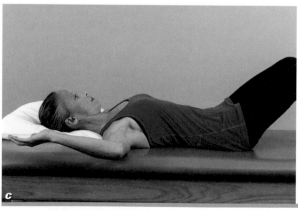
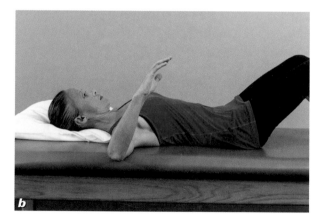

Figure 5.3 Total rotation range of motion in the *(a-b)* dominant and *(c-d)* nondominant shoulder.

the GIRD (glenohumeral internal rotation deficit; see chapter 3 for more detail), may result in an increase of TROM greater than 176° or outside the 5° acceptable window compared to the contralateral shoulder. This may lead to an increased risk of injury due to the increased demands on the dynamic and static stabilizers surrounding the shoulder joint. Further research is needed to elucidate these effects on shoulder injuries. Wilk and colleagues (2012) believe that TROM is a valuable assessment tool and an important component in PROM assessment of throwers' shoulders. This should be incorporated into the thrower's shoulder examination to determine if a ROM discrepancy is present in the athlete.

External rotation deficiency (ERD) is defined as a difference between ER of the throwing shoulder and the nonthrowing shoulder of less than 5°. Therefore, when one is comparing a player's ER PROM from side to side, one would expect to see an ER difference greater than 5°, indicating that the player's ER gain on the throwing side is significant enough to contribute to the demands of throwing, specifically during the late cocking phase of the pitching motion. A pitcher with ER side-to-side differences that are <5° may impart increased stresses on the static stabilizers, thereby contributing to an increased risk of injury over the course of his career (Wilk et al. 2012).

Normative Data

Population-specific normative data are an important consideration for the interpretation of ROM of the overhead athlete. As already mentioned, IR and ER ROM measures performed at 90° of glenohumeral joint abduction are an essential part of the evaluation of the overhead athlete. Combined, these measures create the TROM (Wilk et al. 2012). For the purposes of this book, several key studies with large sport-specific subject populations are presented here, to provide a resource to enhance and facilitate the interpretation of ROM measures for the overhead athlete (table 5.1).

In general, studies involving baseball pitchers show nearly symmetric TROM profiles, characterized by increased dominant arm ER and decreased dominant arm IR (Hurd et al. 2011, Wilk et al. 2012, 2013). This has been reported at the professional level (Ellenbecker et al. 2002, Wilk et al. 2012, 2013) as well as in high school and developmental age players (Hurd et al. 2011, Meister et al. 2005, Shanley et al. 2011). Total rotation ROM in these studies with very large samples sizes is typically within 5° when compared between the dominant and nondominant side. This is in accordance with the recommendation of Wilk and coworkers that TROM in the baseball pitcher should be within the 5° bilateral difference consistently reported in the literature (Wilk et al. 2011a, 2012, 2013).

Ellenbecker and colleagues have reported decreases of 5° to 10° on average in the dominant arm TROM parameter in uninjured elite-level tennis players (see table 5.1) (Ellenbecker et al. 1996, 2002). These differences in TROM are slightly larger than those reported in professional and developmental age throwing athletes (see table 5.1). Similarly, Reeser and colleagues (2012) reported decreases in dominant arm TROM in elite-level volleyball players who were uninjured. These normative data profiles can help clinicians better interpret the actual ROM measures in the overhead athlete in these populations.

Summary of Current Recommendations for Interpreting GIRD and TROM Deficits

Historically, several definitions of the pathologic condition known as GIRD have been used in the literature. A brief summary is provided here to help the reader fully understand this important concept (see also chapters 3 and 7). Global IR deficit is generally defined as the loss in degrees of glenohumeral IR of the dominant shoulder compared with the nondominant shoulder. Calculation of GIRD has been reported by Burkhart and colleagues (2003a, 2003b, 2003c) and others (Myers et al. 2006).

TABLE 5.1 Descriptive Data on Glenohumeral Joint Internal and External Rotation Range of Motion in Overhead Athletes

Dominant arm	Nondominant arm	N	Population and age	Source
ER: 132±1 IR: 52±12 TR: 184	127±11 63±12 190	369	Professional BB pitchers Mean age: 25.6 years	Wilk et al. 2011a
ER: 125.6±11 IR: 53.4±11 TR: 179	117.8±11 61.4±9 179	143	High school BB players Mean age: 15 years	Shanley et al. 2011
ER: 123.8±13 IR: 60.2±13 TR: 184	121.1±14 66.8±12 187	103	High school softball players Mean age: 15 years	Shanley et al. 2011
ER: 143±13 IR: 35.9±9 TR: 178	136±12 41.8±8 178	294	Little League BB players Age range: 8-16 years	Meister et al. 2005
ER: 130 IR: 60 TR: 190	120 75 195	210	High school BB pitchers Mean age: 16.1 years	Hurd et al. 2011
ER: 103.9±9 IR: 39.4±9 TR: 142	99.1±9 52.2±9 151	150	Male elite junior tennis players	Ellenbecker 2014, Ellenbecker et al. 2002
ER: 105.6±7 IR: 41.5±8 TR: 147	101.3±7 52.7±7 154	149	Female elite junior tennis players	Ellenbecker 2014, Ellenbecker et al. 2002
ER: 100±8 IR: 40±8 TR: 140 XARM: 34±6	96±11 50±7 146 42±7	232	Adult male ATP tennis players	Ellenbecker et al. 2015b
XARM: 39.8±7	44.8±5	34	Male elite junior tennis players	Ellenbecker & Kovacs 2013
XARM: 41.3±5	45.2±6	41	Female elite junior tennis players	Ellenbecker & Kovacs 2013

TR = total rotation, XARM = cross arm adduction, BB = baseball, ATP = Association of Tennis Professionals

Adapted, by permission, from R. Manske, K.E. Wilk, G. Davies, T. Ellenbecker, M. Reinold, 2013, "GH motion deficits: Friend or foe?" *International Journal of Sports Physical Therapy* 8(5): 537-553.

Burkhart and associates (2003a, 2003b, 2003c) reported that an acceptable level of GIRD is (1) less than 20° loss of shoulder IR comparing shoulders bilaterally or (2) greater than a 10% loss of the total rotation seen in the nonthrowing shoulder (nondominant shoulder IR + ER ROM) × 10%). Using this determination, for example assuming that the nondominant shoulder has a total arc of motion of 160°, the 10% rule would require only 16° of loss for the determination of GIRD rather than the standard 20° loss typically needed. Burkhart and colleagues (2003a, 2003b, 2003c) have reported that as long as an athlete's GIRD is less than or equal to her ER gain, the throwing shoulder will have no abnormal rotational kinematics and will function properly.

To advance understanding of the current recommendations for GIRD and TROM, the following definitions have been published in a detailed current concepts article by Manske and colleagues (2013). This article introduces the concepts of "anatomical" GIRD and "pathologic" GIRD. A loss of IR can be considered a normal variation observed in asymptomatic overhead athletes. Because of this common finding, it has been suggested that the term anatomical GIRD be used in the asymptomatic overhead athlete. **Anatomical GIRD** (A-GIRD) refers to a normal loss of IR along with adequate ER gain. Despite this normal ROM finding, the term GIRD has continued to have a negative connotation, implying that any side-to-side loss of IR may be pathological or may be a cause of future injury. Therefore a thorough clinical assessment of IR, ER, and TROM is needed before stretching interventions are applied, as in some athletes (i.e., those with A-GIRD) this is an expected and normal adaptation to repetitive overhead throwing.

A second term from the paper by Manske and associates (2013) is **pathologic GIRD**. A shoulder that has IR loss and a concomitant loss of TROM or an increase in ERD would be considered a pathologic glenohumeral internal rotation deficit (P-GIRD). In determining clinically significant P-GIRD, one must also carefully evaluate ER and thus TROM. Wilk and colleagues (2012) reported in 362 healthy throwers that TROM was within 5° for all subjects. Ellenbecker and colleagues (2002) reported on asymptomatic professional baseball pitchers and asymptomatic elite tennis players and reported that TROM was within 5° for the baseball pitchers and within 10° for the elite tennis players. Furthermore, Wilk and colleagues reported that a difference of greater than 5° of TROM correlated with shoulder injuries (2011a).

Clinical Patient Example for Interpreting IR and TROM Measurements

Clinical application of the TROM concept is best demonstrated by a case presentation of a unilaterally dominant upper extremity athlete. If, during the initial evaluation of a high-level baseball pitcher, the clinician finds a ROM pattern of 120° of ER and only 30° of IR, some uncertainty may exist as to whether this represents a ROM deficit in IR that requires rehabilitative intervention via muscle–tendon unit stretching and possibly via the use of specific glenohumeral joint mobilization. However, if measurement of that patient's nondominant extremity rotation reveals 90° of ER and 60° of IR, the current recommendation based on the TROM concept would be to avoid extensive mobilization and passive stretching of the dominant extremity, because the TROM in both extremities is 150° (120° ER + 30° IR = 150° dominant arm total rotation, 90° ER + 60° IR = 150° nondominant arm total rotation). In elite-level tennis players, the total active rotation ROM can be expected to be up to 10° less on the dominant arm before clinical treatment to address IR ROM restriction would be recommended or implemented.

This TROM concept can be used to guide the clinician during rehabilitation, specifically in the area of application of stretching and mobilization, to best determine which glenohumeral joint requires additional mobility and which extremity should not have additional mobility because of the obvious harm induced by increases in capsular mobility and increases in humeral head translation during aggressive upper extremity exertion.

Methods to Improve Shoulder IR ROM in the Throwing Athlete

Now that interpretation of glenohumeral joint ROM has been discussed, this section outlines specific techniques to increase IR ROM in the patient with shoulder dysfunction. This section, addressing the importance of accurate ROM measurement and clinical

the effects of the cross-arm stretch versus the sleeper stretch in a population of recreational athletes, some with significant glenohumeral IR ROM deficiency. Four weeks of stretching produced significantly greater IR gains in the group performing the cross-body stretch as compared with the sleeper stretch. Further research is clearly needed to better characterize the optimal application of these stretches; however, studies have shown improvement in IR ROM with a home stretching program (McClure et al. 2005). Additionally, Laudner and associates (2008) studied the sleeper stretch and found that three consecutive 30-second sleeper stretches produced 3.1° of increased IR in overhead athletes immediately after stretching. Similarly, an independent contract–relax stretching technique using a stretch strap (figure 5.11) has been found to produce increases of 8.26° in IR in uninjured subjects (Ellenbecker et al. 2016). These stretches (sleeper and cross-arm) can be recommended for patients and for overhead athletes to address IR ROM limitation in addition to the procedures recommended here for clinical use. Stretching can also be classified into five types: static stretching, dynamic stretching, low-load long-duration stretching (LLLD), sustained stretching, and static stretching with mobilization.

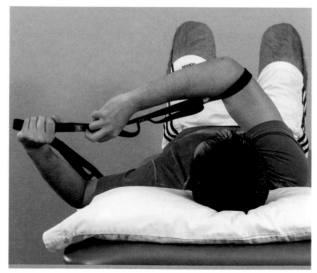

Figure 5.11 Independent cross-arm contract–relax stretch using a stretch strap to improve internal rotation and cross-arm adduction ROM.

SCAPULAR STABILIZATION METHODS AND PROGRESSION

A key component of the early management of rotator cuff pathology is scapular stabilization. Manual techniques are recommended to directly interface the clinician with the patient's scapula to bypass the glenohumeral joint and allow for repetitive scapular exercise without undue stress to the rotator cuff in the early phase. Figure 5.12 shows a specific technique that can be used to manually resist scapular retraction.

Solem-Bertoft and colleagues (1993) have shown the importance of scapular retraction posturing, with reports of a reduction in the width of the subacromial space when scapular protraction posturing was compared with scapular retraction. Activation of the serratus anterior and lower trapezius force couple is imperative to enable scapular upward rotation and stabilization during arm elevation (Kibler 1998). Rhythmic stabilization applied to the proximal aspect of the extremity, progressing to distal with the glenohumeral joint in 80° to 90° of elevation in the scapular plane, can be initiated to provide muscular cocontraction in a functional position. Additionally, with this technique, a protracted scapular position can be used to enhance the activation of the serratus anterior (Decker et al. 1999, Moesley et al. 1992), as several studies have identified decreased muscular activation of this muscle in patients given a diagnosis of glenohumeral impingement and instability (Ludewig & Cook 2000, Warner et al. 1990).

Kibler and colleagues (2008) published several key exercise movements that recruit the serratus anterior and lower trapezius and can be used early in rehabilitation due to the lower levels of elevation inherent in these movements. This minimizes subacromial impingement and capsulolabral stress and makes these movements well tolerated by patients early in rehabilitation. The robbery (figure 5.13) and lawn mower (figure 5.14 on page 116) exercises have extensive EMG verification by Kibler and colleagues (2008) and Tsuruike and Ellenbecker (2015).

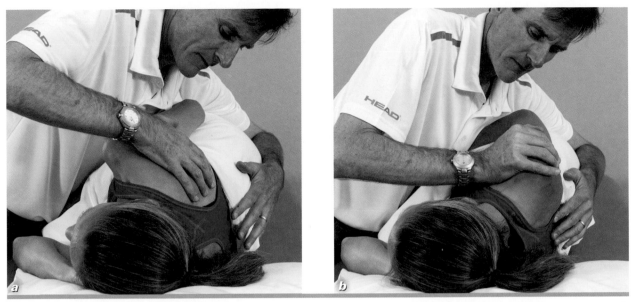

Figure 5.12 Manual scapular retraction technique. Hand placements for increasing *(a)* scapular retraction strength and *(b)* scapular protraction strength.

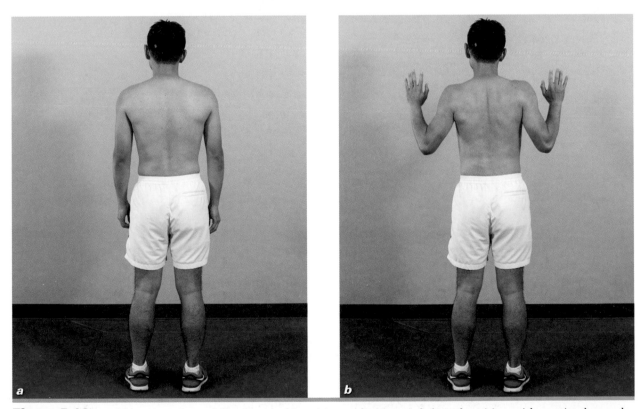

Figure 5.13 Robbery scapular stabilization exercise: *(a)* start position and *(b)* end position with maximal scapular retraction and depression.

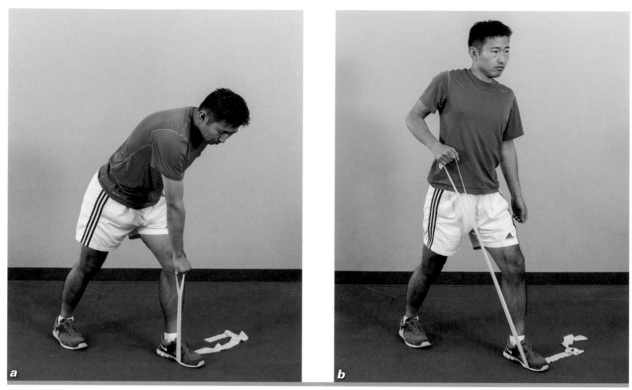

Figure 5.14   Lawn mower exercise for scapular stabilization: *(a)* start position and *(b)* end position.

Figure 5.15 shows an early scapular stabilization exercise utilized by patients during shoulder rehabilitation using elastic resistance. This exercise uses an application of the elastic resistance directly to the scapula bypassing the glenohumeral joint, making early application of this exercise to recruit the trapezius and serratus anterior possible. The patient stands with the arm at his side with the shoulder in external rotation (monitored by observing the hand placed in a "thumb pointing outward" position throughout the duration of the exercise). Against tension in the elastic resistance, the patient then retracts his scapula maximally and takes several steps backward; this increases the resistance, resulting in an isometric contraction of the scapular stabilizers. This position is maintained while the patient returns to the starting position. This exercise

can be utilized early in rehabilitation when the patient is not able to have resistance applied across the glenohumeral joint.

Additional scapular stabilization exercises include ER with retraction (figure 5.16 on page 118), an exercise shown to recruit the lower trapezius at a rate 3.3 times greater than the upper trapezius and to use the important position of scapular retraction (McCabe et al. 2001). The serratus punch performed in supine (figure 5.17 on page 118) has been found to elicit 60% or greater maximum voluntary isometric contraction (MVIC) levels in the serratus anterior musculature (Ekstrom et al. 2003). Multiple seated rowing variations, continued manual scapular protraction–retraction resistance exercise performed by the therapist with hand placements directly on the scapula, and the 90° abducted ER exercise in prone are used to facilitate the

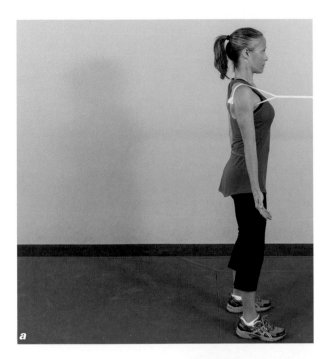 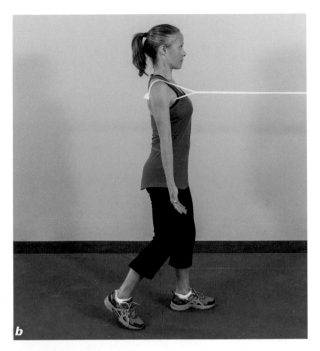

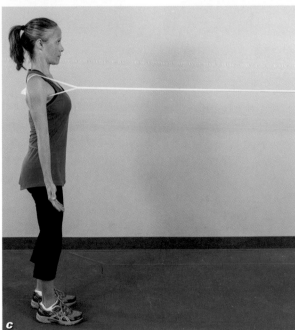

Figure 5.15 Scapular isometric step-out exercise: *(a)* start position, *(b)* stepping back to increase resistance in the elastic band, and *(c)* end position.

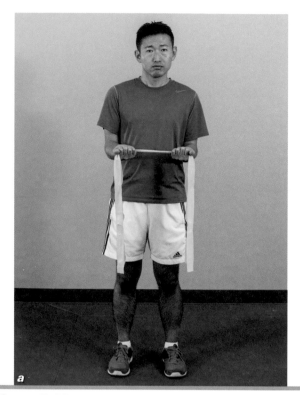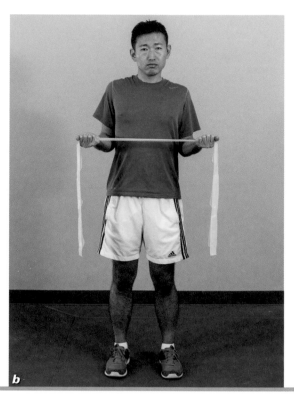

Figure 5.16 External rotation with retraction: *(a)* start position and *(b)* end position.

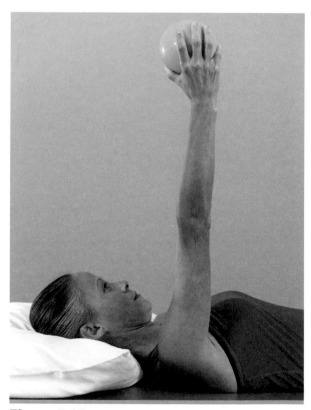

Figure 5.17 Serratus punch exercise.

lower trapezius and other scapular stabilizers during rehabilitation (Ballantyne et al. 1993, Englestad et al. 2001, Reinhold et al. 2004).

Closed chain exercise using the "plus" position, which is characterized by maximal scapular protraction, has been recommended by Moesley and colleagues (1992) and Decker and colleagues (1999) for its inherent maximal serratus anterior recruitment. Closed chain step-ups (figure 5.18), quadruped position rhythmic stabilization (figure 5.19), and variations of the pointer position (unilateral arm and ipsilateral leg extension weight bearing) all are used in endurance-oriented formats (timed sets of 30 seconds or more) to enhance scapular stabilization (Ellenbecker & Davies 2001). Uhl and colleagues (2003) have demonstrated the effects of increased weight bearing and of successive decreases in the number of weight-bearing limbs on muscle activation of the rotator cuff and scapular musculature and have provided guidance regarding closed chain exercise progression in the upper extremity.

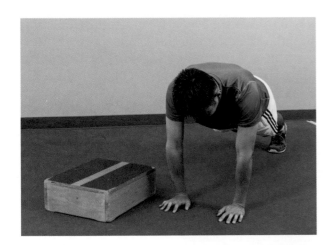

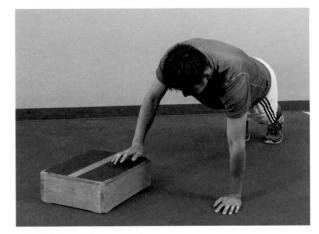

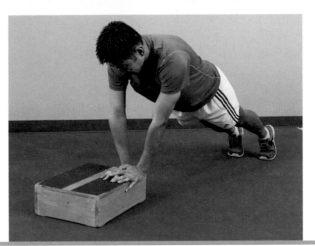

Figure 5.18 Closed chain step-up exercise.

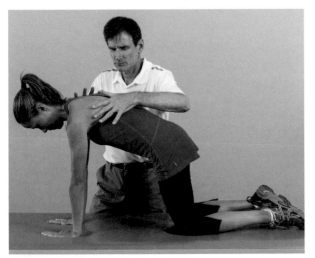

Figure 5.19 Quadruped rhythmic stabilization exercise.

ROTATOR CUFF EXERCISE PROGRESSION

Several key concepts are used to influence decision making during rehabilitation of the shoulder with regard to rotator cuff exercise selection and progression. First and foremost, the exercise movement and position chosen should not place the rotator cuff tendons at risk from anatomical encroachment (subacromial impingement) or tension hypovascularity (Rathburn & Macnab 1970). Secondly, a low-resistance and high-repetition base is recommended to encourage development of local muscular endurance (Fleck & Kraemer 2014), as well as to facilitate greater activation from the rotator cuff relative to the prime mover musculature (Bitter et al. 2007). Finally, the functional progression particularly for the overhead athlete or overhead worker should follow from initial exercise with the arm in the less functional adducted (at the side) position, then ultimately progress to 90° of elevation in the scapular plane, consistent with the functional positioning of the glenohumeral joint during the overhead throwing and serving motions (Ellenbecker & Cools 2010). Whenever possible, EMG studies are used to provide objective evidence regarding the muscular activation and ultimate effectiveness of the movement pattern (exercise) chosen.

Initial Progression

According to Ellenbecker and Davies (2000), an initial resistive exercise progression for shoulder rehabilitation often commences with isometric exercise followed by isotonic exercise and then finally more functional plyometric and isokinetic resistance applications. This allows for increased challenge and specificity in the exercise progression.

One study highlights the importance of early submaximal exercise in increasing local blood flow. Jensen and colleagues (1995) studied the effects of submaximal contractions (5% to 50% MVIC) in the supraspinatus tendon measured with laser Doppler flowmetry. Results showed that even submaximal contractions increased perfusion during all 1-minute contractions but produced a latent hyperemia following the muscular contraction. These findings have provided a rationale for the early use of IR and ER isometrics or submaximal manual resistance in the scapular plane with low levels of elevation to prevent any subacromial contact early in the rehabilitation process. Figure 5.20 shows an early application of isometric exercise for the posterior rotator cuff called "dynamic isometrics," in which elastic resistance is used to provide

known loading in an isometric format as a step is taken by the patient away from the attachment point of the band or tubing to increase resistance. Use of elastic resistance with known, calibrated elongation resistance values allows the clinician to safely and appropriately prescribe isometric exercise dosing for the patient. A towel roll is used under the axilla to most appropriately position the patient's shoulder for rotator cuff exercise (Ellenbecker & Cools 2010, Rathburn & Macnab 1970).

An initial isotonic rotator cuff exercise progression that can be used is shown in figure 5.21. These exercises are based on EMG research showing high levels of posterior rotator cuff activation (Ballantyne et al. 1993, Blackburn et al. 1990, Malanga et al. 1996, Reinhold et al. 2004, Townsend et al. 1991), and they place the shoulder in positions well tolerated by patients with rotator cuff and scapular dysfunction.

Side-lying ER and prone extension with an externally rotated (thumb-out) position are used first, with progressions to prone horizontal abduction and prone ER with scapular retraction following a demonstrated tolerance to the initial two exercises. Prone horizontal abduction is used at 90° of abduction to minimize the effects resulting from subacromial contact (Wuelker et al. 1994). Research has shown that this position creates high levels of supraspinatus muscular activation (Ellenbecker et al. 1988, Fleck & Kraemer 1987, Rathbun & Macnab 1970), making it an alternative to the widely used empty can exercise, which often can cause impingement through the combined inherent movements of IR and elevation. Three sets of 15 to 20 repetitions are recommended to create a fatigue response and improve local muscular endurance (Carter et al. 2007, Niederbracht et al. 2008). The efficacy of these exercises in a four-week training paradigm has been demonstrated, and 8% to 10% increases have been noted in IR and ER strength measured isokinetically in healthy subjects (Niederbracht et al. 2008). Additionally, use of these exercises has resulted in improvement in strength

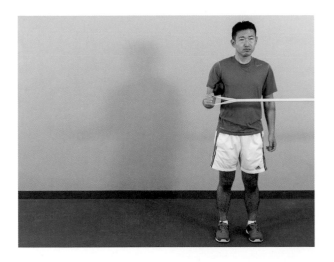
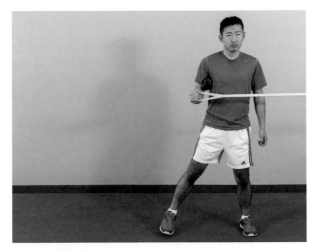
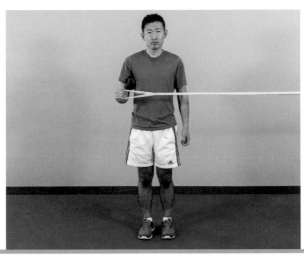

Figure 5.20 External rotation isometric step-outs ("dynamic isometrics").

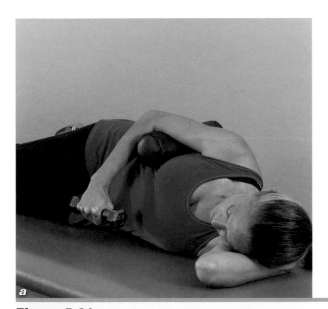
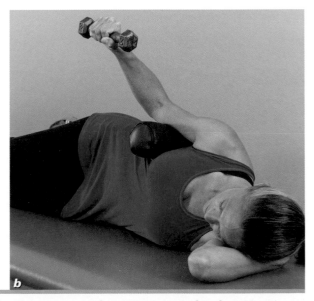

Figure 5.21 Rotator cuff isotonic exercise program: *(a-b)* sidelying external rotation start and end positions.

(continued)

FIGURE 5.21 (*continued*)

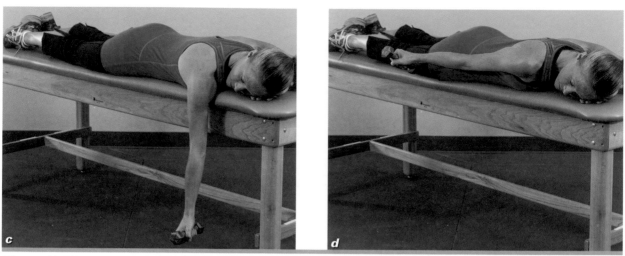

Figure 5.21   Rotator cuff isotonic exercise program: *(c-d)* prone shoulder extension start and end positions.

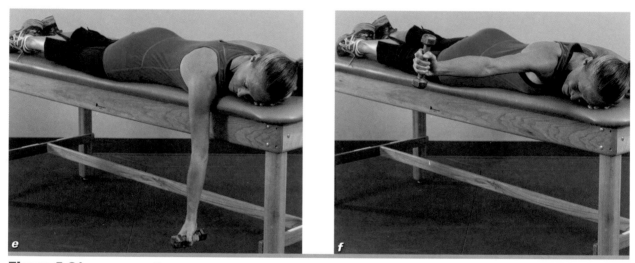

Figure 5.21   Rotator cuff isotonic exercise program: *(e-f)* prone horizontal abduction start and end positions.

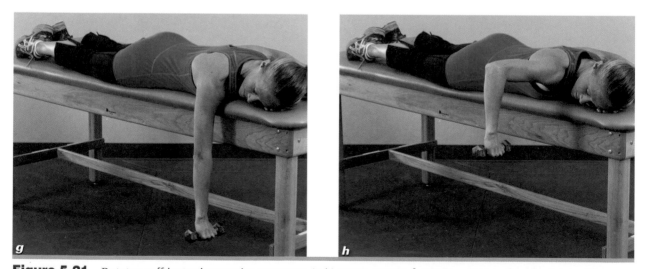

Figure 5.21   Rotator cuff isotonic exercise program: *(g-h)* prone external rotation start and midpoint positions.

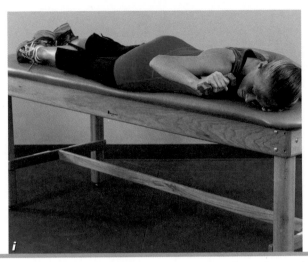

Figure 5.21   Rotator cuff isotonic exercise program: *(i)* prone external rotation end position.

and muscular endurance in both tennis players and overhead athletes in training studies (Fleck & Kraemer 1987, Rathburn & Macnab 1970). Training of the rotator cuff and scapular musculature has resulted in modification and improvement of the ER-to-IR ratio, improved strength, and improved endurance of the rotator cuff as well as performance enhancement (Fleck & Kraemer 1987, Moncrief et al. 2002, Niederbracht et al. 2008, Rathburn & Macnab 1970).

All exercises for ER strengthening in standing and side-lying are performed with the addition of a small towel roll placed in the axilla as pictured in figure 5.22.

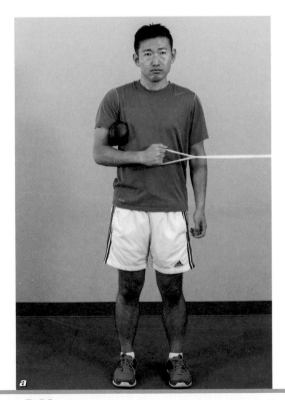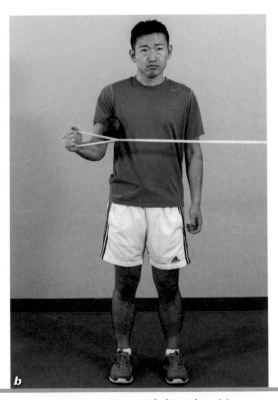

Figure 5.22   External rotation at the side with elastic resistance: *(a)* start position and *(b)* end position.

In addition to assisting in isolation of the exercise and controlling unwanted movements, the towel roll application has been shown to elevate muscular activity by 10% in the infraspinatus muscle when compared with identical exercises performed without towel placement (Reinhold et al. 2004). Another theoretical advantage of the use of a towel roll to place the shoulder in approximately 20° to 30° of abduction is that it prevents the "wringing out" phenomenon shown in cadaver research investigating shoulder microvascularity. Rathburn and Mcnab (1970) showed enhanced blood flow in the supraspinatus tendon when the arm was placed in slight abduction as compared with complete adduction. Finally, another research study further supported the use of a towel roll or pillow between the humerus and the torso under the axilla during a humeral rotational training exercise. Graichen and colleagues (2005) studied 12 healthy shoulders using MRI at 30°, 60°, 90°, 120°, and 150° of abduction. A 15 N force was performed, which resulted in an abduction isometric contraction or an adduction isometric contraction. Adduction isometric muscle contraction produced a significant opening or increase in the subacromial space in all positions of glenohumeral joint abduction. No change in scapular tilting or scapulohumeral rhythm was encountered during abduction or adduction isometric contractions. Results from this research can be applied to the patient with impingement during humeral rotation exercise. Use of the towel roll can facilitate an adduction isometric contraction in patients who may need enhanced subacromial positioning due to impingement during the humeral rotation exercise (Graichen et al. 2005).

Research by Bitter and colleagues (2007) has provided guidance regarding the use of resistive exercise in shoulder rehabilitation. They measured EMG activity of the infraspinatus and middle and posterior deltoid during ER exercise in healthy subjects. Muscular activity was monitored during ER exercise at 10%, 40%, and 70% activation levels (percentage of maximal). This important study found increased relative infraspinatus activity when the resistive exercise level was at 40% of maximal effort, indicating more focused activity from the infraspinatus and less compensatory activation of the deltoid. This study supports the use of lower-intensity strengthening exercise to optimize activation from the rotator cuff and to deemphasize input from the deltoid and other prime movers, which often occurs with higher-intensity resistive loading.

External rotation exercises in neutral (arm at the side) are progressed to the 90° abducted position in the scapular plane for patients who perform overhead sports or repetitive work activities in this position (figure 5.23). Each of these ER-based exercises can be progressed or the challenge increased through the addition of rhythmic stabilization or perturbation (figure 5.24), as well as oscillation (figures 5.25 and 5.26). These perturbations and oscillations ultimately increase the number of contractions and amount of muscular activation to improve local muscular endurance and provide challenge to patients undergoing shoulder rehabilitation.

Progression to the functional position of 90° of abduction in the scapular plane to simulate the throwing and overhead patterning inherent in many sport activities such as serving in tennis and volleyball, as well as daily functions, is based on tolerance of the initial rotator cuff and scapular exercise progression as listed earlier in this chapter. Basset and colleagues (1994) have shown the importance of training the muscle in the position of function based on the change in muscular lever arms and subsequent function in the 90/90 position. Rhythmic stabilization (i.e., perturbations applied to the proximal and distal aspects of the upper extremity) against a therapy ball (figure 5.27) is one example of an early abducted exercise performed with therapist guidance.

The scapular plane position is chosen as an optimal position for this exercise and other exercises in lower planes of elevation in the earlier phase of rehabilitation, as well as with humeral elevation to 90° during this

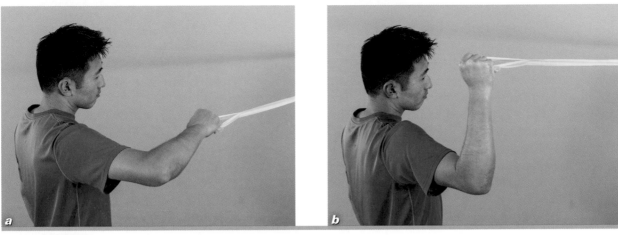

Figure 5.23 External rotation at 90° of elevation in the scapular plane with elastic resistance: *(a)* start position and *(b)* end position.

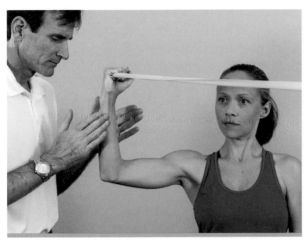

Figure 5.24 External rotation at 90° elevation in the scapular plane with perturbation.

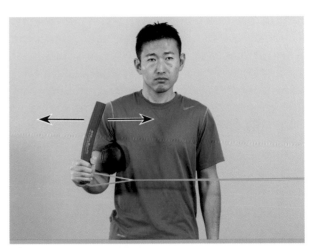

Figure 5.25 External rotation oscillation.

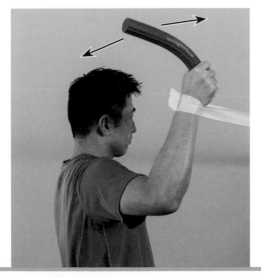

Figure 5.26 Statue of Liberty oscillation exercise.

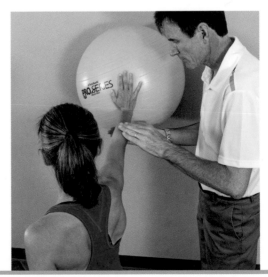

Figure 5.27 Ball-on-the-wall rhythmic stabilization at 90° of elevation in the scapular plane.

phase, for several important reasons. The inherent optimal bony congruency between the humeral head and the glenoid (Saha 1983), as well as the mathematically derived research finding that the rotator cuff is best able to maintain glenohumeral stability with the glenohumeral joint positioned 29.3° anterior to the coronal plane of the body, makes the scapular plane position an optimal position for rehabilitative exercise (Happee & VanDer Helm 1995).

An additional advanced scapular exercise recently published by Castelein et al. (2016) involves an elastic band and starting position with the arms at the side of the body with elbows flexed as shown in figure 5.28a. A slight resistance applied to external rotation is performed by the patient tensing the elastic band and activating the posterior rotator cuff and scapular musculature. The patient then elevates the shoulders together, maintaining the external rotation resistance in the band. The shoulders are elevated to a position of 90° in the scapular plane as pictured in figure 5.28b. High levels of middle and lower tra-

pezius EMG have been reported by Castelein et al. (2016), making this exercise an excellent progression combining scapular activation with the functional movement pattern of elevation.

Wilk and colleagues (2002) have popularized and recommended additional exercises for the rotator cuff and scapular musculature and have packaged them in a program called the Thrower's Ten (see appendix A). A low-resistance, high-repetition format is recommended using the rationale outlined in this chapter as well as key concepts published by Reinold and colleagues (2004).

Additional tools and methods for application of the 90/90 position include the use of the Impulse Trainer (Impulse Training System, Newnan, Georgia) (figure 5.29) to provide ER eccentric overload training in a position of 90° of elevation in the scapular plane and 90° of ER, simulating the functional position used during serving in tennis (Elliott et al. 1986) or throwing in baseball (Fleisig et al. 1995).

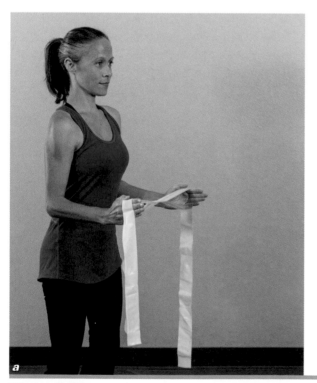 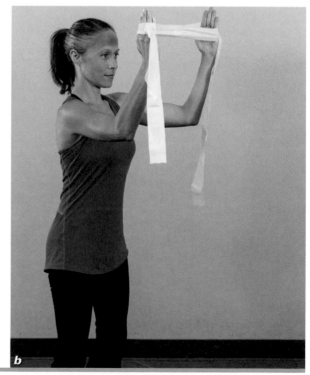

Figure 5.28 External rotation with elevation exercise with elastic resistance: *(a)* start position and *(b)* end position.

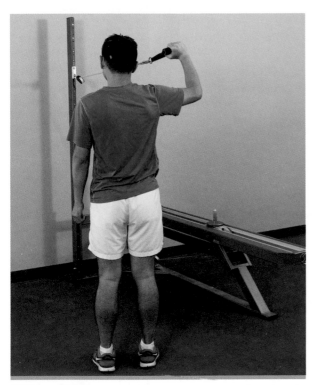

Figure 5.29 External rotation at 90° elevation in the scapular plane using the Impulse machine.

The importance of ER fatigue resistance training has ramifications for the proper biomechanical function of the entire upper extremity kinetic chain. Tsai and colleagues (2003) demonstrated significant scapular positional changes during the early and middle phases of arm elevation—specifically, decreases in posterior scapular tilting and scapular ER following fatigue of the glenohumeral external rotators. In a similar study, Ebaugh and colleagues (2006) used an ER fatigue protocol to fatigue the posterior rotator cuff. Following fatigue of the external rotators, this study found less posterior tilting during subsequent arm elevation, indicating scapular compensations and abnormal movement patterns resulting from rotator cuff fatigue. These studies provide an evidence-based rationale for the significant use of ER-based training for the patient with shoulder dysfunction.

Advanced Thrower's Ten Exercise Program

Overhead throwing athletes typically present with a unique musculoskeletal profile. The overhead thrower exhibits extreme amounts of motion, which result in an inherently unstable glenohumeral complex, thus requiring throwers to rely heavily on their dynamic stabilizers for high-level, symptom-free activity. This unique athletic population demonstrates distinct shoulder pathology that frequently presents a challenge for the clinician. Aggressive strengthening activities that emphasize the restoration of muscle balance, endurance, dynamic stabilization, and symmetry are required to return the throwing athlete to competition. The Advanced Thrower's Ten Exercise Program (Wilk et al. 2011b) provides the standard for comprehensive rehabilitation of the overhead athlete. It functions as a bridge facilitating the transition from rehabilitation to return to competitive throwing by using higher-level principles of dynamic stabilization, neuromuscular control, rotator cuff facilitation, and coordination in the application of throwing-specific exercises in a unique and progressive manner.

The Advanced Thrower's Ten Exercise Program (see appendix B) combines the principles of dynamic stability, coactivation, high-level neuromuscular control, endurance, rotator cuff facilitation, proper posture, core strength-endurance, and coordination in a specific manner designed to enable athletes to progress seamlessly into an interval throwing program and prepare them for a return to sporting participation. The exercises in this program are performed bilaterally to take advantage of neurophysiological overflow, address the whole athlete in the training, and minimize any neurologic insult to the involved extremity or upper quarter. Performing high levels of proprioceptive and neuromuscular control exercises bilaterally serves to enhance the dynamic stability characteristics of the upper quarter and trunk as well as the lumbopelvic complex and lower extremity. The shoulder external rotator, scapular retractor, protractor, and depressor muscles are frequently focused on because of their identifiable weakness in the overhead athlete.

In addition, a stability ball is used during performance of the Advanced Thrower's Ten to further challenge the athlete's position on an unstable surface. While performing each exercise repetition, athletes are positioned in optimal sitting alignment on a stability ball, sitting over their ischial tuberosities, with their feet planted shoulder-width apart and their transverse abdominis engaged. Proper posture and positioning, especially of the scapula, is essential to maximize effective utilization of the exercises in this program. Maintaining a posteriorly tilted, externally rotated, and retracted scapular position is a constant focus. Frequently, athletes are cued until this positioning is maintained continually during all exercises. Manual resistance can also be employed and can be added to any seated stability ball exercise to increase muscle excitation, cocontraction, and dynamic stability; promote endurance; and challenge the fatigability of the rotator cuff muscles.

Additional Advanced Exercises

As the patient tolerates isotonic exercise with 2 to 3 pounds (0.9-1.4 kg) and also can perform rotational training without pain using medium-level elastic resistance, isokinetic rotational exercise is initiated in the modified base position (see figure 5.20). This position places the glenohumeral joint in 30° of flexion and 30° of abduction, and it uses a 30° tilt of the dynamometer relative to the horizontal (figure 5.30) (Davies 1992, Ellenbecker & Davies 2000). This position is well tolerated and allows the patient to progress from submaximal to more maximal levels of resistance at velocities ranging between 120°/sec and 210°/sec for nonathletic patient populations, and between 210°/

sec and 360°/sec during later stages of rehabilitation in more athletic patients. Use of the isokinetic dynamometer is also important to objectively quantify muscular strength levels and, most critically, muscular balance between the internal and external rotators (Davies 1992, Ellenbecker & Davies 2000). Achieving a level of IR and ER strength equal to that of the contralateral extremity is an acceptable initial goal for many patients. However, unilateral increases in IR strength of 15% to 30% have been reported in many descriptive studies of overhead athletes (Ellenbecker & Davies 2000, Ellenbecker & Mattalino 1999, Ellenbecker & Roetert 2003, Wilk et al. 1993); greater rehabilitative emphasis may be required to achieve this level of documented "dominance."

A predominance of IR-ER patterning is used during isokinetic training. This focus on IR-ER exercise is based on an isokinetic

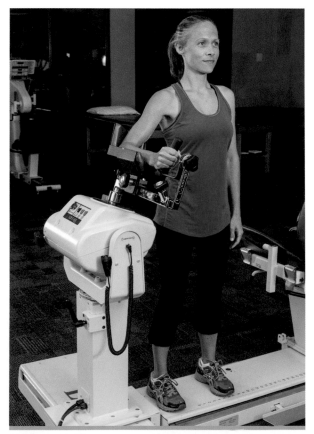

Figure 5.30 Internal and external rotation modified base isokinetic training and testing position.

training study by Quincy and colleagues (2000), who showed that IR-ER training for a period of six weeks not only can produce statistically significant gains in IR and ER strength, but also can improve shoulder extension-flexion and abduction-adduction strength. Training in the patterns of flexion-extension and abduction-adduction over the same six weeks produced only strength gains specific to the direction of training. This overflow of training allows for a more time-efficient and effective focus in the clinic during isokinetic training.

Muscular balance, as defined by the ER/IR ratio, provides objective information for the clinician to ensure that proper strength is present between the anterior and posterior dynamic stabilizers. Ratios in normal, healthy shoulders have been reported at 66% (Davies 1992, Ellenbecker & Davies 2000, Ivey et al. 1985). Emphasis on the development of external rotators (posterior rotator cuff) in rehabilitation for anterior instability has led to the concept of a "posterior dominant" shoulder—a shoulder that essentially has a unilateral strength ratio greater than 66%, with a goal of attaining a ratio of 75% to 80% (Ellenbecker & Davies 2000). Careful monitoring of muscular strength with the use of a dynamometer allows the clinician to specifically observe and focus the rehabilitation program in such a way as to promote the return of muscular balance. Byrum and colleagues (2010) tested ER/IR ratios in professional baseball players and found increases in shoulder injuries requiring surgical management in baseball players who had decreases in the ER/IR ratio (decreased relative ER strength) in the dominant throwing shoulder. This finding provides rationale for close monitoring of this ratio (ER/IR) with HHD and isokinetic testing to determine readiness for return to activity and to measure the dynamic stability of the rotator cuff in rehabilitation and preventive evaluations.

During the end stage of rotator cuff rehabilitation, individuals returning to overhead activities and sports are candidates for advanced isokinetic training using func-

tionally specific rotational training at 90° of abduction in the scapular plane (figure 5.31), with several studies reporting increases in rotator cuff strength and functional overhead sport enhancement following six weeks of isokinetic training with 90° of glenohumeral joint abduction (Moncrief et al. 2002, Mont et al. 1994).

Two advanced versions of elastic resistance exercise are progressed to during the later stages of rehabilitation, especially in overhead athletes and in overhead workers. These include the bilateral external rotation exercise with sustained hold and the simultaneous multivector elastic resistance exercise combining shoulder external rotation with resisted scapular retraction at 90° of abduction (figures 5.32 and 5.33). Both exercises involve the use of elastic resistance in a position of 90° of elevation in the scapular plane to increase posterior rotator cuff and scapular muscle activation. For the sustained hold exercise popularized by Wilk and colleagues in the Advanced Throwers 10 (2011b), one extremity sustains an isometric hold in the position of 90° of external rotation, 90° of abduction in the scapular plane, and 90° of elbow flexion while the other extremity

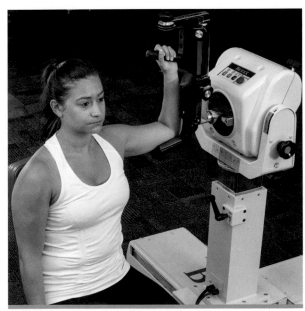

Figure 5.31 Internal and external rotation isokinetic training at 90° of abduction in the scapular plane.

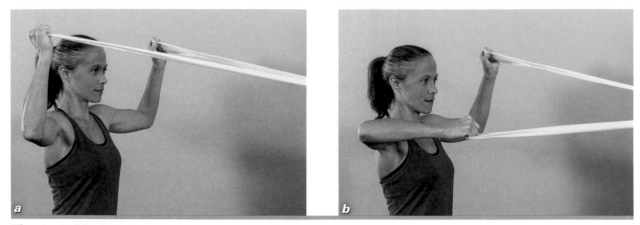

Figure 5.32 Bilateral external rotation with sustained hold: *(a)* starting position and *(b)* unilateral external rotation movement with contralateral sustained hold.

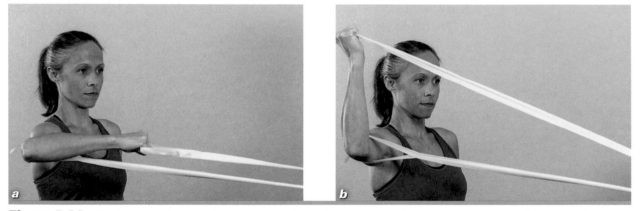

Figure 5.33 Multivector elastic resistance external rotation with scapular retraction exercise: *(a)* start position and *(b)* end position.

performs traditional external rotation. After a preset number of repetitions (10-15 typically), the extremities switch roles for another preselected number of repetitions. The exercise ends with one set of alternating external rotations back and forth between extremities, further challenging the patient's musculature.

For the multivector exercise, one end of the elastic band is placed on the distal aspect of the upper arm just above the elbow and looped such that the other terminal end of the elastic band is placed in the hand to resist external rotation with 90° of scapular plane elevation (figure 5.33*a*). A constant retraction resistance is provided by the proximal portion of the band, increasing the scapular muscle activation during the external rotation exercise. Multiple sets of 15 to 20

repetitions of this exercise are recommended and used in end-stage rehabilitation as well as in preventative conditioning programs for overhead athletes.

Additionally, a plyometric exercise progression is initiated at this time in the rehabilitation progression. Several studies reported in the literature show increases in upper extremity function with plyometric exercise variations (Rathburn & Macnab 1970, Schulte-Edelmann et al. 2005, Vossen et al. 2000). The functional application of the eccentric prestretch, followed by a powerful concentric muscular contraction, closely parallels many upper extremity sport activities and serves as an excellent exercise modality for transitioning the active patient to the interval sport return programs. Figures 5.34 and 5.35 show two plyometric side-lying ER exercises used to develop posterior rotator cuff strength.

Carter and associates (2007) studied the effects of an eight-week training program of plyometric upper extremity exercise and ER strengthening with elastic resistance performed at 90° of glenohumeral joint abduction. They found increased eccentric ER

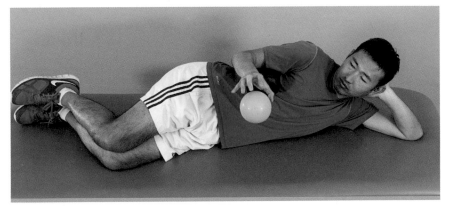

Figure 5.34 Side-lying plyometric external rotation drops.

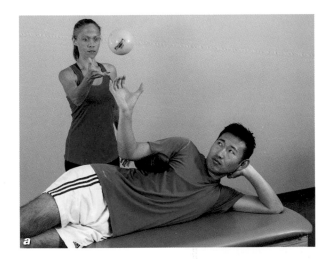

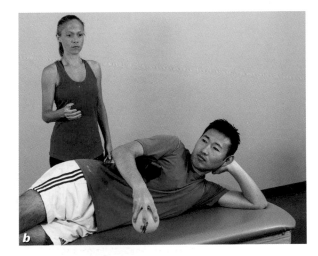

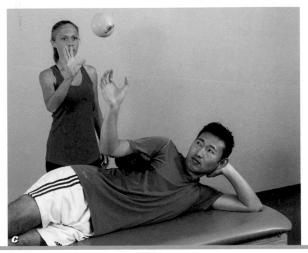

Figure 5.35 Side-lying plyometric external rotation catches: *(a)* partner toss, *(b)* catch and deceleration, and *(c)* concentric throw back to partner.

strength, increased concentric IR strength, and improved throwing velocity in collegiate baseball players, thus showing the positive effects of plyometric and elastic resistance training in overhead athletes. Figures 5.36 and 5.37 demonstrate two recommended plyometric exercises used for overhead athletes. These exercises have been studied by Ellenbecker and colleagues (2015a), who identified high levels of peak EMG activity of the lower trapezius (118-131% MVIC) and infraspinatus (85-103%) during these important exercises.

CONCLUSION

The integration of ROM, scapular stabilization, and rotator cuff exercises forms a crucial and comprehensive part of shoulder rehabilitation. The exercises and techniques detailed in this chapter should guide the rehabilitation professional by providing rationale for and descriptions of high-level interventions for patients with shoulder pathology.

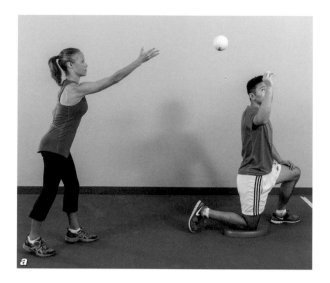

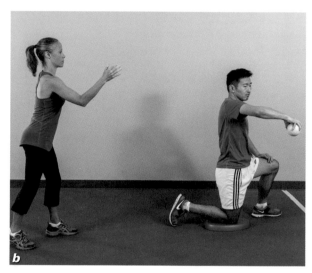

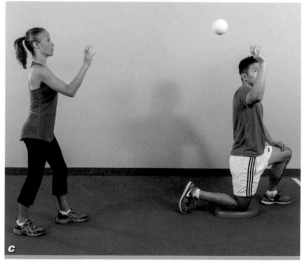

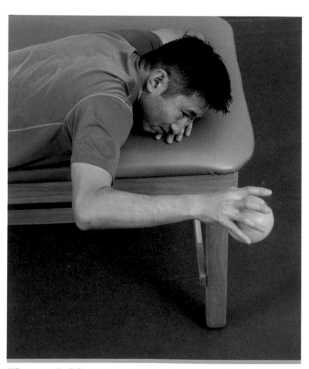

Figure 5.36 Prone 90/90 plyometric drops.

Figure 5.37 Prone 90/90 plyometric reverse catches: *(a)* partner toss, *(b)* catch and deceleration, and *(c)* concentric throw back to partner.

Surgical Repair and Rehabilitation Protocols

The rehabilitation progressions outlined in chapter 5 can guide clinicians through many of the rehabilitation steps used for patients diagnosed with either partial- or full-thickness rotator cuff tears. This chapter covers rotator cuff repair and labral repair.

ROTATOR CUFF REPAIR

Failure of nonoperative rehabilitation, high levels of pain at rest and at night, and significant interruption of daily and recreational or athletic shoulder function are all factors that lead patients to have surgery to address substantial rotator cuff tears (Ellenbecker 2004). However, the success of rehabilitation of full-thickness rotator cuff tears has recently been reported, with rather favorable findings from a rehabilitation perspective. Kuhn and colleagues (2013) studied a cohort of 452 patients with full-thickness rotator cuff tears. Significant improvement was noted between 6 and 12 weeks of nonoperative rehabilitation, with less than 25% of the patients opting to have surgical management for their rotator cuff tear. The tears involved the supraspinatus 70% of the time and the supraspinatus and infraspinatus 21% of the time (91% of the patients in this cohort had a tear of either the supraspinatus or infraspinatus). At two-year follow-up, Kuhn and colleagues (2013) found that 75% of the patients had good or excellent outcomes after nonoperative rehabilitation.

In another study, Kukkonen and colleagues (2014) studied three treatment groups in patients with nontraumatic rotator cuff tears who were 55 years of age or older. The three treatment groups were nonoperative treatment with a physiotherapist; subacromial decompression with postoperative physical therapy; and rotator cuff repair, subacromial decompression, and physical therapy. At one-year follow-up, there was no significant difference between the three groups of patients using the constant score arthroscopic plication. These studies indicate the important role that nonoperative physical therapy can play, although in some patients, operative management is indicated. Most of this section focuses on rotator cuff repair rehabilitation concepts.

Surgical Management

Postoperative treatment for complete rotator cuff tears is based on several principles: tear pattern recognition, secure fixation, and restoration of the footprint. Proper tear pattern recognition is crucial. Many repairs fail because of lack of proper recognition, so a nonanatomical repair is attempted, with increased tension and poor restoration of anatomy (Burkhart et al. 2001).

Complete tear patterns can be broadly divided into two types: crescent-shaped and U-shaped (with several variations). Crescent-shaped tears do not usually retract far from the greater tuberosity and usually are directly repaired back to the greater tuberosity. Their greatest extent is most frequently in a transverse direction to the longitudinal axis of the tendon. They must be debrided to allow high-quality tissue attachment. Adhesion formation usually occurs on both surfaces; these need to be removed to allow complete mobilization and to decrease tension on the repair (Burkhart et al. 2001).

U-shaped tears frequently have their greatest extent in a longitudinal direction to the tendon. The medial point of the tear does not represent retraction but represents the shape that an L-shaped or T-shaped tear assumes with muscle contraction. Mobilization of the two leaves of the tendon, by release of the subacromial and intra-articular adhesions, allows better recognition of the tear pattern. The longitudinal component can be repaired by margin convergence, and the transverse component, now a crescent-shaped tear, can be repaired to the bone. Margin convergence by longitudinal side-to-side closure of the leaves of the tear progressively decreases the strain on the lateral margins of the tear, so that the resulting strain on the lateral transverse margin is within the tolerance for repair (Burkhart et al. 2001).

Suture placement in the tendon is the subject of much study (Burkhart 2000, Fealy et al. 2002). The types of suture placement may be categorized as simple, mattress, or combination (modified Mason-Allen). Although there is literature favoring each

type of suture placement, what is probably more important is how securely the sutures are tied (proper loop security of tendon to bone and knot security within the throws of the knot) and how much load is carried across each suture. Fixation placement should result in proper position of the cuff to bone and optimum pullout strength of the fixation device or construct. Suture anchors should be placed at a 45° angle to increase the anchor's resistance to pullout. For single-row repairs, the suture anchors are placed within 4 to 5 mm of the articular margin. More recently, double-row and suture bridge repairs have been advocated to maximize suture placement and load per suture and to maximize fixation placement. The rows consist of medial suture anchors and lateral bone tunnels or medial and lateral suture anchors (Fealy et al. 2002). Clinical reports demonstrate good results with either of these techniques. The double-row and suture bridge (also referred to as the **transosseous equivalent**) repairs also appear to result in the closest reapproximation of the total geometry of the rotator cuff footprint. Most repairs replicate the width, but not the size, of the original insertion. By allowing a larger, more physiological area of contact, these double-row and suture bridge repair techniques have a theoretical ability to increase healing potential and ultimate tensile strength of the repair construct (Park et al. 2007). The supraspinatus footprint can be defined as the area on the greater tuberosity of the insertion of the supraspinatus and is typically estimated in size as 12 mm anterior to posterior and 24 mm in a medial to lateral orientation (Mochizuki et al. 2009).

Postsurgical Rehabilitation Protocols

The preceding sections have outlined several important concepts of arthroscopic rotator cuff repair that have significant ramifications in postsurgical rehabilitation. Figure 6.1 presents a postsurgical rehabilitation protocol following arthroscopic rotator cuff

FIGURE 6.1 Protocol for Arthroscopic Rotator Cuff Repair

GENERAL GUIDELINES

- Progression of resistive exercise and ROM is dependent on patient tolerance.
- Resistance exercise should not be performed with specific shoulder joint pain or pain over the incision site.
- A sling is provided to the patient for support as needed with daily activities and to wear at night. The patient is weaned from the sling as tolerated.
- Early home exercises are given to the patient following surgery, including stomach rubs, sawing, and gripping activity.
- Progression to active ROM against gravity and duration of sling use are predicated on the size of the rotator cuff tear, quality of the tissue, and fixation.

POSTOPERATIVE WEEKS 1 AND 2

1. Early PROM to patient tolerance during the first four to six weeks:
   a. Flexion
   b. Scapular and coronal plane abduction
   c. Internal–external rotation with 90° to 45° abduction
2. Submaximal isometric IR-ER, flexion-extension, and adduction.
3. Mobilization of the glenohumeral joint and scapulothoracic joint. Passive stretching of elbow, forearm, and wrist to terminal ranges.
4. Side-lying scapular protraction–retractio n resistance to encourage early serratus anterior and lower trapezius activation and endurance.
5. Home exercise instructions:
   a. Instruction in PROM and AAROM home exercises with T-bar, pulleys, or opposite-arm assistance in supine position using ROM to patient tolerance
   b. Instruction in weight bearing (closed chain) Codman exercise over a ball or countertop or table
   c. Theraputty for grip strength maintenance

POSTOPERATIVE WEEK 3

1. Continue shoulder ROM and isometric strength program from previous weeks to patient tolerance. Progress patient to AAROM.
2. Add upper body ergometer if available.
3. Begin active scapular strengthening exercises and continue side-lying manual scapular stabilization exercise:
   a. Scapular retraction
   b. Scapular retraction with depression
4. Begin resistive exercise for total arm strength using positions with glenohumeral joint completely supported:
   a. Biceps curls
   b. Triceps curls
   c. Wrist curls—flexion, extension, radial and ulnar deviation
5. Begin submaximal rhythmic stabilization using the balance point position (90°-100° of elevation) in supine position to initiate dynamic stabilization.

(continued)

FIGURE 6.1 *(continued)*

POSTOPERATIVE WEEKS 5 AND 6

1. Initiate isotonic resistance exercise focusing on the following movements:
    a. Side-lying ER
    b. Prone extension
    c. Prone horizontal abduction (limited range to 45°)
    d. Supine IR
    e. Flexion to 90°

    Note: A low-resistance, high-repetition (i.e., 30 repetitions) format is recommended using no resistance initially (i.e., weight of the arm).

2. Progression to full PROM and AROM in all planes including ER and IR in neutral adduction progressing from the 90° abducted position used initially postoperatively.
3. External rotation oscillation (resisted ER with towel roll under axilla and oscillation device).
4. Home exercise program for strengthening the rotator cuff and scapular musculature with isotonic weights or elastic tubing.

POSTOPERATIVE WEEK 8

1. Begin closed chain step-ups and quadruped rhythmic stabilization exercise.
2. Initiate upper extremity plyometric chest passes and functional two-hand rotation tennis groundstroke or golf swing simulation using small exercise ball, progressing to light medicine ball as tolerated.

POSTOPERATIVE WEEK 10

1. Initiation of submaximal isokinetic exercise for IR-ER in the modified neutral position.

    Criteria for progression to isokinetic exercise:
    a. Patient has IR-ER ROM greater than that used during the isokinetic exercise.
    b. Patient can complete isotonic exercise program pain-free with a 2- to 3-pound (0.9-1.4 kg) weight or medium-resistance surgical tubing or an elastic resistance band.
2. Progression to 90° abducted rotational training in patients returning to overhead work or sport activity.
    a. Prone ER
    b. Standing ER-IR with 90° abduction in the scapular plane
    c. Statue of Liberty (ER oscillation)

POSTOPERATIVE WEEK 12 (3 MONTHS)

1. Progression to maximal isokinetics in IR-ER and isokinetic testing to assess strength in modified base 30/30/30 position. Formal documentation of AROM, PROM, and administration of shoulder rating scales.
2. Begin interval return programs if these criteria have been met:
    a. Internal–external rotation strength minimum of 85% of contralateral extremity
    b. External/internal rotation ratio 60% or higher
    c. Pain-free ROM
    d. Negative impingement and instability signs during clinical examination

POSTOPERATIVE WEEK 16 (4 MONTHS)

1. Isokinetic reevaluation, documentation of AROM and PROM, and shoulder rating scales.
2. Progression continues for return to full upper extremity sport activity (e.g., throwing, serving in tennis).
3. Preparation for discharge from formal physical therapy to home program phase.

AROM = active range of motion; AAROM = active assistive range of motion.

repair of a medium-sized tear. Initial postsurgical rehabilitation focuses on ROM to prevent capsular adhesions while protecting surgically repaired tissues. Some postsurgical rehabilitation protocols call for specific ROM limitations to be applied during the first six weeks of rehabilitation.

Several basic science studies have been published that provide a rationale for the safe application of glenohumeral joint ROM and the movements that allow joint excursion, as well as capsular lengthening, while safe and protective inherent tensions are produced in the repaired tendon. Hatakeyama and coworkers (2001) used a cadaveric model to repair 1 × 2 cm supraspinatus tears and studied the effects of humeral rotation ROM on tension in the supraspinatus at 30° of elevation in the coronal, scapular, and sagittal planes. Results showed that compared with tension in a position of neutral rotation, 30° and 60° of ER actually showed a decrease in tension within the supraspinatus muscle–tendon unit. In contrast, 30° and 60° of IR showed increases in tension within the supraspinatus tendon. This study provides important insight into the ability to perform early PROM in the directions of ER following rotator cuff repair. Additionally, because most patients are placed in positions of IR following surgery during the period of immobilization, movement of the shoulder into IR is performed despite the increased tension identified by Hatakeyama and colleagues (2001). One additional finding of clinical relevance in the study by Hatakeyama and associates (2001) was the comparison of the intrinsic tensile load in the repaired supraspinatus tendon between the frontal or coronal plane, the

scapular plane, and the sagittal plane during humeral rotation. Significantly higher loading was present in the supraspinatus tendon during humeral rotation in the sagittal plane as compared with both the frontal and scapular planes. Therefore, based on this important basic science study, early PROM is performed into the directions of both external and internal humeral rotation, using the scapular plane position to minimize tensile loading in the repaired tendon (Hatakeyama et al. 2001) (figure 6.2).

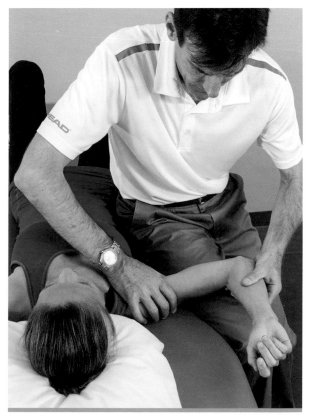

Figure 6.2   External rotation at 90° of abduction in the scapular plane used following rotator cuff repair.

Another basic science study provides guidance for ROM application in the early postoperative phase. Muraki and colleagues (2006) studied the effects of passive motion on tensile loading of the supraspinatus tendon in cadavers, in a study similar to the one conducted by Hatakeyama and colleagues (2001). They found no significant increases in strain during the movement of cross-arm adduction in either the supraspinatus or the infraspinatus tendon at 60° of elevation. However, IR performed at 30° and 60° of elevation did place increased tension on the inferior-most portion of the infraspinatus tendon over the resting or neutral position. This study provides additional guidance for clinicians in the selection of safe ROM positions following surgery. It also shows the importance of knowing the degree of tendon involvement and repair, as posteriorly based rotator cuff repairs (those involving the infraspinatus and teres minor) may be subjected to increased tensile loads if early IR is applied during postoperative rehabilitation.

Additional research by Muraki and associates (2007) addressed the effect of joint mobilization on the repaired rotator cuff (supraspinatus) tendon. Their findings showed that the application of joint mobilization with 30° of abduction produced less tensile loading in the repaired rotator cuff tendon than was present in a reference position with the shoulder joint at rest in 0° of abduction. Therefore, joint mobilization should not be performed with the shoulder placed in 0° of abduction but rather with the shoulder in elevation in the scapular plane, thereby minimizing tendon stress and allowing for mobilizations to be applied safely during the rehabilitation program following rotator cuff repair (Hatakeyama et al. 2001, Muraki et al. 2007).

One of the most significant current debates in rotator cuff repair rehabilitation is the concept of early versus delayed range of motion following rotator cuff repair. A systematic review in 2009 found insufficient evidence to provide an evidence-based conclusion or recommendation regarding immobilization versus early passive ROM for rotator cuff repair rehabilitation (Arndt et al. 2012).

Four randomized controlled trials (RCTs) have been published comparing early passive ROM to sling immobilization following arthroscopic rotator cuff repair (Cuff et al. 2012, Keener et al. 2014, Kim et al. 2012, Lee et al. 2012). A meta-analysis identified the important findings from these RCTs for clinical application (Riboh et al. 2014). Advocates of early passive ROM following surgery cite the most common complication following arthroscopic rotator cuff repair (postoperative stiffness) as the primary rationale for early mobilization and movement (Brislin et al. 2007, Namdari et al. 2010); opponents cite the high incidence of re-tear (Galatz et al. 2004, Tashjian et al. 2010). The meta-analysis (Riboh et al. 2014) shows that early postoperative passive ROM results in substantial increases in shoulder flexion at 3, 6, and 12 months after surgery compared with immobilization. External rotation ROM also increased across the early passive ROM groups; however, this increase was only significant at 3 months after surgery. Perhaps most important, early passive ROM did not result in increased rotator cuff re-tear rates at a minimum follow-up of one year. The studies included in this analysis excluded massive rotator cuff tears. Continued outcomes research and investigational studies will help identify both optimal healing times and immobilization periods as surgical fixation and rehabilitation methods continue to refine and improve in the future.

One key element in the rehabilitation process following rotator cuff repair lies in the progression from passive-based ROM applications to active assistive and active ROM. There is some disagreement as to the degree of muscular activation that occurs during commonly used rehabilitation activities; this can be clarified by a review of the appropriate literature. Research by McCann and colleagues (1993) provides clear delineation of the degree of muscular activation of the supraspinatus during supine assisted ROM and seated elevation with the use of a pulley. Although both activities arguably produce low levels of inherent muscular activation in the supraspinatus, the upright pulley activity produces significantly more muscular activity as compared with the supine activities studied by McCann and colleagues (1993).

Additionally, research by Ellsworth and associates (2006) has quantified levels of muscular activation during Codman's pendulum exercise. Their study shows minimal levels of muscular activation in the rotator cuff musculature during this exercise; however, the exercise cannot be considered passive because the musculature is truly activated, especially in individuals with shoulder pathology. Additionally, many therapists do not recommend the use of weight application in the hand during pendulum exercises because of the potential for unwanted anterior translation. Ellsworth and colleagues (2006) found that muscular activity in the rotator cuff musculature was not changed between the performance of pendulum exercises with and without weight application. Pendulum exercises without weight have the same effect on muscular activity as those performed with weight application; thus the use of pendulum exercises in the early postsurgery phase may be questioned in cases in which only passive movements may be indicated.

These studies provide objective guidance for the early application of assisted ROM activities that can be used safely in early postsurgical rehabilitation following rotator cuff repair. Rehabilitation in the first two to four weeks following rotator cuff repair typically consists of the use of truly passive—as well as several minimally active or active assistive—exercises for the rotator cuff such as active assisted elevation, overhead pulleys, and pendulums. Additionally, the balance point position (90° of shoulder flexion) is used in the supine position, with the patient cued to perform small active motions of flexion-extension from the 90° starting position to recruit rotator cuff and scapular muscular activity (figure 6.3). These exercises, coupled with early scapular stabilization via manual resistance techniques emphasizing

direct hand contacts on the scapula, are recommended to bypass force application to the rotator cuff and to optimize trapezius, rhomboid, and serratus anterior muscular activation. Kibler and colleagues (2008) have published EMG quantification of low-level closed chain exercise such as weight shifting on a rocker board and have highlighted the low levels (10%) of activation of the rotator cuff and the scapular musculature during application.

Progression to resistive exercise for the rotator cuff and the scapular musculature typically occurs in a time interval approximating six weeks following surgery, when early theoretical healing is assumed in the repaired tissues. Significant variation exists in the literature regarding the time course for this initiation of resistive exercise

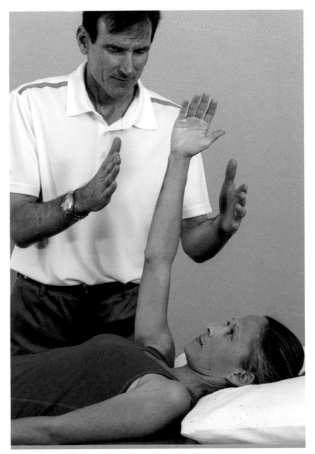

Figure 6.3 Balance point position at 90° of elevation.

(Timmerman et al. 1994) and is based on several factors. These factors include, but are not limited to, tear size, tear type, tissue quality, concomitant surgical procedures, and patient health status and age.

Clinical application of resistive exercise during this critical stage of rehabilitation is guided both by published literature detailing the level of muscular activity within individual muscles of the rotator cuff and scapular stabilizers and by patients who demonstrate exercise tolerance. These studies (discussed in chapter 5) provide the rationale behind the determination of optimal exercise movement patterns to produce the desired level of muscular activation in the rotator cuff and scapular stabilizers. The application of very low resistance levels in a repetitive format is recommended for safety and for relative protection of the repaired tissues, as well as to improve local muscular endurance. Multiple sets of 15 to 20 repetitions have been recommended and described in several studies to improve muscular strength in the

rotator cuff and scapular stabilizing musculature (Malliou et al. 2004, Wang et al. 1999). Exercise patterns using shorter lever arms, as well as maintaining the glenohumeral joint in positions of less than 90° of elevation and anterior to the coronal plane of the body, are theorized to reduce the risks of both compressive irritation and capsular loading and attenuation during performance. Additionally, early focus on the rotator cuff and scapular stabilizers without emphasis on larger prime mover muscles such as the deltoid, pectorals, and upper trapezius is recommended to minimize unwanted joint shear and inappropriate arthrokinematics, in addition to attempting to optimize ER-IR muscle balance (Lee & An 2002, Malliou et al. 2004). The upper extremity Ranger (Rehab Innovations, Omaha, Nebraska) is used to provide assistance with elevation—to prevent and minimize scapular compensation by providing optimal leveraging and assist with shoulder elevation during this phase of the rehabilitation (figure 6.4).

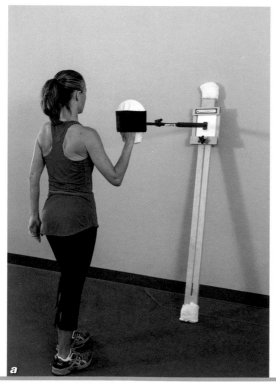 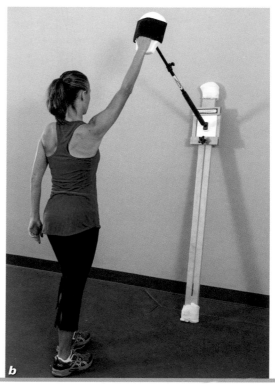

Figure 6.4 Upper extremity Ranger device used to assist with initial elevation of the shoulder following rotator cuff repair: *(a)* start position and *(b)* end position.

One specific exercise that has been described extensively in the literature is the empty can exercise (scapular plane elevation with an internally rotated [thumb down] extremity position; see chapter 3 for more detail). Although EMG studies have shown high levels of activation of the supraspinatus during the empty can exercise (Malanga et al. 1996, Thigpen et al. 2006), the combined movements of elevation and IR have produced clinically disappointing results in practical application, as well as the common occurrence of patterns of substitution and improper biomechanical execution (Thigpen et al. 2006). Increases in scapular IR and anterior tilting have been shown when the empty can is compared with the full can (scapular plane elevation with ER) exercise using motion analysis. Movement patterns characterized by scapular IR and anterior tilting theoretically decrease the subacromial space, and could jeopardize the ability to apply repetitive movement patterns required for strength acquisition needed during shoulder rehabilitation (Thigpen et al. 2006).

Specific exercise application for the scapular stabilizers focuses on the lower trapezius and serratus anterior musculature. Donatelli and Ekstrom (2003) and Kibler and colleagues (2008) have summarized the upper extremity exercise movement patterns that elicit high levels of activation of these important force couple components responsible for scapular stabilization. Progression from early manual resistive patterns to exercise patterns with elastic resistance and light dumbbells is an important part of the rehabilitation protocol following rotator cuff repair. Wang and coworkers (1999) have shown improvements in muscular strength and positive changes in scapulohumeral rhythm following six weeks of training using elastic resistance exercise. The use of resistive exercise patterns emphasizing scapular retraction and external humeral rotation is emphasized to optimize scapular stabilization and promote muscular balance during shoulder rehabilitation. Later stages of postoperative rotator cuff repair rehabilitation are similar to the progressions outlined in the earlier sections of this book and are presented in figure 6.1 for further clarification

Short-term follow-up of patients after both mini-open and all-arthroscopic rotator cuff repair shows the return of nearly full range of active and passive motion, with deficits in muscular strength ranging from 10% to 30% in IR and ER compared with the uninjured extremity (Ellenbecker et al. 2006). Greater deficits following mini-open and all-arthroscopic rotator cuff repair have been reported in the posterior rotator cuff (external rotators) despite particular emphasis on these structures during postsurgical rehabilitation.

LABRAL REPAIR

The inherently complicated nature of injuries involving the superior aspect of the glenoid labrum can present a substantial clinical challenge. Successful return to unrestricted function requires integrating the appropriate diagnosis, surgical management, and rehabilitation in a coordinated effort. The advent of new arthroscopic techniques has helped to provide a better understanding of normal labral anatomy, capsulolabral anomalies, and the pathomechanics of conditions involving this structure. Likewise, these techniques have drastically improved the surgical treatment options available to successfully address these pathologies. Andrews and colleagues (1985) originally described the detachment of the superior labrum in a subset of throwing athletes. Later, Snyder and colleagues (1995) introduced the term SLAP lesion, indicating an injury located within the superior labrum extending anterior to posterior. They originally classified these lesions into four distinct categories based on the type of lesion present, emphasizing that this lesion may disrupt the origin of the long head of the biceps brachii (Snyder et al. 1990). Subsequent authors have added additional classification categories and specific subtypes, further expanding on the four originally described categories (Gartsman & Hammerman 2000, Maffet et al. 1995,

Morgan et al. 1998). Based on these subtle differences in labral pathology, an appropriate treatment plan may be developed to adequately address the specific pathology present.

It has become clear that symptomatic superior labral lesions and detachments can be treated effectively with either arthroscopic debridement or repair, depending on the specific type of pathology present (Field & Savoie 1993, Pagnani et al. 1995a, 1995b, Reinold et al. 2002, Snyder & Kollias 1997, Williams et al. 1994). To ensure a successful outcome it is critical to carefully follow a postoperative rehabilitation program based on an accurate diagnosis that specifies the extent of superior labral pathology.

Nonoperative Rehabilitation

When designing a nonoperative rehabilitation program for individuals who have a SLAP lesion, it is important to consider the type of SLAP lesion, extent of the lesion, and concomitant lesions. SLAP lesions that involve detachment of the glenoid labrum such as types II, IV, and VI through X are often unable to successfully rehab without surgery to repair the lesion. Type I and possibly type III lesions can be successfully managed nonoperatively. Concomitant lesions such as rotator partial tears or cuff fraying and long head of the biceps involvement can further complicate the rehabilitation process.

The rehabilitation program should include reducing the patient's inflammation and pain, restoring normal motion (especially IR), and reestablishing normal capsular mobility. Furthermore, acceptable ER/IR muscular ratios need to be restored along with an improvement in scapular position and muscular strength; this would include strengthening of the lower trapezius, middle trapezius, and rhomboids. It is imperative to restore normal scapular posture and position as a necessary component to the rehabilitation program. Once these objectives are achieved, the patient may begin a gradual return to sport activities.

Success with nonoperative rehabilitation was studied in 39 patients by Edwards and colleagues (2010), who demonstrated during a three-year follow-up that 51% of patients were classified as treatment failures, requiring surgical management of their SLAP lesion. Of the remaining patients who had successful rehabilitative outcomes, only 66% of overhead athletes were able to return to successful overhead throwing. This study shows that an initial trial of nonoperative rehabilitation may be indicated in patients with superior labral injury but that successful return to overhead sports is not always possible without surgical management. Further research on nonoperative treatment of SLAP lesions is clearly needed to better understand the role that nonoperative rehabilitation can play and also to enable identification of patients who may be optimal candidates for this type of treatment.

Surgical Management

Nonoperative management of SLAP lesions may be unsuccessful, particularly with type II and type IV lesions with labral instability and underlying shoulder instability. Therefore, surgical intervention is most often warranted to repair the labral lesion while addressing any concomitant pathology. In the event that an athlete does undergo conservative rehabilitation, many of the principles discussed in the following sections may be applied.

Experience suggests that a type I SLAP lesion may represent age-related fraying of the superior labrum and does not necessarily require specific treatment. Often the overhead athlete may exhibit fraying of the superior and posterior labrum due to internal impingement (Walch et al. 1992). Isolated debridement of labral fraying has not been shown to reliably relieve symptoms over the long term (Altchek et al. 1992, Davies et al. 2004). However, if symptoms are progressive or warrant surgical intervention, type I SLAP lesions are generally debrided back to a stable labral rim.

Type III SLAP lesions should also be excised and debrided back to a stable rim, much like some bucket-handle meniscus tears in the knee. The exception to this is a type III lesion involving a Buford complex, which should be treated as a type II SLAP lesion (Snyder et al. 1990).

The outcomes following debridement (without repair) of unstable type II and IV SLAP lesions have been poor; thus these should be repaired to restore the normal anatomy (Altchek et al. 1992, Davies et al. 2004). In the presence of a type II SLAP lesion, the superior labrum should be reattached to the glenoid and the biceps anchor stabilized (figure 6.5). The type II lesion is often stabilized using suture anchors. Treatment of type IV SLAP lesions is generally based on the extent to which the biceps anchor is involved. When biceps involvement is less than approximately 30% of the entire anchor, the torn tissue is typically resected and the superior labrum reattached. If the biceps tear is more substantial, a side-to-side repair of the biceps tendon, in addition to reattachment of the superior labrum, is generally performed. However, if the biceps tear is extensive enough to substantially alter the biceps origin, a biceps **tenodesis** (reattachment of the bicep long head tendon distal to the native attachment

on the supraglenoid tubercle of the scapula [glenoid]) is more practical than a direct repair. In addition to the treatment of the SLAP lesion, associated rotator cuff pathology or glenohumeral joint instability should be independently evaluated and treated at the time of surgery.

The goal of surgical repair of a SLAP lesion is to obtain a strong repair that allows the patient to aggressively rehabilitate the shoulder and return to full activities or sport competition. Using arthroscopic surgical techniques, the superior labrum is mobilized along the entire area of detachment using a 4.5 mm motorized shaver to take down any fibrous adhesions. This area usually extends from approximately the 11 to the 1 o'clock positions of the glenoid (in a right shoulder). The bony area of attachment is abraded to create a bleeding bed to facilitate healing. The repair surface of the labrum is also gently debrided to stimulate a healing response. Two suture anchors are usually adequate to secure the biceps anchor and superior labrum. Some surgeons prefer to use bioabsorbable suture anchors with a number 2 braided nonabsorbable suture loaded on the eyelet. The number of anchors used is based on the size of the SLAP lesion present. The suture anchors are positioned so that each one splits the difference between the biceps and the normal area of labral insertion, usually 11:30 and 12:30 on a clock face. The suture anchors are placed at the junction of the articular cartilage and cortical bone. The security of anchor fixation is tested with a firm pull on the sutures. Once the suture anchors are in place, one end of each suture is passed through the labrum. The surgeon may choose to incorporate some of the biceps tendon near the junction of the biceps and labrum, if necessary, to secure the biceps anchor. Arthroscopic knot-tying techniques are used. In general, the placement of anchors and tying knots progresses from posterior to anterior.

The outcomes following repair of unstable SLAP II and IV lesions have been good, with satisfactory results in over 80% of patients in the majority of published articles (Pagnani et

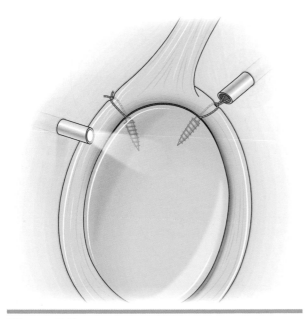

Figure 6.5 SLAP II repair using suture anchors.

al. 1995a, 1995b, Stetson & Templin 2002). Reinold and colleagues (2003) reported that 87% of athletes undergoing thermal capsulorraphy (TACS) with concomitant debridement of a SLAP lesion and 84% of athletes with a concomitant SLAP repair returned to competition with good to excellent outcomes using a shoulder scoring scale known as the Modified Athletic Shoulder Outcome Scale.

Postsurgical Rehabilitation Protocols

The specific rehabilitation program following surgical intervention involving the superior glenoid labrum is dependent on the severity of the pathology and should specifically match the type of SLAP lesion, the exact surgical procedure performed (debridement vs. repair), and other possible concomitant procedures performed, because of the underlying glenohumeral joint instability that is often present. Overall, emphasis should be placed on restoring and enhancing dynamic stability of the glenohumeral joint while at the same time ensuring that adverse stresses are not applied to healing tissue.

Before rehabilitation, it is imperative that a thorough subjective and clinical exam be performed to determine the exact mechanism and nature of labral pathology. For patients who sustained a SLAP lesion via a compressive injury, such as a fall on an outstretched hand, weight-bearing exercises should be avoided to minimize compression and shear on the superior labrum. Patients with traction injuries should avoid heavy resisted or excessive eccentric biceps contractions. Furthermore, patients with peel-back lesions, such as overhead athletes, should avoid excessive amounts of shoulder ER while the SLAP lesion is healing. Thus, the mechanism of injury is an important factor to individually assess when one is determining appropriate rehabilitation guidelines for each patient.

Although the efficacy of rehabilitation following SLAP repairs has not been documented, the following sections overview guidelines based on clinical experience and basic science studies on the mechanics of the glenoid labrum and pathomechanics of SLAP lesions (Burkhart & Morgan 1998, Nam & Snyder 2003, Powell et al. 2004, Reinold et al. 2003, Rodosky et al. 1994, Shepard et al. 2004, Vangsness et al. 1994, Wilk et al. 2001b).

Rehabilitation Following Debridement of Type I and III SLAP Lesions

Type I and type III SLAP lesions normally undergo a simple arthroscopic debridement of the frayed labrum without an anatomic repair. Figure 6.6 outlines the rehabilitation program following this type of procedure. This program can be somewhat aggressive in restoring motion and function, because the biceps–labral anchor is stable and intact.

The rate of progression during the course of postoperative rehabilitation is based on the presence and extent of concomitant lesions. If, for example, significant rotator cuff fraying (partial-thickness tear) is present and has been treated with arthroscopic debridement, the rehabilitative program must be appropriately adapted. Generally, a sling is worn for comfort during the first three or four days following surgery. **Active assistive range of motion** (AAROM) with the assistance of the therapist guiding the motion and PROM exercises are initiated immediately following surgery, with full PROM expected within 10 to 14 days postoperatively. Flexion ROM is performed to tolerance. External rotation and IR in the scapular plane are initiated at 45° of glenohumeral abduction and advanced to 90° of abduction, usually by postoperative day 4 or 5. Range of motion exercises may be performed early because an anatomical repair has not been performed.

Isometric strengthening in all planes of shoulder motion is performed submaximally and pain-free during the first seven days after surgery to retard muscular atrophy. Light isotonic strengthening for the shoulder and scapular musculature (with the exception of the biceps) is initiated approximately eight

PHASE I: MOTION PHASE (DAYS 1 TO 10)

Goals
- Reestablish nonpainful ROM
- Retard muscular atrophy
- Decrease pain and inflammation

Range of Motion
- Pendulum exercise
- PROM-AAROM rope and pulley
  - Flexion-extension
  - Abduction-adduction
  - External–internal rotation (begin at 0° AB, progress to 45° AB, then 90° AB)
- Self-stretches (capsular stretches)

Exercises
- Isometrics

Note: No biceps isometrics for five to seven days post-op.

- May initiate tubing for ER-IR at 0° AB late phase (usually 7-10 days post-op)

Decrease Pain and Inflammation
- Ice
- NSAIDs
- Modalities

PHASE II: INTERMEDIATE PHASE (WEEKS 2–3)

Goals
- Regain and improve muscular strength
- Normalize arthrokinematics
- Improve neuromuscular control of shoulder complex

Criteria to Progress to Phase II
- Full PROM
- Minimal pain and tenderness
- "Good" MMT of IR, ER, flexion

Week 2

Exercises
- Initiate isotonic program with dumbbells
  - Shoulder musculature
  - Scapulothoracic
  - Tubing ER-IR at 0° abduction
  - Side-lying ER
  - Prone rowing ER
  - Proprioceptive neuromuscular facilitation manual resistance with dynamic stabilization
- Normalize arthrokinematics of shoulder complex
  - Joint mobilization
  - Continue stretching of shoulder (ER-IR at 90° of abduction)
- Initiate neuromuscular control exercises
- Initiate proprioception training
- Initiate trunk exercises
- Initiate UE endurance exercises

Decrease Pain and Inflammation
Continue use of modalities, ice, as needed

Week 3

Exercises
- Thrower's Ten program
- Emphasize rotator cuff and scapular strengthening
- Dynamic stabilization drills

(continued)

FIGURE 6.6 *(continued)*

PHASE III: DYNAMIC STRENGTHENING PHASE— ADVANCED STRENGTHENING PHASE (WEEKS 4-6)

Goals
- Improve strength, power, endurance
- Improve neuromuscular control
- Prepare athlete to begin to throw

Criteria to Enter Phase III
- Full nonpainful AROM and PROM
- No pain or tenderness
- Strength 70% compared to contralateral side

Exercises
- Continue Thrower's Ten program
- Continue dumbbell strengthening (supraspinatus, deltoid)

- Initiate tubing exercises in the 90/90 position for ER-IR (slow–fast sets)
- Exercises for scapulothoracic musculature
- Tubing exercises for biceps
- Initiate plyometrics (two-hand drills, progressing to one-hand drills)
- Diagonal patterns (PNF)
- Initiate isokinetic strengthening
- Continue endurance exercises: neuromuscular control exercises
- Continue proprioception exercises

PHASE IV: RETURN TO ACTIVITY PHASE (WEEK 7 AND BEYOND)

Goals

Progressively increase activities to prepare patient for full functional return

Criteria to Progress to Phase IV
- Full PROM
- No pain or tenderness
- Isokinetic test results for ER/IR muscle balance and bilateral comparison
- Pain-free clinical exam

Exercises
- Initiate interval sport program (e.g., throwing, tennis)
- Continue all exercises as in phase III (throw and train on same day, LE and ROM on opposite days)
- Progress interval program

Follow-Up Visits
- Isokinetic tests
- Clinical exam

AROM = active range of motion; AAROM = active assistive range of motion; AB = abduction; NSAIDs = nonsteroidal anti-inflammatory medications; UE = upper e ; LE = lower extremity.

days following surgery. This includes ER-IR exercise tubing, side-lying ER, prone rowing, prone horizontal abduction, and prone ER. Active elevation exercises, such as scapular plane elevation (full can) and lateral raises, are also included. Weighted resistance begins at 0.45 kg (1 pound) and advances by 0.45 kg per week in a gradual, controlled, progressive resistance fashion. This progression is used to gradually challenge the musculature. Light biceps resistance is usually not initiated until two weeks following surgery in an attempt to prevent debridement site irritation. Furthermore, caution is warranted regarding early overaggressive elbow flexion and forearm supination exercises, particularly eccentric exercises.

As the strengthening program progresses after this type of surgical procedure, the emphasis of rehabilitative interventions should be on obtaining muscular balance and promoting dynamic shoulder stability. This is accomplished through a variety of manual resistance and end-range rhythmic stabilization drills performed in conjunction with isotonic strengthening and core stabilization exercises. The primary goal of these drills is to reestablish dynamic humeral head control, especially if the pathomechanics of the labral lesion was due to excessive glenohumeral laxity.

The individual is advanced to controlled weight training activities between postoperative weeks 4 and 6. The patient is instructed on proper technique, such as avoiding excessive shoulder extension during bench press and seated rows, to minimize strain on the shoulder. Plyometric exercises are initiated between weeks 4 and 5 to train the upper extremity to both absorb external forces and develop forces. Two-hand plyometrics such as chest pass, side throws, and overhead throws are performed initially, progressing to include one-hand drills such as baseball throws in 7 to 10 days. The athlete is allowed to begin a gradual return to sport-specific activities between postoperative weeks 7 and 10, typically using an interval sport program. The rate of return to overhead sports is often dependent on the extent of concomitant injuries. For example, an athlete with rotator cuff debridement involving 20% to 30% penetration of the rotator cuff will usually begin an interval sport program following these guidelines, while an athlete with more extensive pathology may need to delay starting the interval sport program for up to four months. The aim of an interval sport program is to ensure that the athlete uses a gradual increase in applied loads to the healing tissues (Reinold et al. 2002). The start date for initiating any interval sport program is often varied based on the time of year, the goals of the patient, and the competitive athletic season. The ultimate success of return to high-level activity following this procedure is dependent on the individual's ability to dynamically stabilize the glenohumeral joint during the performance of high-demand activities; thus appropriate and adequate rehabilitation is paramount.

Criteria to begin an interval return to sport activity include minimal pain, full ROM, adequate strength and dynamic stability, and

an appropriate rehabilitation progression as previously described (Pagnani et al. 1995a, 1995b). To determine if the patient has adequate strength, isokinetic testing can be performed with the goals of ER peak torque/body weight ratios of 18% to 23%, ER/IR ratio of 66% to 76%, and ER/abduction ratio of 67% to 75% at 180°/sec (Reinold et al. 2004, Wilk et al. 1997, 2001b, 2004).

Rehabilitation Following Repair of Type II SLAP Lesions

Overhead throwing athletes commonly present with a type II SLAP lesion with the biceps tendon detached from the glenoid rim. Frequently, a peel-back lesion is also present. The initial rehabilitative concern is to ensure that forces and loads on the repaired labrum are appropriately controlled. It is important to determine the extent of the lesion and understand its exact location and the number of suture anchors in constructing an appropriate rehabilitation program. For instance, the rate of rehabilitation progression would be slower for a SLAP repair completed with three anchors compared to a one-anchor repair, based on the extent of the pathology and tissue involvement. Postoperative rehabilitation is delayed to allow healing of the more extensive anatomical repair required to reattach the biceps tendon anchor in a type II lesion in comparison to type I lesions (figure 6.7).

The patient is instructed to sleep in a shoulder immobilizer and wear a sling during the daytime for the first four weeks following surgery to protect the healing structures from excessive amounts of motion. Gradual ROM in a protective range is performed for the first four weeks below 90° of elevation to avoid strain on the labral repair (Wilk et al. 1997). During the first two weeks, IR and ER ROM exercises are performed passively in the scapular plane to approximatcly 10° to 15° of ER and 45° of IR. Initial ER ROM is performed cautiously to minimize strain on the labrum through the peel-back mechanism. Internal and external rotation ROM activities are progressed to 90° of shoulder

FIGURE 6.7 Protocol Following Arthroscopic Type II SLAP Repair

PHASE I: IMMEDIATE POSTOPERATIVE PHASE, "PROTECTED MOTION" (DAY 1 TO WEEK 6)

Goals
- Protect the anatomic repair
- Prevent negative effects of immobilization
- Promote dynamic stability
- Diminish pain and inflammation

Weeks 0 to 2
- Sling for four weeks
- Sleep in immobilizer for four weeks
- Elbow–hand PROM
- Hand gripping exercises
- Passive and gentle shoulder AAROM exercise
  - Flexion to 60° (week 2: flexion to 75°)
  - Elevation in scapular plane to 60°
- External–internal rotation with arm in scapular plane
  - External rotation to 10° to 15°
  - Internal rotation to 45°

Note: No active ER or extension or abduction.
- Submaximal isometrics for shoulder musculature
- No isolated biceps contractions
- Cryotherapy, modalities as indicated

Weeks 3 and 4
- Discontinue use of sling at four weeks
- Sleep in immobilizer until week 4
- Continue gentle ROM exercises (PROM and AAROM)
  - Flexion to 90°
  - Abduction to 75° to 85°
  - External rotation in scapular plane to 25° to 30°
  - Internal rotation in scapular plane to 55° to 60°

Note: Rate of progression based on evaluation of the patient.
- No active ER, extension, or elevation
- Initiate rhythmic stabilization drills
- Initiate proprioception training
- Tubing ER-IR at 0° abduction
- Continue isometrics
- Continue use of cryotherapy

Weeks 5 and 6
- Gradually improve ROM
  - Flexion to 145°
  - External rotation at 45° abduction: 45° to 50°
  - Internal rotation at 45° abduction: 55° to 60°
- May initiate stretching exercises
- May initiate light (easy) ROM at 90° abduction
- Continue tubing ER-IR (arm at side)
- Proprioceptive neuromuscular facilitation manual resistance
- Initiate active shoulder abduction (without resistance)
- Initiate full can exercise (weight of arm)
- Initiate prone rowing, prone horizontal abduction
- No biceps strengthening

PHASE II: INTERMEDIATE PHASE, MODERATE PROTECTION PHASE (WEEKS 7–12)

Goals
- Gradually restore full ROM (week 10)
- Preserve the integrity of the surgical repair
- Restore muscular strength and balance

Weeks 7 to 9

- Gradually progress ROM:
  - Flexion to 180°
  - External rotation at 90° abduction: 90° to 95°
  - Internal rotation at 90° abduction: 70° to 75°

- Continue to progress isotonic strengthening program
- Continue PNF strengthening
- Initiate Thrower's Ten program
- May begin AROM biceps

Weeks 10 to 12

- May initiate slightly more aggressive strengthening
- Progress ER to thrower's motion

External rotation at 90° abduction: 110° to 115° in throwers

- Progress isotonic strengthening exercises
- Continue all stretching exercises

Note: Progress ROM to functional demands (i.e., overhead athlete).

- Continue all strengthening exercises

PHASE III: MINIMAL PROTECTION PHASE (WEEKS 12–20)

Goals

- Establish and maintain full PROM and AROM
- Improve muscular strength, power, and endurance
- Gradually initiate functional activities

Criteria to Enter Phase III

- Full nonpainful AROM
- Satisfactory stability
- Muscular strength (graded good or better)
- No pain or tenderness

Weeks 12 to 16

- Continue all stretching exercises (capsular stretches)
- Maintain thrower's motion (especially ER)
- May begin resisted biceps and forearm supination exercises
- Continue strengthening exercises:

- Thrower's Ten program or fundamental exercises
- Proprioceptive neuromuscular facilitation manual resistance
- Endurance training
- Initiate light plyometric program
- Restricted sport activities (light swimming, half golf swings)

Weeks 16 to 20

- Continue all exercises already listed
- Continue all stretching
- Continue Thrower's Ten program
- Continue plyometric program

- Initiate interval sport program (throwing and so on)

Note: See interval throwing program in chapter 8.

PHASE IV: ADVANCED STRENGTHENING PHASE (WEEKS 20–26)

Goals

- Enhance muscular strength, power, and endurance
- Progress functional activities
- Maintain shoulder mobility

Criteria to Enter Phase IV

- Full nonpainful AROM
- Satisfactory static stability
- Muscular strength 75% to 80% of contralateral side
- No pain or tenderness

(continued)

FIGURE 6.7 (continued)

Weeks 20 to 26

- Continue flexibility exercises
- Continue isotonic strengthening program
- Proprioceptive neuromuscular facilitation manual resistance patterns
- Plyometric strengthening
- Progress interval sport programs

PHASE V: RETURN TO ACTIVITY PHASE (MONTHS 6 TO 9)

Goals
- Gradual return to sport activities
- Maintain strength, mobility, and stability

Criteria to Enter Phase V
- Full functional ROM
- Muscular performance isokinetic (fulfills criteria)

AROM = active range of motion.

- Satisfactory shoulder stability
- No pain or tenderness

Exercises
- Gradually progress sport activities to unrestricted participation
- Continue stretching and strengthening program

---

abduction at week 4. Motion is gradually increased to restore full ROM (90°-100° of ER at 90° of abduction) by eight weeks and progressed to thrower's motion (approximately 115°-120° of ER) through week 12. Restoration of motion is usually accomplished with minimal difficulty.

Isometric exercises are performed immediately postoperatively. Exercises are initially performed with rhythmic stabilization drills for ER-IR and flexion-extension. These rhythmic stabilizations theoretically promote dynamic stabilization and cocontraction of the shoulder and rotator cuff musculature (Wilk & Arrigo 1993, Wilk et al. 2001a, 2001b, 2002, 2004). This concept is important when one is considering the underlying glenohumeral joint instability often observed with SLAP lesions. Rhythmic stabilizations may also be performed with manual resistance ER exercises by incorporating the alternating isometric contractions within sets of ER (figure 6.8). Other exercises designed to promote proprioception, dynamic stability, and neuromuscular control include joint repositioning exercises and PNF drills.

External–internal rotation exercise tubing is initiated in weeks 3 to 4 and progressed to include lateral raises, full can, prone rowing,

and prone horizontal abduction by week 6. As the patient progresses, a full isotonic exercise program, such as the Advanced Thrower's Ten program in appendix B (Wilk & Arrigo 1993, Wilk et al. 2001a, 2001b, 2002), is initiated by weeks 7 to 8. Emphasis is placed on strengthening exercises for the external rotators and scapular stabilizations, such as side-lying ER, prone rowing, and prone horizontal abduction (Reinold et al. 2004). No resisted biceps activity (either elbow flexion or forearm supination) is allowed for the first eight weeks to protect healing of the biceps anchor. Neuromuscular control drills are integrated as tolerated to enhance dynamic stability of the shoulder. These include rhythmic stabilization and perturbation drills incorporated into manual resistance and exercise tubing exercises (figure 6.9).

Aggressive strengthening of the biceps is avoided for 12 weeks following surgery. Furthermore, weight-bearing exercises are typically not performed for at least 8 weeks to avoid compression and shearing forces on the healing labrum. Two-hand plyometrics, as well as more advanced strengthening activities, are allowed between 10 and 12 weeks, progressing to the initiation of an

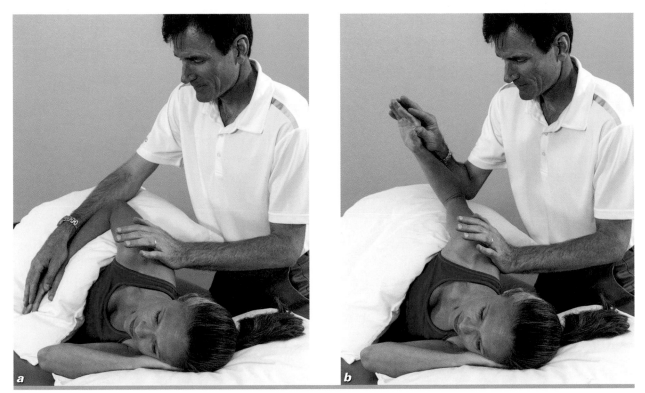

Figure 6.8 Manual resistance external rotation and end-range rhythmic stabilizations. *(a)* The clinician may resist external rotation as well as scapular retraction with the proximal hand. *(b)* End-range rhythmic stabilizations and perturbations may be incorporated to enhance neuromuscular control.

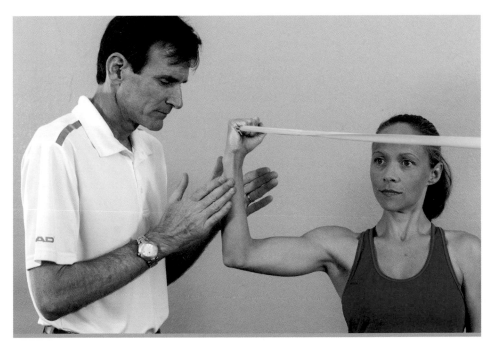

Figure 6.9 Perturbation and rhythmic stabilization drills incorporated into external rotation at 90° abduction with exercise tubing.

interval sport program at postoperative week 16. The same criteria described previously are used to determine whether to begin an interval sport program. Return to play following the surgical repair of a type II SLAP lesion typically occurs at approximately 9 to 12 months following surgery.

Often a type II SLAP repair may be performed with a concomitant glenohumeral stabilization procedure, such as a thermal capsular shrinkage, arthroscopic plication, or Bankart repair. In these instances the rehabilitation program must be a combined approach that considers the healing constraints inherent to both procedures. The reader is encouraged to review several articles to learn more about these approaches (Wilk 1999, Wilk et al. 2001b, 2002, 2004).

Rehabilitation Following Repair of Type IV SLAP Lesions

The surgical repair of a type IV SLAP lesion with either a biceps repair, biceps resection of frayed area, or tenodesis calls for much the same postoperative rehabilitation course as outlined for a type II lesion, in that the ROM and exercise activities are progressed similarly. However, there are substantial differences related to controlling both active and resistive biceps activity based on the extent of bicipital involvement. In cases in which the biceps is resected, biceps muscular contractions may begin between six and eight weeks postsurgery. Conversely, in the cases of repaired biceps tears or biceps tenodesis, no resisted or active biceps exercise is recommended until three months following surgery, when the soft tissue is most likely healed. Light isotonic strengthening for elbow flexion is initiated between weeks 12 and 16 postoperatively and progresses gradually as tolerated from that point. Full resisted biceps activity is not incorporated until weeks 16 to 20. Progression to sport-specific activities, such as plyometrics and interval sport programs, follows guidelines similar to those outlined for type II SLAP repairs.

Rehabilitation Following Bankart Reconstructions

A Bankart lesion, which is found in as many as 85% of dislocations (Gill et al. 1997), is described as a labral detachment that occurs at between 2 o'clock and 6 o'clock on a right shoulder and between the 6 and 10 o'clock positions on a left shoulder. This anterior inferior detachment decreases glenohumeral joint stability by interrupting the continuity of the glenoid labrum and compromising the glenohumeral capsular ligaments (Speer et al. 1994). Detachment of the anterior inferior glenoid labrum creates increases in anterior and inferior humeral head translation, a pattern commonly seen in patients with glenohumeral joint instability (Speer et al. 1994).

Initial Bankart reconstructions were performed via an open incision and led to very strong repairs with fewer failures (redislocations) than less invasive arthroscopic techniques (Lenters et al. 2007, Ozturk et al. 2013). However, in systematic reviews, arthroscopic Bankart reconstructions have been found to restore greater levels of function postoperatively via less invasive surgical exposures (Friedman et al. 2014, Lenters et al. 2007). Open Bankart reconstructions violate the subscapularis and anterior capsule required for access to the anterior inferior labrum to repair the detached labrum to the glenoid. Greater postoperative scarring in the repaired anterior capsule and subscapularis is thought to provide a stronger repair, often recommended in contact sport athletes and laborers, but has been reported to jeopardize ER ROM reattainment and limit function for overhead activities, especially throwing (Ozturk et al. 2013). Redislocation or failure rates for both arthroscopic and open Bankart reconstructions vary in the literature from 0% to 60% (Friedman et al. 2014). With the evolution of arthroscopic techniques after the introduction of suture anchors in labral stabilization, arthroscopic stabilization outcomes have improved, with recent reports of failure from these procedures ranging between 4% and 21% in outcome reviews.

Often performed concomitantly with the repair of the Bankart lesion are procedures to address anterior capsular laxity and redundancy such as capsular plication. Knowledge of the specific procedures and extent of anterior capsular shortening or modification is important for rehabilitation professionals, to better understand the ROM limitations and rates of progression that can be expected in patients postoperatively. A thorough and comprehensive postoperative initial evaluation is needed to document capsular laxity, accessory and physiological glenohumeral joint mobility, and underlying mobility status (i.e., Beighton hypermobility index) to develop the optimal treatment plan and determine the rate of progression in the rehabilitation protocol (figure 6.10). Reports on return to sport following arthroscopic Bankart reconstruction in young athletic (<25 years of age) patients is 87% (Ozturk et al. 2013). Patients at greatest risk for redislocation (failure) following arthroscopic stabilization are those with increased generalized ligamentous laxity, anterior glenoid bone loss, Hill-Sachs lesion, and multiple (>5) instability episodes.

Figure 6.10 outlines rehabilitation techniques and progressions following an arthroscopic Bankart reconstruction. Several important variables warrant further discussion specific to the rehabilitation of patients following arthroscopic Bankart reconstruction. Sling use is typical for the first four to six weeks and is dictated and regulated by the referring surgeon. Referral to physical therapy following surgery in many centers occurs after the first 10 to 14 days of sling immobilization. Initial ROM is typically limited in the direction of ER to protect the anterior capsule and the anterior inferior labral repair (Ellenbecker & Mattalino, 1999, Ellenbecker et al. 2011). Initial ER ROM is performed in the first 30° to 45° of scapular plane elevation, using a range of 30° to 45° of ER (Ellenbecker et al. 2011).

Basic science research can be used to guide the progression of ROM following Bankart reconstruction. Black and associates (1997) identified a low-tension zone in the intact anterior capsule in the range of 0° to 46° in the adducted shoulder in cadaveric specimens. This 46° window would allow motion with little increased stress in the anterior capsule and capsulolabral junction, making the recommendation in the protocol for 30° to 45° of ER ROM safe for early postoperative rehabilitation. Penna and associates (2008), in a similar cadaveric study, investigated stress imparted to a Bankart reconstruction during forward flexion, abduction, and ER in adduction, as well as ER with abduction. Stresses reported were much smaller than previously expected in all ranges of motion studied, indicating safe ROM application early in rehabilitation with limited potential negative stress to the Bankart reconstruction. The one exception was a significant increase in stress on the anterior labral reconstruction during the combined movements of ER and glenohumeral abduction (Penna et al. 2008). Therefore, based on the results of this study and prior recommendations (Ellenbecker et al. 2011), early ROM in the first six weeks following Bankart reconstruction should not include the motion of ER combined with abduction. Early ER up to 45° can be safely applied without jeopardizing the labral repair in the rehabilitation process; however, this ER should not be performed in an abducted shoulder but rather with the shoulder in adduction near the body. The scapular plane should be used for positioning during ER, further limiting anterior capsular stress during application of ER ROM (Saha 1983).

Initiation of early rotator cuff and scapular strengthening is indicated and, in contrast to the guarded and protected strengthening approaches needed following rotator cuff repair, patients following Bankart reconstruction can follow early, submaximal progressions of rotator cuff and scapular exercise. One additional emphasis for consideration by the rehabilitation professional is the use of exercise movements and positions in the initial rehabilitation weeks where minimal stresses are imparted to the anterior capsule and labral structures. These include positions with ER in the abducted shoulder; use of the coronal plane, which has greater

FIGURE 6.10 Protocol Following Arthroscopic Bankart Reconstruction

PHASE I: IMMOBILIZATION (WEEKS 1 AND 2)

- No ROM of the glenohumeral joint.
- Patient to wear sling for comfort as needed.
- Emphasis on ROM of elbow, forearm, and wrist.
- Strengthening of elbow extension-flexion, forearm pronation-supination, and wrist flexion-extension. Theraputty for grip strengthening.

Note: Elbow flexion resistance contraindicated with SLAP lesion repair for first six to eight weeks post-op.

- Scapular mobilization and active elevation and retraction. Manual resistance to scapula with protection of glenohumeral joint emphasizing patterns of protraction and retraction.
- Modalities to control pain in shoulder as indicated.

PHASE II: INITIATION OF MOVEMENT (WEEKS 3 AND 4)

- Continue with preceding exercise guidelines.
- Begin PROM of the glenohumeral joint as tolerated, including ER with 30° to 45° of scapular plane elevation. Range of motion is limited to 30° to 45° of ER to protect the anterior capsule. No stretching, PROM only. Initiation of active antigravity motion as tolerated. Active ROM is to patient tolerance unless otherwise specified.
- Limit stress on anterior capsule. No anterior accessory mobilizations. Include posterior glide mobilization for posterior capsule tightness, and caudal glide to assist with elevation if significant restrictions are encountered on clinical examination.
- Rhythmic stabilization techniques in open chain environment.
- Begin manual resistive exercise for shoulder IR-ER in a submaximal fashion through a non-compromising ROM. Progression to light, submaximal isotonic rotator cuff exercises based on patient tolerance to manual strengthening exercises.
- Begin upper body ergometer for upper extremity endurance as tolerated.

PHASE III (WEEKS 4 THROUGH 8)

- Continue with AROM-PROM to terminal ranges as indicated. Continued inclusion of posterior glide and cross-arm adduction stretching and mobilization is essential to stress the posterior capsule and tight posterior muscle–tendon units.
- Advancement of rotator cuff and scapular resistive exercise in the form of surgical tubing and light isotonic weights.
- Movement patterns to emphasize:
  - External rotation in varying positions of abduction and flexion
  - Prone horizontal abduction
  - Prone extension
  - Internal rotation
- Continue scapular and distal upper extremity strengthening exercise in a low-resistance, high-repetition format.
- Scapular patterns to emphasize:
  - Protraction-retraction
  - Depression

- Initiate upper extremity plyometric program progressing from Swiss ball to weighted medicine balls as tolerated. Chest passes are the initial movement, with progression after 8 to 10 weeks post-op to diagonals and eventually throwing simulation. Emphasize posterior rotator cuff deceleration-type plyometrics in the 8- to 10-week post-op phase.

PHASE IV (WEEKS 9 THROUGH 12)

- Begin isokinetic exercise in the modified neutral position at intermediate and fast contractile velocities.
- Criteria for progression to isokinetics:
  - Completion of isotonic exercise with a minimum of a 2.5- to 3-pound (1-1.4 kg) weight or medium elastic resistance band
  - Pain-free ROM in the isokinetic training movement pattern
- Isokinetic test performed after two or three successful sessions of isokinetic exercise; modified neutral (30/30/30) test position.
- Progression to 90° abducted isokinetic and isotonic functional strengthening for the rotator cuff (shoulder IR-ER) based on patient tolerance.
- Continue with scapular strengthening and ROM exercises listed in earlier stages.

PHASE VI: RETURN TO FULL ACTIVITY

Return to full activity is predicated on physician's evaluation, isokinetic strength parameters, functional ROM, and tolerance to interval sport return programs.

anterior capsular tension than the scapular plane; and using ranges of motion below 90° of elevation to minimize subacromial contact (Flatow et al. 1994). These rotator cuff and scapular exercise progressions are presented in detail in chapter 5.

After six weeks post-op, patients are progressed to terminal ranges of motion in all planes, including gradual increases in ER (figure 6.10). These increases include both advances in actual ER ROM and gradual progression of the amount of abduction in which ER is performed. This would begin in the first 30° to 45° of abduction in the scapular plane, then progress between weeks 6 and 12 to 90° of elevation in the scapular plane and eventually in the coronal plane. Each of these graded increases in position increases stress on the anterior capsular and labral repair, allowing patients to return to overhead reaching and eventually throwing activities. Alongside ROM progression are increases in intensity and positional challenges with strengthening exercises, including the 90° elevated rotational exercises that simulate sport-specific demands and prepare the patient for an eventual return to full activity.

CONCLUSION

A wide variety of pathology may affect the rotator cuff and labrum. Clinical examination is often difficult due to the numerous injury mechanisms and various extents of rotator cuff and labral pathology. Proper identification of the exact mechanism and the specific severity of pathology is vital to accurately diagnose and manage these injuries. Surgical procedures to address SLAP lesions vary from minimal debridement to extensive labral repair. It is suggested that postoperative rehabilitation be based on the specific injury and surgical procedure performed, as well as an understanding of basic science related to injury and tissue healing of the rotator cuff and labrum. Rehabilitation places emphasis on gradually restoring ROM, strength, and dynamic stability of the glenohumeral joint while controlling forces. The aim is for the patient to return to full functional activities as quickly and safely as possible.

IV

RETURN TO SPORT

The final and possibly most important part of the rehabilitation of an athlete following shoulder injury is the return to sport phase. This is often overlooked; instead it is assumed that athletes will know, unguided, how to return to their prior level of sport activity. Part IV offers detailed information on key markers used to return shoulder patients back to functional activity, as well as the specific programs that can be followed to provide the needed guidance for patients during this critical time frame in their rehabilitation from shoulder injury. The interval sport return programs presented in this part of the book will guide injured athletes through a step-wise progression of steadily increased sport-specific demands to ultimately return them to full participation in the sport. The sequence of sport-specific stressors is ordered and applied to most successfully allow for adaptation and reintegration with regard to the specific movement patterns and loading characteristic in common sport activities that patients return to following shoulder injury.

Clinical Decision Making for Return to Sport

"When can I start throwing [or serving, or batting, or golfing, or swimming] again?" This is the question almost every physician, athletic trainer, and physical therapist cringes over when hearing it from any athlete recovering from a shoulder injury. And it is almost always the first question out of any patient's mouth following an injury or surgery to the shoulder. Typically the clinical issue is that answering the question is not at all simple, and trying to put a concrete time frame on what is a complex, multifactorial decision, particularly immediately after surgery, seems daunting. This chapter provides a set of clinically proven objective criteria that can be used to effectively determine when to begin an interval sport return program (described in chapter 8) and how to implement and progress the program to ensure a successful return to throwing following shoulder injury or surgery.

KEY CRITERIA FOR A RETURN TO SPORT EVALUATION

The overhead throwing and serving motions are highly skilled movements performed at extremely high velocity, which requires flexibility, muscular strength, coordination, synchronicity, and neuromuscular control (Wilk et al. 2002). The throwing and serving motions place extraordinary demands on the shoulder joint (see chapter 2). It is because of these high repetitively applied forces that the shoulder is the most commonly injured joint in professional baseball pitchers (Conte et al. 2009). Because of these complex elements, returning an overhead athlete back to competition successfully can be a difficult process requiring a skilled, adept approach to the process of initiating and progressing the functional return.

This chapter discusses the clinical decision-making process for the overhead throwing athlete. Similar steps and decision making would apply for overhead athletes in tennis, as well as golf, swimming, and other arm-dominant sport activities. It is beyond the scope of this book and the space available to apply this detailed discussion to every sport, however. Extensive information on biomechanics and clinical evaluation is presented earlier in this book (chapters 2 and 3), which will assist the clinician in applying the model and information discussed in this chapter to other overhead and arm-dominant athletes. Athletes are motivated to resume high-level training drills and unrestricted athletics as soon as possible; it is therefore crucial that a set of objective measurable criteria be established to allow a reasonable sequential progression through the rehabilitation program and back to sport. It is the clinician's role to determine, to the best of her ability, when an athlete may safely advance from one phase of the rehabilitation program to the next. This is especially true when one is treating a complex area like the shoulder and the patient is returning to an activity as demanding as throwing. The patient's ability to successfully move through each phase of the rehabilitation program is a key factor in determining when higher-level training and return to throwing may begin. Specific criteria for the advancement and progression through a standardized four-phase rehabilitation program are an important element in formulating an efficacious rehabilitation program for any throwing athlete. The phases, goals, and progression criteria for each of the four phases in a thrower's rehabilitation program are detailed in figure 7.1. The patient is allowed to progress from one phase of the program to the next only when all of the criteria have been met; therefore, the time required for program progression will vary between individuals but will always be objectively controlled by fulfillment of the specific criteria outlined. As patients progress through the later phases of the rehabilitation program, the clinician must determine when they may safely begin a throwing progression and ultimately unrestricted athletics.

A critical need exists for a well-defined set of testing criteria focused on establishing a progressive and purposeful path to safely and effectively return athletes to competitive sport. Postoperative time frames alone are grossly insufficient to determine when a patient should begin throwing, let alone to guide return to unrestricted activity. Likewise, no single measure is sufficient to determine athletic readiness. Athletic function is not one activity or element and should not be treated as such in the determination of something as critical as return to throwing following shoulder injury or surgery. Returning the throwing patient to unrestricted athletic participation should involve a careful progression of the key functional elements necessary for athletic performance that are then tested, measured, and advanced in a sequential, criteria-driven manner.

The evaluation and testing criteria used to determine when an interval throwing program can safely begin are outlined in figure 7.2 on page 163. The criteria are divided into four categories: healing time frames, clinical examination, isokinetic testing, and functional testing. This battery of tests has been shown to be a successful set of assessment elements to use to determine activity readiness before introducing the demanding functional athletic element of throwing, to reduce the risk of reinjury, and to promote psychological confidence in the throwing athlete.

Healing Time Frames

The initial criterion that must be respected is the minimum amount of time required to allow for adequate healing of the injured, repaired, or reconstructed structures. Nonoperative healing constraints for internal impingement and anterior instability range from 8 to 12 weeks following the initiation of a formal rehabilitation program. Throwing program readiness following arthroscopic decompression and partial-thickness rotator cuff debridement is generally considered to be between 12 and 16 weeks after surgery.

PHASE 1: ACUTE PHASE

Goals
- Diminish pain and inflammation
- Normalize motion
- Delay muscular atrophy
- Reestablish dynamic stability (muscular balance)
- Control functional stress, strain

Exercises and Modalities
- Cryotherapy, iontophoresis, ultrasound, electrical stimulation
- Flexibility and stretching for posterior shoulder muscles to improve shoulder IR and horizontal adduction
- Rotator cuff strengthening (especially external rotator muscles)
- Scapular muscle strengthening (especially retractor and depressor muscles)
- Dynamic stabilization exercises (rhythmic stabilization)
- Weight-bearing exercises
- Proprioception training
- Abstinence from throwing

PHASE 2: INTERMEDIATE PHASE

Goals
- Progress strengthening exercises
- Restore muscular balance
- Enhance dynamic stability
- Control flexibility and stretches

Exercises and Modalities
- Continue stretching and flexibility (especially shoulder IR and horizontal adduction)
- Progress isotonic strengthening
  - Complete shoulder program
  - Thrower's Ten program
- Rhythmic stabilization drills
- Initiate core lumbopelvic region strengthening program
- Initiate leg lower extremity program

PHASE 3: ADVANCED STRENGTHENING PHASE

Goals
- Aggressive strengthening
- Progress neuromuscular control
- Improve strength, power, and endurance

(continued)

FIGURE 7.1 *(continued)*

Exercises and Modalities
- Flexibility and stretching
- Rhythmic stabilization drills
- Advanced Thrower's Ten program
- Initiate plyometric program
- Initiate endurance drills
- Initiate short-distance throwing program

PHASE 4: RETURN TO ACTIVITY PHASE

Goals
- Progress to throwing program
- Return to competitive throwing
- Continue strengthening and flexibility drills

Exercises
- Stretching and flexibility drills
- Thrower's Ten program
- Plyometric program
- Progress interval throwing program to competitive throwing

Interval throwing is appropriate to consider following arthroscopic debridement of type I and III SLAP lesions as quickly as 8 weeks following surgery. In contrast, interval throwing is not considered after type II SLAP repairs until 16 to 20 weeks following surgery. Arthroscopic capsulolabral repairs can be assessed with regard to beginning throwing between 16 and 18 weeks after surgery; starting an interval throwing program after capsulolabral repairs or anterior capsular shift procedures can be considered as early as 14 weeks following surgery.

Clinical Examination

The athlete must exhibit the appropriate ROM specific to a throwing athlete, and this motion must be fully available and nonpainful. Most throwers exhibit excessive ER and limited IR of their throwing shoulder compared to the nonthrowing shoulder when measured at 90° of abduction (Bigliani et al. 1997, Brown et al. 1988, Burkhart et al. 2003, Johnson 1996, Wilk & Arrigo 1992). This loss of IR in the throwing shoulder is referred to as GIRD (see chapters 3 and 5 for more detail) and has been shown to be an osseous adaptation of the humerus into greater retroversion secondary to the stresses of throwing (Chant et al. 2007, Crockett et al. 2002, Paine 1994, Pieper 1998). Pitchers exhibit greater throwing shoulder ER than position players (Bigliani et al. 1997, Brown et al. 1988, Johnson 1996, Wilk et al. 1993). Brown and colleagues (1988) showed that professional pitchers exhibited a mean of 141° ± 15° of shoulder ER measured at 90° of abduction, which was 9° more than the ER of their nonthrowing shoulder and 9° greater than the throwing shoulder ER of position players. Reagan and associates (2002) reported on the ROM of professional baseball pitchers, noting that ER averaged 136.9° ± 14.7° and IR 40.1° ± 9.6° when passively assessed at 90° of abduction. In pitchers, the passive ER is approximately 9° greater in the throwing shoulder, and for passive IR, values were 8.5° greater in the nonthrowing shoulder.

Most important is the concept that Wilk and colleagues (2002) referred to as TROM of the shoulder (see chapters 3 and 5 for

FIGURE 7.2 Criteria to Initiate an Interval Throwing Program

1. Appropriate time frame to allow surgery or injury site to heal
2. Satisfactory clinical examination
   - Full nonpainful ROM (appropriate and necessary ROM)
   - Acceptable muscular strength (especially of rotator cuff, scapular, and core muscles)
   - Special tests with acceptable results (subluxation–relocation test, SLAP tests)
   - Physician approval of initiation of throwing program
3. Satisfactory isokinetic test (if appropriate to perform)
   - PT/BW ratio for ER and IR:
     External rotation PT/BW at 180°/sec: 18% to 23%
     Internal rotation PT/BW at 180°/sec: 26% to 32%
   - External/internal rotation ratio:
     68% to 72% at 180 °/sec
   - Bilateral comparison:
     External rotation comparison: 95% or greater
     Internal rotation comparison: 110-115% or greater
   - Endurance ratios:
     10% to 15% decrease in PT for ER and IR from first three reps to last three reps
4. Satisfactory functional tests
   - Single-leg squat, 10 reps without loss of balance (squat to 45°-50°)
   - Prone ball flips for 30 seconds (satisfactory number and no pain)
   - 1-pound (0.45 kg) PlyoBall throws from 20 feet (6 m) into PlyoBack—15 baseball throws with normal mechanics and no pain
   - 2-pound (0.90 kg) PlyoBall throws against wall (10 reps) with rhythmic stabilizations at reps 5 and 10 (perform standing baseball-style throws)

PT/BW: peak torque/body weight ratio.

more detail). This combination of ER and IR when measured in 90° of shoulder abduction provides a total arc of available motion. This arc is within 7° in a side-to-side comparison, with the total rotational arc of motion being 176.3° ± 16° in both the throwing and nonthrowing shoulders (Wilk et al. 2002). Therefore it is imperative that full passive ER greater than that measured on the nonthrowing shoulder be restored and that the total arc of rotational motion available be equal (±7°) between shoulders before the start of a throwing program.

Muscular strength of the rotator cuff, scapular, and core muscles must be acceptable before the start of an interval throwing program. Because of the limited usefulness of MMT in the healthy athletic population, the use of an HHD to assess rotator cuff and scapular strength is recommended (figure 7.3).

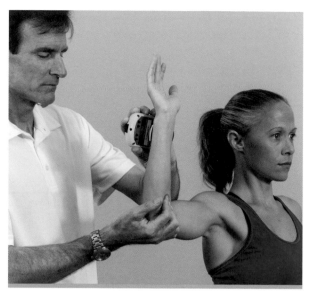

Figure 7.3 Handheld dynamometer testing of ER strength in 90° abduction.

At a minimum, testing of the shoulder should be performed in the positions of abduction, adduction (scapular plane with internal and external humeral orientation; also called **scaption**), ER, and IR at the side, as well as in 90° of abduction, and also in all four planes of scapular motion. These tests should be evaluated for bilateral comparisons and unilateral agonist-to-antagonist ratios (ER/IR ratio, abduction/adduction ratio). Although no large data sample currently exists for these assessments in the overhead athlete in the present literature, ratios similar to those presented for isokinetic testing provide clinical guidelines for appropriate values in these comparisons. Additionally, to assess core control, the front plank and unilateral side planks should be performed for 60-second bouts and assessed for control and ability to hold without substitution. Careful monitoring of scapular control is again recommended during these prolonged positional core challenges to identify significant scapular prominence on the involved (rehabilitating) side during these maneuvers. This provides valuable insight into the athlete's ability to stabilize the scapula and use the scapular stabilizing force couples to con-trol scapular motion during a weight-bearing challenge.

Special test examination should be negative with an absence of provocation or pain or apprehension. Routinely, tests are performed to eliminate any sign of subacromial impingement, SLAP provocation, anterior instability, and internal impingement (all of these tests are outlined extensively in chapter 3). The Hawkins test is used to assess subacromial impingement. The biceps load test, pronated biceps load test, and resisted ER with supination test are performed to test the integrity of the glenoid labrum because of their high sensitivity for detection of SLAP involvement in the overhead athlete (Myers et al. 2005). Finally, the subluxation–relocation test is used to test for the presence of internal impingement and for joint stability assessment.

The final element of the clinical examination is physician clearance to begin throwing. If the athlete is under the care of a physician or surgeon, approval to initiate a throwing program from that person should be obtained before the start of the throwing progression.

Isokinetic Testing

When available, isokinetic testing of the shoulder should be performed because it has been shown to be an effective tool to assist in determining readiness to initiate throwing. Wilk and colleagues (1995, 2009) have reported on the effectiveness of a standardized isokinetic assessment of the throwing shoulder, demonstrating that ER strength of the throwing shoulder in pitchers was significantly weaker by 6% and that IR was significantly stronger by 3% than compared to the nonthrowing side on a Biodex isokinetic dynamometer. Additionally, they demonstrated that adduction of the throwing shoulder was significantly stronger than that of the nonthrowing shoulder by 9% to 10% (Wilk et al. 2009).

Critical assessment parameters are outlined in figure 7.2 for peak torque to body weight ratios of both ER and IR, ER/IR muscle ratios, bilateral comparisons of ER and IR, and ER and IR endurance ratios for the throwing athlete for isokinetic test interpretation on a Biodex isokinetic dynamometer.

Functional Testing

When the injured thrower is being returned to functional performance, four functional tests must be satisfactorily completed before the start of any interval throwing program. These elements assist in determining overall balance, core and lower extremity strength, and shoulder complex readiness for the high-demand act of throwing.

- Single-leg squats for 10 repetitions to 45° to 50° are performed to assess balance, trunk control, and lower extremity strength. The individual should maintain good alignment, balance, and control bilaterally for each of 10 consecutive repetitions.

- Prone 90/90 plyometric drops are performed on the throwing side for 30 seconds (refer to figure 5.36 in chapter 5). A minimum of 25 flips should be performed pain-free without substitution in the 30-second testing bout.

- Baseball throws into the plyometric rebounder from a 20-foot (6 m) distance using a 1-pound (0.45 kg) plyometrics ball are also assessed (figure 7.4). The athlete should be able to perform 15 throws delivered pain-free with normal throwing mechanics.

- Finally, baseball-style 2-pound (0.9 kg) plyometric throws into the wall are performed and assessed for 10 repetitions, with rhythmic stabilizations performed at repetitions 5 and 10 of the test (figure 7.5). This manually assesses control of the shoulder complex, arm, and trunk when external forces are imparted during the throwing activity. The athlete should be capable of completing these throws pain-free without losing control or balance during the test.

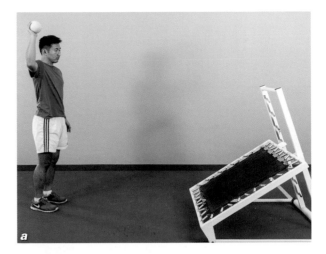

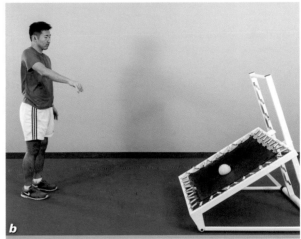

Figure 7.4 Baseball throws into a plyometric rebounder: *(a)* start position in 90/90 position and *(b)* follow-through position prior to ball return off rebounder.

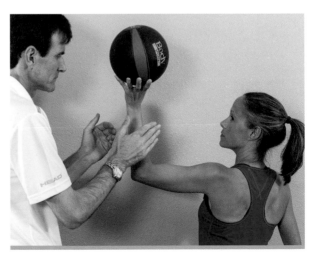

Figure 7.5 Internal rotation medicine ball plyometric wall throws with rhythmic stabilization.

INTERVAL THROWING PROGRAM

Once the athlete has progressed through an appropriate rehabilitation progression and is able to fulfill the criteria detailed here and outlined in figure 7.2, an interval throwing program can safely begin. An interval throwing program is designed to gradually increase the quantity, distance, intensity, and type of throws needed to ensure gradual restoration of normal arm strength and throwing ability. The interval throwing program is discussed in greater detail in the next chapter.

CONCLUSION

The throwing athlete presents with a unique musculoskeletal profile that includes ROM, postural, and strength changes that are functional adaptations to the process of throwing. This unique presentation leads to unique pathologies and imposes equally distinctive rehabilitation and return to throwing requirements. The use of a defined set of criteria to determine when it is appropriate to begin throwing and a regimented return to throwing program are essential to returning the throwing athlete to unrestricted symptom-free activity following shoulder injury or surgery.

Interval Return to Sport Programs

One of the most often overlooked and underemphasized aspects of the rehabilitation process following shoulder injury is the return to activity phase or interval return to sport program. Failure to integrate an interval return to sport program into the rehabilitation of an athlete following shoulder injury or surgery can result in reinjury and delay an effective return.

OBJECTIVE CRITERIA

Consistent with the information provided in chapter 7, the objective conditions or criteria for beginning an interval return to sport program are as follows:

- Pain-free tolerance of the previously presented resistive exercise progressions for the scapula, rotator cuff, and distal upper extremity musculature
- Negative clinical exam including impingement and provocational testing for instability (i.e., negative impingement and instability tests such as the subluxation–relocation test)

- Objective documentation of rotator cuff at a minimum level equal to that of the contralateral extremity with either manual assessment, HHD, or isokinetic testing
- Grip strength measured with a dynamometer equal to or greater than that of the contralateral side with no pain provocation
- Functional range of shoulder motion with a particular focus on the restoration of proper TROM and cross-arm adduction ROM

TENNIS PROGRAM

Characteristics of interval sport return programs include alternate-day performance, as well as gradual progressions of intensity and repetitions of sport activities. The interval tennis program, for example, initially uses a foam ball, progressing to a series of low-compression tennis balls (both used in teaching tennis to young children). These balls are recommended for use during the initial phase of the return to tennis program and are thought to result in a decrease in impact stress and increased tolerance to early tennis-specific activity. Additionally, performing the interval program under supervision, either during physical therapy sessions or with a knowledgeable tennis teaching professional or coach, allows for the biomechanical evaluation of technique and guards against overzealous intensity levels, which can be a common mistake in well-intentioned, motivated athletes, especially adolescents. Using the return program on alternate days, with rest between sessions, allows for recovery and decreases the risk of reinjury.

An interval tennis program has been published previously (Ellenbecker et al. 2006), and a modified version is shown in figure 8.1. It includes updated information on the use of the various tennis ball progressions and takes the player through a series advancing from groundstrokes to volleys and finally serves and overheads. It is recommended that the athlete's racket and string type and tension be evaluated by a qualified tennis teaching professional, as certain racket and string characteristics may be indicated for athletes returning from shoulder injury.

Concepts similar to those for the interval tennis program are involved in the interval throwing programs included in this chapter. As with the interval tennis program, having the athlete's throwing mechanics evaluated using video and by a qualified coach or biomechanist is a very important part of the return to activity phase of the rehabilitation process. Integrating the program with physical therapy or placing it under the auspices of a knowledgeable coach is recommended.

BASEBALL AND SOFTBALL PROGRAM

The interval sport return program for baseball and softball (throwing) is designed to gradually return motion and strength to (and confidence in) the throwing arm after injury or surgery by slowly progressing through graduated throwing distances. The program begins upon clearance by the athlete's physician to resume throwing and is performed under the supervision of the rehabilitation team (physician, physical therapist, and athletic trainer). The program is set up to minimize the chance of reinjury and emphasize prethrowing warm-up and stretching. In development of the interval throwing program (ITP), the following factors are considered most important:

- The act of throwing the baseball involves the transfer of energy from the feet through the legs, pelvis, and trunk and out the shoulder through the elbow and hand. Therefore, any return to throwing after injury must include attention to the entire body.
- The chance for reinjury is lessened by a graduated progression of interval throwing.
- Proper warm-up is essential.
- Most injuries occur as the result of fatigue.
- Proper throwing mechanics lessen the incidence of reinjury.
- Baseline requirements for throwing include these:
  - Pain-free ROM
  - Adequate muscle power
  - Adequate muscle resistance to fatigue

Because of individual variability among throwing athletes, there is no set timetable for completion of the program. Most athletes, by nature, are highly competitive individuals and wish to return to competition at the earliest possible moment. While this is a necessary quality in all athletes, the proper channeling of the athlete's energies into a strictly controlled throwing program is essential to lessen the chance of reinjury during the rehabilitation process. The athlete may tend to want to increase the intensity of the throwing program. This will increase the incidence of reinjury and may greatly retard the rehabilitation process. The recommendation

FIGURE 8.1 **Interval Return to Sport Program for Tennis**

GUIDELINES

- Begin at stage indicated by your physical therapist or doctor.
- Do not progress or continue program if joint pain is present.
- Always stretch your shoulder, elbow, and wrist before and after the interval program, and perform a whole-body dynamic warm-up before performing the interval tennis program.
- Play on alternate days, giving your body a recovery day between sessions.
- Do not use a wallboard or backboard, as this leads to exaggerated muscle contraction without rest between strokes. Ball feeds or a ball machine is preferred.
- Ice your injured arm after each session of the interval tennis program.
- It is highly recommended that you have your stroke mechanics formally evaluated by a USPTA tennis teaching professional.
- The initial phases of this program use foam or low-compression tennis balls. These are recommended before you hit with an actual tennis ball to minimize joint loading and impact forces.
- Do not attempt to impart heavy topspin or underspin to your groundstrokes until later stages in the interval program.
- Contact your physical therapist or doctor if you have questions or problems with the interval program.
- Do not continue to play if you encounter localized joint pain.

PROGRAM

Perform each stage a specified number of times based on patient history and signs and symptoms before progressing to the next stage. Do not progress to the next stage if you had pain or excessive fatigue on your previous outing—remain at the previous stage until you can perform that part of the program without fatigue or pain.

Stage 1
   a. Have a partner feed 20 forehand groundstrokes to you from the net using a foam ball. (Partner must use a slow, looping feed that results in a waist-high ball bounce for player contact.)
   b. Have a partner feed 20 backhand groundstrokes with a foam ball.
   c. Rest 5 minutes.
   d. Repeat 20 forehand and backhand feeds.

Stage 2
Repeat stage 1 with a low-compression ball (orange ball; Penn Racquet Sports, Phoenix, AZ).

Stage 3
Repeat stage 1 with a low-compression ball (green ball; Penn Racquet Sports, Phoenix, AZ).

Stage 4
Repeat stage 1 with a regulation tennis ball.

Stage 5
   a. Begin as in the previous stages, with partner feeding 10 forehands and 10 backhands from the net as a warm-up. Use an orange or green ball to warm up and continue to use the green ball for the first session or two throughout this stage to decrease ball impact stress.
   b. Rally with partner from baseline, hitting controlled groundstrokes until you have hit 50 to 60 strokes. (Alternate between forehands and backhands and allow 20 to 30 seconds rest after every two or three rallies.)

(continued)

FIGURE 8.1 *(continued)*

    c.   Rest 5 minutes.

    d.   Repeat the rally instructions for another 50 to 60 strokes.

Stage 6

    a.   Rally groundstrokes (forehands and backhands) from the baseline for 15 to 20 minutes.

    b.   Rest 5 minutes.

    c.   Hit 10 to 15 forehand and 10 to 15 backhand volleys, emphasizing a contact point in front of your body.

    d.   Rally groundstrokes for 15 to 20 additional minutes from the baseline.

    e.   Hit 10 to 15 forehand and backhand volleys.

Pre-Serve Interval (Perform Before Stage 7)
Note: *This can be performed off court and is meant solely to determine readiness for progression to stage 7 of the interval tennis program.*

    a.   *After stretching, with racket in hand, perform serving motion for 10 to 15 repetitions without a ball or any ball contact.*

    b.   *Using a foam ball, hit 10 to 15 serves without concern for the performance result (focus only on form, contact point, and the presence or absence of symptoms).*

    c.   *If this is successful and pain-free, progress to stage 7.*

Stage 7

    a.   Hit groundstrokes for 20 to 30 minutes, mixing in volleys using an 80% groundstroke/20% volley format.

    b.   Perform 5 to 10 simulated serves without a ball.

    c.   Perform 5 to 10 serves using a foam ball or low-compression ball (orange ball).

    d.   Perform 10 to 15 serves using a standard tennis ball at approximately 75% effort.

Note: It is important to hit flat or slice serves, not kick serves, in the initial phase of the interval tennis program.

    e.   Finish with 10 to 15 minutes of groundstrokes.

Stage 8

    a.   Hit 30 minutes of groundstrokes, mixing in volleys using an 80% groundstroke/20% volley format.

    b.   Perform 5 to 10 serves using a foam ball or low-compression ball (orange ball).

    c.   Perform 10 to 15 serves using a standard tennis ball at approximately 75% effort.

    d.   Rest 5 minutes.

    e.   Perform 10 to 15 additional serves as in *c.*

    f.   Finish with 15 to 20 minutes of groundstrokes.

Stage 9

    a.   Repeat stage 8, increasing the number of serves to 20 to 25 instead of 10 to 15.

    b.   Before resting between serving sessions, have a partner feed easy short lobs for you to attempt four or five controlled overheads.

Stage 10

Before attempting match play, complete stages 1 to 10 without pain or excess fatigue in the upper extremity. Continue to increase the amount of time rallying with groundstrokes and volleys, in addition to increasing the number of serves per workout, until you can perform 60 to 80 serves overall, interspersed throughout a workout. Initiate kick serves once you have completed the initial stages of the program. Remember that an average of up to 120 serves can be performed in a singles tennis match; therefore be prepared to gradually increase the number of serves in the interval program before engaging in full competitive play.

is to follow the program exactly, as this is the safest route to return to competition.

During the recovery process the athlete will probably experience soreness and a dull, diffuse aching sensation in the muscles and tendons. If the athlete experiences sharp pain, particularly in the joint, all throwing activity should be stopped until this pain ceases. If the pain continues, he should contact his physician.

Weight Training

The athlete should supplement the ITP with a high-repetition, low-weight exercise program. Strengthening should address a good balance between anterior and posterior musculature so that the shoulder will not be predisposed to injury. Special emphasis must be given to posterior rotator cuff musculature for any strengthening program. Weight training does not increase throwing velocity, but it increases the resistance of the arm to fatigue and injury. The athlete should do weight training on the same day as throwing but after the throwing has been completed; the day in between should be used for flexibility exercises and a recovery period. A weight training pattern or routine should be stressed at this point as a "maintenance program." This pattern can and should accompany the athlete into and throughout the season as a deterrent to further injury. It must be emphasized that weight training is of no benefit unless accompanied by a sound flexibility program.

Individual Variability

The ITP is designed so that each level is achieved without pain or complications before the next level is initiated. This sets up a progression in which the athlete achieves a goal before advancing, rather than advancing according to a specific time frame. Because of this design, the ITP may be used for different levels of skills and abilities compared to those characteristic of high school to professional levels. Pro-

gression will vary from person to person throughout the ITP. As an example, one athlete may wish to use alternate days throwing with or without using weights in between; another athlete may have to throw every third or fourth day due to pain or swelling. The athlete should be reminded to listen to her body, since pain signifies when it may be necessary to slow down. Again, completion of the steps of the ITP will vary from person to person. There is no set timetable with regard to days to completion.

Warm-Up

Performing one set of 10 repetitions is recommended before starting the ITP. Jogging may also assist in warm-up. Jogging increases blood flow to the muscles and joints, thus increasing their flexibility and decreasing the chance of reinjury. Since the amount of warm-up will vary from person to person, the athlete should jog until a light sweat develops, then progress to stretching.

Stretching

Since throwing involves all muscles in the body, all muscle groups should be stretched before throwing. This should be done in a systematic fashion beginning with the legs and including the trunk, back, neck, and arms. Continue with capsular stretches and L-bar ROM exercises.

Throwing Mechanics

A critical aspect of the ITP is maintenance of proper throwing mechanics throughout the advancement. Use of the crow hop method simulates the throwing act, allowing emphasis on the proper body mechanics. This throwing method should be adopted during the performance of the interval throwing program. Throwing flat-footed encourages improper body mechanics, placing increased stress on the throwing arm and therefore predisposing the arm to reinjury. The pitching coach and sport biomechanist (if available) may be valuable allies of the rehabilitation team with their knowledge of throwing mechanics.

Components of the crow hop method are first a hop and then a skip, followed by the throw. The velocity of the throw is determined by the distance, whereas the ball should have only enough momentum to travel each selected distance. Again, empha-sis should be placed on proper throwing mechanics to decrease the chance of reinjury.

Throwing

Using the crow hop method, the athlete should begin warm-up throws at a comfortable distance (approximately 30-45 feet [9.1-13.7 m]) and then progress to the distance indicated in the first column of table 8.1.

TABLE 8.1 Interval Throwing Program

45 ft (13.7 m) phase	60 ft (18.3 m) phase	90 ft (27.4 m) phase	120 ft (36.6 m) phase
Step 1: A) Warm-up throwing B) 45 ft (25 throws) C) Rest 3-5 min D) Warm-up throwing E) 45 ft (25 throws)	Step 3: A) Warm-up throwing B) 60 ft (25 throws) C) Rest 3-5 min D) Warm-up throwing E) 60 ft (25 throws)	Step 5: A) 60 ft (10 throws) B) 90 ft (20 throws) C) Rest 3-5 min D) 60 ft (10 throws) E) 90 ft (20 throws)	Step 7: A) 60 ft (5-7 throws) B) 90 ft (5-7 throws) C) 120 ft (15 throws) D) Rest 3-5 min E) 60 ft (5-7 throws) F) 90 ft (5-7 throws) G) 120 ft (15 throws)
Step 2: A) Warm-up throwing B) 45 ft (25 throws) C) Rest 3-5 min D) Warm-up throwing E) 45 ft (25 throws) F) Rest 3-5 min G) Warm-up throwing H) 45 ft (25 throws)	Step 4: A) Warm-up throwing B) 60 ft (25 throws) C) Rest 3-5 min D) Warm-up throwing E) 60 ft (25 throws) F) Rest 3-5 min G) Warm-up throwing H) 60 ft (25 throws)	Step 6: A) 60 ft (7 throws) B) 90 ft (18 throws) C) Rest 3-5 min D) 60 ft (7 throws) E) 90 ft (18 throws) F) Rest 3-5 min G) 60 ft (7 throws) H) 90 ft (18 throws)	Step 8: A) 60 ft (5 throws) B) 90 ft (10 throws) C) 120 ft (15 throws) D) Rest 3-5 min E) 60 ft (5 throws) F) 90 ft (10 throws) G) 120 ft (15 throws) H) Rest 3-5 min I) 60 ft (5 throws) J) 90 ft (10 throws) K) 120 ft (15 throws)

Flat throwing (for pitchers only)

A) Throw 60 ft (10-15 throws)
B) Throw 90 ft (10 throws)
C) Throw 120 ft (10 throws)
D) Throw 60 ft (flat ground) using pitching mechanics (20-30 throws)
E) Rest 3-5 min
F) Throw 60-90 ft (10-15 throws)
G) Throw 60 ft (flat ground) using pitching mechanics (20 throws)

The throwing program should be performed every other day, with one day of rest between steps, unless otherwise specified by the physician. Perform each step two or three times before progressing to the next step. For pitchers, progression to the throwing off the mound ITP shown in figure 8.2 follows the successful completion of the phases listed here.

Adapted with permissions of Journal of Orthopaedic & Sports Physical Therapy®, from *Journal of Orthopaedic Sports Physical Therapy*, "Interval sport programs: Guidelines for baseball, tennis, and golf," Michael M. Reinold, Kevin E. Wilk, Jamie Reed, Ken Crenshaw, and James R. Andrews, 32(6): 293-298, 2002, permission conveyed through Copyright clearance Center, Inc.

The program consists of throwing at each step two or three times without pain or symptoms before progressing to the next step. The object of each phase is for the athlete to be able to throw the ball without pain the specified number of feet (45 feet [13.7 m], 60 feet [18.3 m], 90 feet [27.4 m], 120 feet [36.6 m], 150 feet [45.7 m], and 180 feet [54.9 m]), 75 times at each distance. After the athlete can throw at the prescribed distance without pain he will be ready for throwing from flat ground 60 feet, 6 inches using normal pitching mechanics or return to his position. At this point, full strength in the arm and confidence should be restored.

It is important to stress the crow hop method and proper mechanics with each throw. Just as the advancement to this point has been gradual and progressive, the return to unrestricted throwing must follow the same principles. A pitcher should first throw only fastballs at 50%, progressing to 75% and to 100%. At this time, he may start more stressful pitches such as breaking balls. The position player should simulate a game situation, again progressing at 50%, then 75%, then 100%. Once again, athletes who have increased pain, particularly at the joint, should back off from the throwing program and re-advance as tolerated, under the direction of the rehabilitation team.

Batting

Depending on the type of injury the athlete has, the time of return to batting should be determined by the physician. Stress placed on the arm in the batting motion is very different from that in the throwing motion. Return to unrestricted use of the bat should follow the same progression guidelines as in the return to throwing training program. Begin with dry swings, progressing to hitting off the tee, then hitting to soft tossing and finally live pitching.

After the completion of the ITP in table 8.1 and after the athlete can throw to the prescribed distance without pain, she will be ready for the more position-specific ITP, which includes throwing off the mound or return to the respective position (figure 8.2). At this point, full strength in the athlete's arm and confidence should be restored.

FIGURE 8.2 Interval Throwing Program—Throwing Off the Mound

STAGE 1: FASTBALLS ONLY

Step 1
- Interval throwing (use interval throwing 120-foot [36.6 m] phase as warm-up)
- 15 throws off mound at 50% (except for steps 12, 13, 14).

Step 2
- Interval throwing
- 30 throws off mound at 50%

Step 3
- Interval throwing
- 45 throws off mound at 50%

Step 4
- Interval throwing
- 60 throws off mound at 50%

Step 5
- Interval throwing (use speed gun to aid in effort control)
- 70 throws off mound at 50%

Step 6
- 45 throws off mound at 50%
- 30 throws off mound at 75%

Step 7
- 30 throws off mound at 50%
- 45 throws off mound at 75%

Step 8
- 65 throws off mound at 75%
- 10 throws off mound at 50%

(continued)

FIGURE 8.2 *(continued)*

STAGE 2: FASTBALLS ONLY

Step 9
- 60 throws off mound at 75%
- 15 throws in batting practice

Step 10
- 50 to 60 throws off mound at 75%
- 30 throws in batting practice

Step 11
- 45 to 50 throws off mound at 75%
- 45 throws in batting practice

STAGE 3

Step 12
- 30 throws off mound at 75% (warm-up)
- 15 throws off mound at 50% (breaking balls)
- 45 to 60 throws in batting practice (fastballs only)

Step 13
- 30 throws off mound at 75% (warm-up)
- 30 breaking balls at 75%
- 30 throws in batting practice

Step 14
- 30 throws off mound at 75% (warm-up)
- 60 to 90 throws in batting practice (gradually increase breaking balls)

Step 15
- Simulated game: progressing by 15 throws per workout (pitch count)

For pitchers, successful completion of the ITP shown in table 8.1 is required before starting the program shown in this figure.

Adapted with permissions of Journal of Orthopaedic & Sports Physical Therapy®, from *Journal of Orthopaedic Sports Physical Therapy*, "Interval sport programs: Guidelines for baseball, tennis, and golf," Michael M. Reinold, Kevin E. Wilk, Jamie Reed, Ken Crenshaw, and James R. Andrews, 32(6): 293-298, 2002, permission conveyed through Copyright clearance Center, Inc.

If the athlete is a catcher, then a specific ITP is progressed to one more specific to the position. See table 8.2 for the three-step process to get the catcher back to the demands of an actual game.

Windmill softball pitchers have a specialized ITP (figure 8.3) for their rehabilitation program following the successful completion of the initial ITP (see table 8.1). It is important to have them throw from the mound every other day, three days per week, and to continue the resistance exercises, stretching, hitting drills, and other throwing drills previously mentioned.

TABLE 8.2   Interval Throwing Program for Catchers

Step 1	Warm-up throwing at 180 ft (54.9 m) phase 20 throws from squat position to pitcher 10 throws to each base at 50% intensity from squat
Step 2	Warm-up throwing at 180 ft (54.9 m) phase 40 throws from squat position to pitcher 15 throws to each base at 50% intensity from squat
Step 3	Warm-up throwing at 180 ft (54.9 m) phase 40 throws from squat position to pitcher 10 throws to each base at 75% intensity from squat
Step 4	Simulated game including fielding bunts, throws to bases, and throws to the mound

Adapted from Reinold et al. 2002.

FIGURE 8.3   Interval Throwing Program for Windmill Softball Pitchers

STEP 1

- Warm-up at 100-foot (30.5 m) phase
- 20 windmills at 50% intensity

STEP 2

- Warm-up at 100-foot phase
- 30 windmills at 50% intensity

STEP 3

- Warm-up at 100-foot phase
- 40 windmills at 50% intensity
- 15 windmills at 75% intensity

STEP 4

- Warm-up at 100-foot phase
- 20 windmills at 50% intensity
- 35 windmills at 75% intensity

STEP 5

- Warm-up at 100-foot phase
- 50 windmills at 75% intensity
- 15 windmills at 50% intensity

STEP 6

- Warm-up at 100-foot phase
- 60 windmills at 75% intensity
- 15 batting practice throws

STEP 7

- Warm-up at 100-foot phase
- 40 windmills at 75% intensity
- 10 to 15 windmills at 90% intensity
- 20 breaking balls at 50% intensity
- 30 batting practice throws

STEP 8

- Warm-up at 100-foot phase
- 30 windmills at 75% intensity
- 10 to 15 windmills at 90% to 100%
- 30 breaking balls at 75% intensity
- 30 batting practice throws

STEP 9

- Simulated game
- Gradually increase number of breaking balls and total number of pitches

STEP 10

- Competition
- Gradually return to competition
- May use pitch count if necessary

For softball pitchers, successful completion of the ITP shown in table 8.1 is required before starting the program shown in this figure.

Based on Reinold, Wilk, Reed, Crenshaw, and Andrews 2002.

FIGURE 8.4 *(continued)*

    2. No butterfly.

    3. Kicking sets without board.

    4. Use breaststroke more often.

  g. Other

    1. Return from stabilization procedure: Protect anterior capsule.

    2. Can be back in the water in 6 weeks, but with involved arm by the side and using fins or zoomers. Must have compliant patient and permission from MD.

    3. Modified freestyle allowed at 12-16 weeks.

    4. No backstroke for the first 6-8 weeks back in the water and, upon return to backstroke, use fins or zoomers.

    5. No backstroke or regular starts for at least 3 months after return to water.

GOLF PROGRAM

The interval golf program can be followed after injury or surgery for a graduated and successful return to golf.

General guidelines for an interval sport return program for golf include the following:

- Always emphasize proper golf swing mechanics.

- Allow one day of rest between sessions.

- Have the golfer perform a thorough complete body warm-up and active stretching routine before training.

- The athlete must perform the program as outlined for each day without complications before advancing to the next step.

- Although minor discomfort is expected intermittently, the athlete should avoid swinging the golf club through pain.

- If pain or swelling persists, discontinue the program until the individual has been examined by a medical professional. Resume the program at the step preceding the offending step.

The program, seen in table 8.3, requires preconditioning not only of the shoulder and scapular region but also of the entire kinetic chain, with a particular focus on core training and trunk rotation. Graduated steps are taken to all sequentially increased loading to the shoulder during this program. It is imperative that the athlete's mechanics be closely evaluated by a certified and qualified golf teaching professional to minimize the risk of injury and to improve performance.

CONCLUSION

Any athlete using an interval sport return program in conjunction with a structured rehabilitation program should be able to return to full competition status, minimizing any chance of reinjury. The program and its progression should be modified to meet the specific needs of each individual athlete. A comprehensive program consisting of a maintenance strength and flexibility program, appropriate warm-up and cool-down procedures, proper mechanics, and a progressive interval sport return program will allow the athlete to safely return to competition.

TABLE 8.3   Interval Return to Sport Program for Golf

	Day 1	Day 2	Day 3
Week 1	10 putts 10 chips Rest 15 chips	15 putts 15 chips Rest 25 chips	20 putts 20 chips Rest 20 putts 20 chips Rest 10 chips 10 short irons
Week 2	20 chips 10 short irons Rest 10 short irons	20 chips 15 short irons Rest 10 short irons 15 chips	15 short irons 10 medium irons Rest 20 short irons 15 chips
Week 3	15 short irons 10 medium irons Rest 5 long irons 15 short irons Rest 20 chips	15 short irons 10 medium irons 10 long irons Rest 10 short irons 10 medium irons 5 long irons 5 woods	15 short irons 10 medium irons 10 long irons Rest 10 short irons 10 medium irons 10 long irons 10 woods
Week 4	15 short irons 10 medium irons 10 long irons 10 drives Rest Repeat above	Play 9 holes	Play 9 holes
Week 5	Play 9 holes	Play 9 holes	Play 18 holes

Chips = pitching wedge; short irons = 9, 8; medium irons = 7, 6, 5; long irons = 4, 3, 2; woods = 3, 5; drives = driver.

Adapted with permissions of Journal of Orthopaedic & Sports Physical Therapy®, from *Journal of Orthopaedic Sports Physical Therapy,* "Interval sport programs: Guidelines for baseball, tennis, and golf," Michael M. Reinold, Kevin E. Wilk, Jamie Reed, Ken Crenshaw, and James R. Andrews, 32(6): 293-298, 2002, permission conveyed through Copyright clearance Center, Inc.

Appendix A
Thrower's Ten Exercise Program

The Thrower's Ten program is designed to exercise the major muscles necessary for throwing. The goal was to create an organized and efficient exercise program.

All the exercises included are specific to the thrower and are designed to improve strength, power, and endurance of the shoulder complex musculature.

External Rotation at 0° Abduction: Stand with involved elbow fixed at side, elbow at 90°, and involved arm across front of body. Grip tubing handle while the other end of tubing is fixed. Pull out arm, keeping elbow at side. Return tubing slowly and in a controlled manner. Perform _____ sets of _____ repetitions _____ times daily.

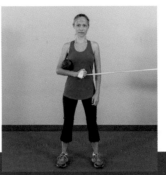 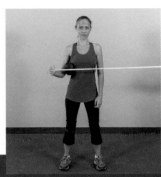

External Rotation at 90° Abduction: Stand with shoulder abducted 90°. Grip tubing handle while the other end is fixed straight ahead, slightly lower than the shoulder. Keeping shoulder abducted, rotate shoulder back, keeping elbow at 90°. Return tubing and hand to start position.
I. Slow-speed sets (slow and controlled): Perform _____ sets of _____ repetitions _____ times daily.
II. Fast-speed sets: Perform _____ sets of _____ repetitions _____ times daily.

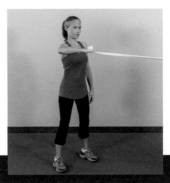 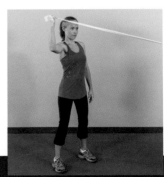

Internal Rotation at 0° Abduction: Stand with elbow at side fixed at 90° and shoulder rotated out. Grip tubing handle while other end of tubing is fixed. Pull arm across body, keeping elbow at side. Return tubing in a slow and controlled manner. Perform _____ sets of _____ repetitions _____ times daily.

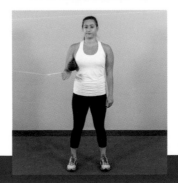 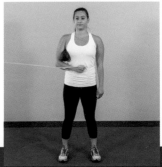

Internal Rotation at 90° Abduction: Stand with shoulder abducted to 90°, externally rotated 90°, and elbow bent to 90°. Keeping shoulder abducted, rotate shoulder forward, keeping elbow bent at 90°. Return tubing and hand to start position.

I. Slow-speed sets (slow and controlled): Perform _____ sets of _____ repetitions _____ times daily.

II. Fast-speed sets: Perform _____ sets of _____ repetitions _____ times daily.

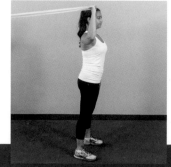
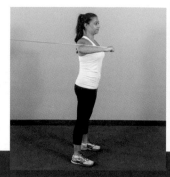

Shoulder Abduction to 90°: Stand with arm at side, elbow straight, and palm against side. Raise arm to the side, palm down, until arm reaches 90° (shoulder level). Perform _____ sets of _____ repetitions _____ times daily.

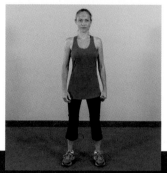
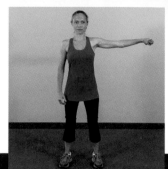

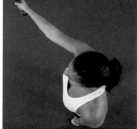

Scaption, ER "Full Can": Stand with elbow straight and thumb up. Raise arm to shoulder level at 30° angle in front of body. Do not go above shoulder height. Hold 2 seconds and lower slowly.

Perform _____ sets of _____ repetitions _____ times daily.

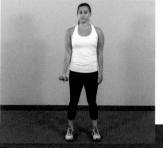
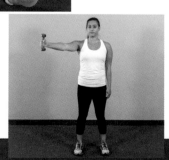

Side-Lying ER: Lie on uninvolved side, with involved arm at side of body and elbow bent to 90°. Keeping the elbow of involved arm fixed to side, raise arm. Hold 2 seconds and lower slowly. Perform _____ sets of _____ repetitions _____ times daily.

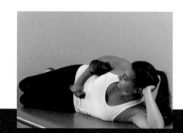
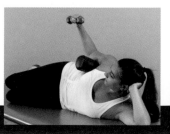

Prone Horizontal Abduction (Neutral): Lie on table, facedown, with involved arm hanging straight to the floor and palm facing down. Raise arm out to the side, parallel to the floor. Hold 2 seconds and lower slowly. Perform _____ sets of _____ repetitions _____ times daily.

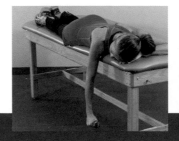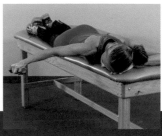

Prone Horizontal Abduction (Full ER, 100° Abduction): Lie on table facedown, with involved arm hanging straight to the floor and thumb rotated up (hitchhiker). Raise arm out to the side with arm slightly in front of shoulder, parallel to the floor. Hold 2 seconds and lower slowly. Perform _____ sets of _____ repetitions _____ times daily.

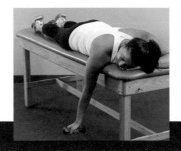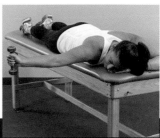

Prone Rowing: Lie on your stomach with your involved arm hanging over the side of the table, dumbbell in hand and elbow straight. Slowly raise arm, bending elbow, and bring dumbbell as high as possible. Hold at the top for 2 seconds, then slowly lower. Perform _____ sets of _____ repetitions _____ times daily.

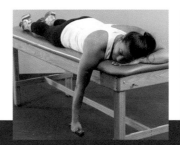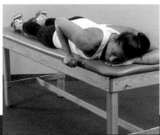

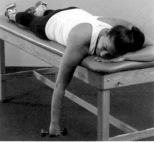

Prone Rowing Into ER: Lie on your stomach with your involved arm hanging over the side of the table, dumbbell in hand and elbow straight. Slowly raise arm, bending elbow, up to the level of the table. Pause 1 second. Then rotate shoulder upward until dumbbell is even with the table, keeping elbow at 90°. Hold at the top for 2 seconds, then slowly lower, taking 2 to 3 seconds. Perform _____ sets of _____ repetitions _____ times daily.

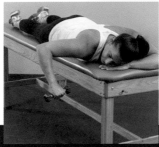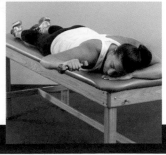

Rows at 90° Abduction, Seated on Stability Ball: Sit on stability ball with both arms straight ahead, grasping tubing. Keeping arms at shoulder height, bend elbows and pull tubing toward the body until elbows are at shoulder level and directly out to both sides (90° abduction). Hold position for 2 seconds, then slowly return to starting position. Perform _____ sets of _____ repetitions _____ times daily.

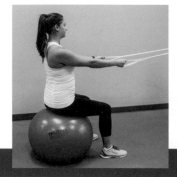

Rows Into ER at 90° Abduction, Seated on Stability Ball: Sit on stability ball with both arms straight ahead, grasping tubing. Keeping arms at shoulder height, bend elbows and pull tubing toward the body until elbows are at shoulder level and directly out to both sides (90° abduction). Hold for 1 second, then rotate shoulder upward until arm is at 90° of ER and abduction. Hold at top for 2 seconds, then return slowly to starting position. Perform _____ sets of _____ repetitions _____ times daily.

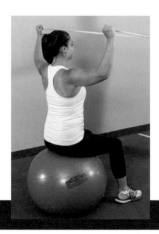

Lower Trap, Seated on Stability Ball: Sit on stability ball with both arms fixed at side and elbows bent to 90°, thumbs facing upward. Grasp tubing with both hands and rotate both shoulders outward (ER), rotating thumbs until parallel with floor. Hold for 2 seconds, then return to starting position. Perform _____ sets of _____ repetitions _____ times daily.

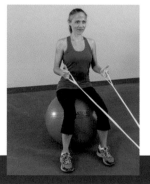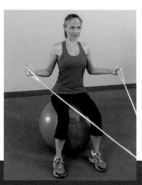

Elbow Flexion: Standing with arm against side and palm facing inward, bend elbow upward, turning palm up as you progress. Hold 2 seconds and lower slowly. Perform _____ sets of _____ repetitions _____ times daily.

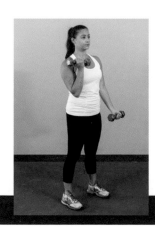

Elbow Extension, Tricep Push-Downs: Stand with arms against side, elbows bent to 90°, facing cable column machine. Grasp handles of short bar and pull down until elbows straighten. Hold at bottom for 2 seconds, then slowly return to starting position. Perform _____ sets of _____ repetitions _____ times daily.

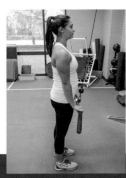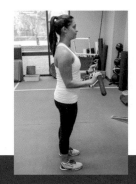

Wrist Extension: Supporting the forearm and with palm facing downward, raise weight in hand as far as possible. Hold 2 seconds and lower slowly. Perform _____ sets of _____ repetitions _____ times daily.

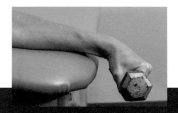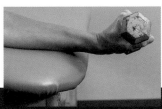

Wrist Flexion: Supporting the forearm and with palm facing upward, lower a weight in the hand as far as possible and then curl it up as high as possible. Hold for 2 seconds and lower slowly.

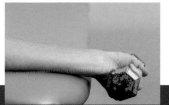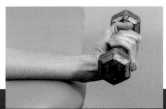

Supination: Have forearm supported on table with wrist in neutral position. Using a weight or hammer, rotate your forearm and wrist to a position such that your palm is facing upward (as pictured). Hold for a 2 count and return to starting position. Perform _____ sets of _____ repetitions _____ times daily.

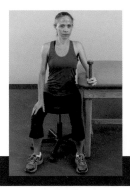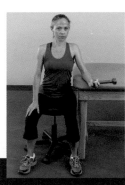

Pronation: Forearm should be supported on a table with wrist in neutral position. Using a weight or hammer, rotate your forearm and wrist to a position such that your palm is facing downward (as pictured). Hold for a 2 count and return to starting position. Perform _____ sets of _____ repetitions _____ times daily.

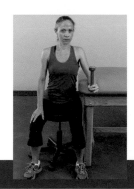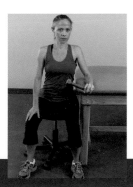

Appendix B
Advanced Thrower's Ten Exercise Program

Overhead throwing athletes typically present with a unique musculoskeletal profile. The overhead thrower exhibits extreme amounts of motion; these result in an inherently unstable glenohumeral complex, thus requiring throwers to rely heavily on their dynamic stabilizers for high-level, symptom-free activity. This unique athletic population demonstrates distinct shoulder pathology that frequently presents a challenge for the clinician. Aggressive strengthening activities that emphasize the restoration of muscle balance and symmetry are required to return the throwing athlete to competition. The Advanced Thrower's Ten Exercise Program provides the standard for comprehensive rehabilitation of the overhead athlete. It functions as a bridge facilitating the transition from rehabilitation to return to competitive throwing by using higher-level principles of dynamic stabilization, neuromuscular control, rotator cuff facilitation, and coordination in the application of throwing-specific exercises in a unique and progressive manner.

The Advanced Thrower's Ten Exercise Program combines the principles of dynamic stability, coactivation, high-level neuromuscular control, endurance, rotator cuff (RTC) facilitation, proper posture, core strength-endurance, and coordination in a specific manner designed to enable athletes to progress seamlessly into an interval throwing program and prepare them for a return to sporting participation. The exercises in this program are performed bilaterally to take advantage of neurophysiologic overflow, address the whole athlete in the training, and minimize any neurologic insult to the involved extremity or upper quarter. Performing high levels of proprioceptive and neuromuscular control exercises bilaterally serves to enhance the dynamic stability characteristics of the upper quarter and trunk as well as the lumbopelvic complex and lower extremity. The shoulder external rotator, scapular retractor and protractor, and depressor muscles are a frequent focus because of their identifiable weakness in the overhead athlete.

The Advanced Thrower's Ten Exercise Program places demands on the shoulder and emphasizes progressive challenges to the postural muscles and the endurance-fatigability of the musculature via the application of sustained holds and alternating arm movements with sustained hold techniques. Muscle fatigue has been associated with a decrease in neuromuscular control, and the Advanced Thrower's Ten Exercise Program emphasizes endurance training not only of the shoulder and scapulothoracic musculature but also of the stabilizing musculature responsible for maintaining appropriate body and leg position during throwing. The exercise volume goal of the program is designed to challenge the endurance of the athlete's shoulder and to gradually increase shoulder proprioception and neuromuscular control. The alternating movement patterns incorporated into this program challenge shoulder and scapular neuromuscular control while facilitating the RTC by using alternating dynamic and sustained hold sequences during exercise performance. Exercise activities completed in this fashion not only address strength, dynamic stability, and proprioception but also promote the type of high-level endurance required to return an athlete to a high-demand, repetitive sporting activity such as throwing.

An athlete is typically instructed to perform 10 repetitions of each sequence (movement pattern) for each exercise in the Advanced Thrower's Ten program. The sequence described for each exercise is performed twice. These exercise sets are performed without rest between sets. The pattern incorporated during performance of this program follows a sequential progression that integrates three specific movement patterns. A bilateral isotonic movement set is performed first, followed by a unilateral isotonic movement of the involved arm with a contralateral sustained hold of the uninvolved arm; then a third set alternates repetitions between a sustained isometric hold and an active isotonic movement pattern from arm to arm. Incorporating sustained holds challenges the athlete to maintain a fixed elevated arm position while the opposite extremity performs isotonic dumbbell or resistance tubing exercise movements.

In addition, a stability ball is used during the performance of the Advanced Thrower's Ten Exercise Program to further challenge the athlete's position on an unstable surface. While performing each exercise repetition, athletes are positioned in good sitting alignment on a stability ball, sitting over their ischial tuberosities, with their feet planted shoulder-width apart and their transverse abdominis engaged. Proper posture and positioning, especially of the scapula, is essential to maximal effective utilization of the exercises in this program. Maintaining a posteriorly tilted, externally rotated, and retracted scapular position is a constant focus. Frequently, athletes are cued until this positioning is maintained continually during all exercises. Manual resistance can also be employed and can be added to any of the seated stability ball exercises to increase muscle excitation, cocontraction, and dynamic stability, as well as promote endurance and challenge the fatigability of the RTC muscles.

External Rotation at 0° Abduction: Sit on stability ball with elbow at side fixed at 90° and involved arm across front of body. Grip tubing and pull out arm while keeping elbow at side. Return tubing in a slow and controlled manner. Perform _____ sets of _____ repetitions _____ times daily.

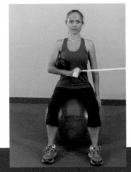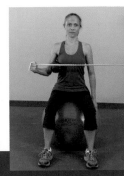

Internal Rotation at 0° Abduction: Sit on stability ball with elbow at side fixed to 90° and shoulder rotated out. Grip tubing and pull arm across body, keeping elbow at side. Return tubing in a slow and controlled fashion. Perform _____ sets of _____ repetitions _____ times daily.

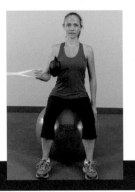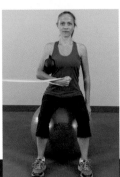

External Rotation at 0° Abduction With Sustained Hold: Sit on stability ball with elbow at side fixed at 90° and involved arm across front of body, with uninvolved arm at side, elbow straight, and palm against side. Raise uninvolved arm to the side, thumb up, until arm reaches 90° (shoulder level). Sustain uninvolved arm position while involved arm grips tubing and pulls out, keeping elbow at side. Return tubing in a slow and controlled manner. Perform _____ sets of _____ repetitions _____ times daily.

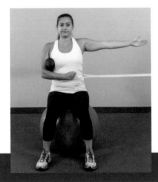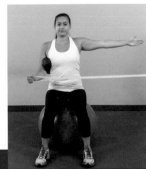

Internal Rotation at 0° Abduction With Sustained Hold: Sit on stability ball with elbow at side fixed at 90° and shoulder rotated out, with uninvolved arm at side, elbow straight, and palm against side. Raise uninvolved arm to the side, thumb up, until arm reaches 90° (shoulder level). Sustain uninvolved arm position while involved arms grips tubing and pulls arm across body, keeping elbow at side. Return tubing in a slow and controlled manner. Perform _____ sets of _____ repetitions _____ times daily.

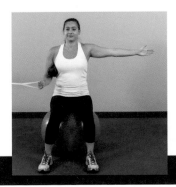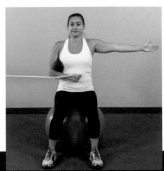

Shoulder Abduction to 90° With Sustained Hold:

First Set: Sit on ball with both arms at side, elbows straight, and palms against sides. Raise both arms to the side, thumbs up, until both arms reach 90° (shoulder level).

Second Set: Sit on ball with both arms at side, elbows straight, and palms against sides. Raise both arms to the side, thumbs up, until both arms reach 90°. Return involved arm to side and repeat motion while uninvolved arm sustains position for duration of the set. Repeat for uninvolved side with sustained hold of involved side.

Third Set: Sit on ball with both arms at side, elbows straight, and palms against sides. Raise

both arms to the side until both arms reach 90°. Alternate returning each arm to side while opposite arm sustains its position at shoulder level. Perform _____ sets of _____ repetitions _____ times daily.

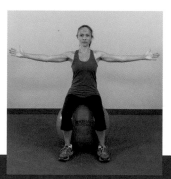 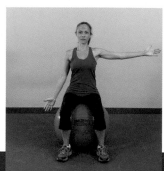

Scaption, ER "Full Can":

First Set: Seated on ball with both arms at side, elbow straight and thumb up. Raise both arms to shoulder level at 30° angle in front of body. Do not go above shoulder height. Hold for 2 seconds and lower slowly.

Second Set: Sit on ball with both arms at side, elbow straight, and thumbs up. Raise both arms to shoulder level at 30° angle in front of body. Return involved arm to side and repeat motion while uninvolved arm sustains position for duration of set. Repeat for uninvolved side with sustained hold of involved arm.

Third Set: Sit on ball with both arms at side, elbow straight, and thumbs up. Raise both arms

to shoulder level at 30° angle in front of body. Alternate returning each arm to side while opposite arm sustains its position at shoulder level. Perform _____ sets of _____ repetitions _____ times daily.

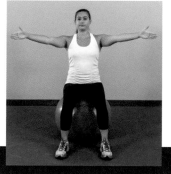 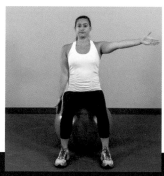

Side-Lying ER: Lie on uninvolved side, with involved arm at side of body and elbow bent to 90°. Keeping the elbow of involved arm fixed to side, raise arm with dumbbell in hand. Hold for 2 seconds and lower back to starting position. Perform _____ sets of _____ repetitions _____ times daily.

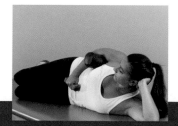 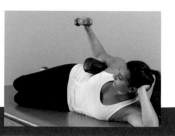

Prone Horizontal Abduction:

First Set: Lie prone on stability ball facedown, with both arms hanging straight to floor and palms facing down. Raise both arms out to the side, parallel to the floor, hold for 2 seconds, then lower slowly back to starting position.

Second Set: Lie prone on stability ball facedown, with both arms hanging straight to floor and palms facing down. Raise both arms out to the side, parallel to the floor. Return involved arm to starting position and repeat motion while uninvolved arm sustains hold parallel to floor for duration of set. Repeat for uninvolved arm.

Third Set: Lie prone on stability ball facedown, with both arms hanging straight to floor and palms facing down. Raise both arms out to the side, parallel to the floor. Alternate returning each arm to starting position while opposite arm sustains hold position. Perform _____ sets of _____ repetitions _____ times daily.

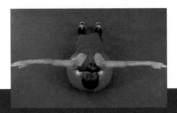

Prone Horizontal Abduction (Full ER, 100° Abduction):

First Set: Lie on stability ball facedown, with both arms hanging straight to floor and thumbs rotated up (hitchhiker). Raise arms out to side with arms slightly in front of shoulders, parallel to the floor. Hold 2 seconds at top and lower slowly.

Second Set: Lie on stability ball facedown, with both arms hanging straight to floor and thumbs rotated up (hitchhiker). Raise arms out to side with arms slightly in front of shoulders, parallel to the floor. Return involved arm to starting position and repeat motion while uninvolved arm sustains position parallel to floor. Repeat for uninvolved arm.

Third Set: Lie on stability ball facedown, with both arms hanging straight to floor and thumbs rotated up (hitchhiker). Raise arms out to side with arms slightly in front of shoulders, parallel to the floor. Alternate returning each arm to starting position while opposite arm sustains hold position. Perform _____ sets of _____ repetitions _____ times daily.

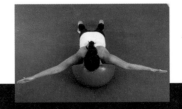
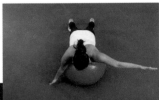

Prone Row: Lie on stability ball facedown, with both arms hanging to floor, dumbbells in hand, and elbows straight. Slowly raise each arm, bending elbows, bringing dumbbells as high as possible. Perform _____ sets of _____ repetitions _____ times daily.

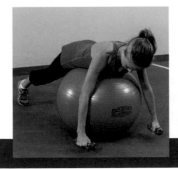
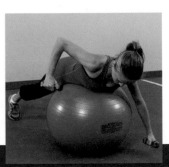

Prone Row Into ER:

First Set: Lie on stability ball, with both arms hanging to floor, dumbbells in each hand and elbows straight. Slowly raise both arms, bending elbows, up to the level of the top of the stability ball. Pause 1 second, then rotate shoulders upward until dumbbells are parallel to floor, keeping elbow at 90°. Hold at top for 2 seconds, then slowly return back to starting position.

Second Set: Lie on stability ball facedown, with both arms hanging to floor, dumbbells in each hand and elbows straight. Slowly raise both arms, bending elbows, up to the level of the top of the stability ball. Pause 1 second, then rotate shoulders upward until dumbbells are parallel to floor, keeping elbow at go. Return involved arm to starting position and repeat motion while opposite arm sustains position at the top. Repeat for uninvolved arm.

Third Set: Lie on stability ball facedown with both arms hanging to floor, dumbbells in each hand and elbows straight. Slowly raise both arms, bending elbows, up to the level of the top of the stability ball. Pause 1 second, then rotate shoulders upward until dumbbells are parallel to floor, keeping elbow at 90°. Alternate returning each arm to starting position while opposite arm sustains hold position. Perform _____ sets of _____ repetitions _____ times daily.

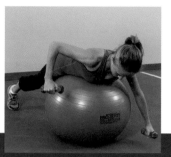 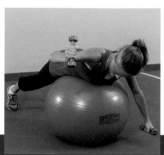

Seated Scapular Retraction Into ER:

First Set: Sit on stability ball with both arms straight ahead, grasping tubing. Keeping arms at shoulder height, bend elbows and pull tubing toward the body until elbows are at shoulder level and directly out to both sides (90° abduction). Hold for 1 second, then rotate shoulder upward until arm is at 90° of ER and abduction. Hold at top for 2 seconds, then return slowly to starting position.

Second Set: Sit on stability ball, with both arms straight ahead, grasping tubing. Keeping arms at shoulder height, bend elbows and pull tubing toward the body until elbows are at shoulder level and directly out to both sides (90° abduction). Hold for 1 second, then rotate shoulder upward until arm is at 90° of ER and abduction. Return involved arm to starting position while uninvolved arm holds position at top. Repeat for uninvolved arm.

Third Set: Sit on stability ball, with both arms straight ahead, grasping tubing. Keeping arms straight ahead, grasping tubing. Keeping arms at shoulder height, bend elbows and pull tubing toward the body until elbows are at shoulder level and directly out to both sides (90° abduction). Hold for 1 second, then rotate shoulder upward until arm is at 90° of ER and abduction. Alternate returning each arm to starting position while opposite arm sustains hold position at top. Perform _____ sets of _____ repetitions _____ times daily.

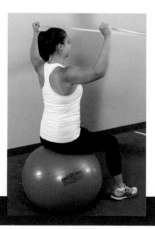

Seated Low Trap: Sit on stability ball, with both arms fixed at side and elbows bent to 90°, thumbs facing upward. Grasp tubing with both hands and rotate both shoulders outward (ER), rotating thumbs until parallel with floor. Hold for 2 seconds, then return to starting position. Perform _____ sets of _____ repetitions _____ times daily.

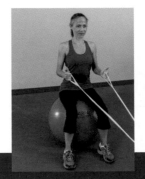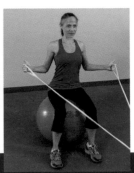

Seated Neuromuscular Control: Sit on stability ball with involved arm at side, elbow flexed to 90°. If preferred, a towel roll can be used under involved arm during this exercise. Resistance is applied to top of shoulder as shoulder is shrugged up against resistance. Resistance is then applied to bottom of towel roll as shoulder moves downward against resistance. Resistance is next applied to front of shoulder as shoulder moves forward against resistance. Apply resistance to back of shoulder as shoulder moves back against resistance and scapulas are pinched together. Perform _____ sets of _____ repetitions _____ times daily.

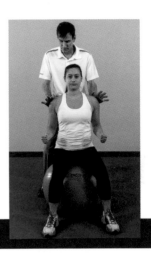

Tilt Board Push-Ups: Start in down position with arms in comfortable position, both hands no more than shoulder-width apart, on tilt board. Keeping body in a straight line, push up as high as possible, rolling shoulders forward after elbows are straight. Return slowly to starting position. Perform _____ sets of _____ repetitions _____ times daily.

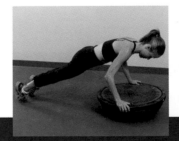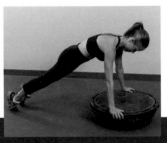

Elbow Flexion (Bicep Curl): Sitting on stability ball with both arms facing inward, bend elbow upward, turning palm up as you progress. Hold for 2 seconds at top and lower slowly. Perform _____ sets of _____ repetitions _____ times daily.

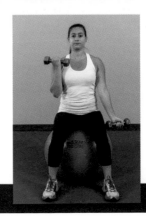

Elbow Extension (Triceps): Sitting on stability ball, raise involved arm overhead. Provide support at elbow from uninvolved hand (not pictured). Straighten arm overhead. Hold for 2 seconds and lower slowly. Repeat for uninvolved arm. Perform _____ sets of _____ repetitions _____ times daily.

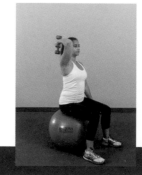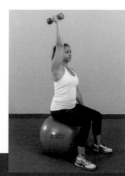

Wrist Extension: Supporting the forearm and with palm facing downward, raise weight in hand as far as possible. Hold for 2 seconds and lower slowly. Perform _____ sets of _____ repetitions _____ times daily.

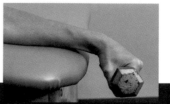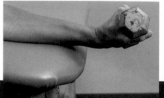

Wrist Flexion: Supporting the forearm and with palm facing upward, lower a weight in hand as far as possible and then curl it up as high as possible. Hold for 2 seconds and lower slowly. Perform _____ sets of _____ repetitions _____ times daily.

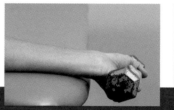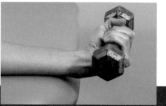

Wrist Supination: Forearm is supported on table with wrist in neutral position. Using a weight or hammer, rotate your forearm and wrist to a position such that your palm is facing upward (as pictured). Hold for 2 seconds and return to starting position. Perform _____ sets of _____ repetitions _____ times daily.

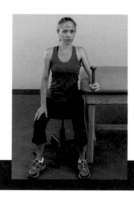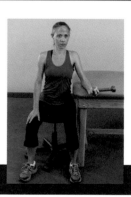

Wrist Pronation: Forearm is supported on table with wrist in neutral position. Using a weight or hammer, rotate your forearm and wrist to a position such that your palm is facing downward (as pictured). Hold for 2 seconds and return to starting position. Perform _____ sets of _____ repetitions _____ times daily.

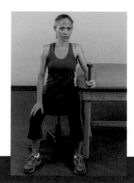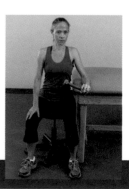

From T.S. Ellenbecker and K.E. Wilk, 2017, *Sport therapy for the shoulder: Evaluation, rehabilitation, and return to sport* (Champaign, IL: Human Kinetics). Adapted from American Sports Medicine Institute and Champion Sports Medicine.

References

Chapter 1

Abbott LC, Lucas DB. The function of the clavicle: its surgical significance. *Ann Surg.* 1954:140:583-597.

Basmajian JV, Bazant FJ. Factors preventing downward dislocation of the adducted shoulder joint. *J Bone Joint Surg Am.* 1959;41-A:1182-1186.

Bassett R, Browne A, Morrey BF, et al. Glenohumeral muscle force and moment mechanics in a position of shoulder instability. *J Biomech.* 1990;23:405-415.

Bateman JE. *The Shoulder and Neck.* Philadelphia: Saunders; 1971.

Bearn JG. Direct observations on the function of the capsule of the sternoclavicular joint in clavicular support. *J Anat.* 1967;101:159-170.

Bechtol CO. Biomechanics of the shoulder. *Clin Orthop.* 1980;46:37-41.

Bigliani LU, Morrison DS, April EW. The morphology of the acromion and its relationship to rotator cuff tears. *Orthop Trans.* 1986;10:228.

Boileau P, Baque F, Valerio L, et al. Isolated arthroscopic biceps tentomy or tendodesis improves symptoms in patients with massive irreparable rotator cuff tears. *J Bone Joint Surg Am.* 2007;89:747-757.

Bost FC, Inman VTG. The pathological changes in recurrent dislocations of the shoulder. *J Bone Joint Surg.* 1942;24:595-613.

Brewer BJ. Aging of the rotator cuff. *Am J Sports Med.* 1979;7:102-110.

Brown MK, Warren RF. Ligamentous control of shoulder stability based on selective cutting and static translation experiments. *Clin Sports Med.* 1991;10:4.

Clark JM, Harryman DT 2nd. Tendons, ligaments, and the capsule of the rotator cuff. *J Bone Joint Surg Am.* 1992;74:713-725.

Codman EA. *The Shoulder.* Boston: Thomas Todd; 1934.

Comtet JJ, Herberg G, Naasan IA. Biomechanical basis of transfers for shoulder paralysis. *Hand Clin.* 1989;5:1-14.

Conte S, Requa RF, Garrick JG. Disability days in major league baseball. *Am J Sports Med.* 2001;29(4):431-436.

Cooper DE, Arnoczky SP, O'Brien SJ, Warren RF, DiCarlo E, Allen AA. Anatomy, histology, and vascularity of the glenoid labrum: An anatomical study. *J Bone Joint Surgery.* 1992;74A:46-52.

Crockett HC, Gross LB, Wilk KE, et al. Osseous adaptation and range of motion at the glenohumeral joint in professional baseball pitchers. *Am J Sports Med.* 2002;30:20-26.

Curtis AS, Burbank KM, Tierney JJ, et al. The insertional footprint of the rotator cuff: an anatomic study. *Arthroscopy.* 2006;22:609.

Cyprien JM, Vasey HM, Burdet A, et al. Humeral retrotorsion and glenohumeral relationship in the normal shoulder and in recurrent anterior dislocation (scapulometry). *Clin Orthop.* 1983;175:8-17.

DeLuca CJ, Forrest WJ. Force analysis of individual muscles acting simultaneously on the shoulder joint during isometric abduction. *J Biomech.* 1973;6:385-393.

Dempster WT. Mechanisms of shoulder movement. *Arch Phys Med Rehabil.* 1965;46:49-70.

DePalma AF. *Surgery of the Shoulder.* 2nd ed. Philadelphia: Lippincott; 1973.

DePalma A, Callery G, Bennet G. Variational anatomy and degenerative lesions of the shoulder joint. In: Blount W, Banks S. eds. *The A.A.O.S. Instructional Course Lectures.* Vol VI. Ann Arbor, MI: J W Edwards; 1949:255.

Dugas JR, Campbell DA, Warren RF, et al. Anatomy and dimensions of rotator cuff insertions. *J Shoulder Elbow Surg.* 2002;11:498-503.

Dvir Z, Berme N. The shoulder complex in elevation of the arm: mechanism approach. *J Biomech.* 1978;11:219-225.

Fealy S, Dodeo SA, Dicarlo EF, O'Brien SJ. The developmental anatomy of the glenohumeral joint. *J Shoulder Elbow Surg.* 2000;9:217-222.

Ferrari DA. Capsular ligaments of the shoulder: anatomical and functional study of the anterior superior capsule. *Am J Sports Med.* 1990;18:20-24.

Fitzpatrick MJ, Powell SE, Tibone JE, Warren RF. The anatomy, pathology, and definitive treatment of rotator interval lesions: current concepts. *Arthroscopy.* 2003;19:70-79.

Flatow EL, Soslowsky LJ, Ticker JB, et al. Excursion of the rotator cuff under the acromion. Patterns of subacromial contact. *Am J Sports Med.* 1994;22:779-788.

Fleisig GS, Andrews JA, Dillman CJ, Escamilllia RF. Kinetics of baseball pitching with implications about injury. *Am J Sports Med.* 1995;23(2):234-239.

Frankel VH, Nordin M. *Basic Biomechanics of the Skeletal System.* Philadelphia: Lea & Febiger; 1980.

Gagey O, Bonfait H, Gillot C, et al. Anatomic basis of ligamentous control of elevation of the shoulder (reference position of the shoulder joint). *Surg Radiol Anat.* 1987;9:19-26.

Harryman DT, Sidles JA, Harris SL, Matsen FA. The role of the rotator interval capsule in passive motion and stability of the shoulder. *J Bone Joint Surg Am.* 1992;74:53-66.

Hovelius L, Olosson A, Sandstrom B, et al. Non-operative treatment of primary anterior shoulder dislocation in patients forty years of age or younger. A prospective 25 year follow-up study. *J Bone Joint Surg Am.* 2008;90(5):945-952.

Howell SM, Imobersteg AM, Seger DH, Marone PJ. Clarification of the role of the supraspinatus muscle in shoulder function. *J Bone Joint Surg Am.* 1986;68:398-404.

Huber WP, Putz RV. Periarticular fiber system of the shoulder joint. *Arthroscopy.* 1997;13:680-691.

Hunt SA, Kwon YW, Zuckerman JD. The rotator interval: anatomy, pathology, and strategies for treatment. *J Am Acad Orthop Surg.* 2007;15:4:218-227.

Hurchler C, Wulker N, Mendilia M. The effect of negative intraarticular pressure and rotator cuff force on glenohumeral translation during simulated active elevation. *Clin Biomech.* 2000;15:306-314.

Inman VT, Saunders JB, Abbott LC. Observations on the function of the shoulder joint. *J Bone Joint Surg Am.* 1944;26(1):1-30.

Johnston TB. The movements of the shoulder-joint: a plea for the use of the "plane of the scapula" as the plane of reference for movements occurring at the humeroscapular joint. *Br J Surg.* 1937;25:252-160.

Jost B, Koch PP, Gerber C. Anatomy and functional aspects of the rotator interval. *J Shoulder Elbow Surg.* 2000;9:336-341.

Kaltsas DS. Comparative study of the properties of the shoulder joint capsule with those of other joint capsules. *Clin Orthop.* 1983;173:20-26.

Kazar B, Relouszky E. Prognosis of primary dislocation of the shoulder. *Acta Orthop Scand.* 1969;40:216-219.

Kelley DL. *Kinesiological Fundamentals of Motion Description.* Englewood Cliffs, NJ: Prentice Hall; 1971.

Kelly AM, Drakos MC, Fealy S, et al. Arthroscopic release of the long head of the biceps tendon: functional outcome and clinical results. *Am J Sports Med.* 2005;33:208-213.

Kent BE. Functional anatomy of the shoulder complex. *Phys Ther.* 1971;51:947.

Kessler RM, Hertling D. *Management of Common Musculoskeletal Disorders: Physical Therapy Principles and Methods.* New York: Harper & Row; 1983.

Kovacs M, Ellenbecker TS, Kibler WB, Roetert EP, Lubbers P. Injury trends in American competitive junior tennis players. *Journal of Medicine and Science in Tennis.* 2014;18(1).

Kumar VP, Satku K, Balasubramaniam P. The role of the long head of biceps brachii in the stabilization of the head of the humerus. *Clin Orthop.* 1989;244:172-175.

Lambert AE. A rare variation in the pectoralis minor muscle. *Anat Rec.* 1925;31:193.

Laumann U. Kinesiology of the shoulder joint. In: Kolbel R, ed. *Shoulder Replacement.* Berlin: Springer-Verlag; 1987.

Lieberson F. Os acromiale—a contested anomaly. *J Bone Joint Surg.* 1937;19:683-689.

Ljungren AE. Clavicular function. *Acta Orthop Scand.* 1979;50:261-268.

Lucas DB. Biomechanics of the shoulder joint. *Arch Surg.* 1973;107:425-432.

Matsen FA, Harryman DT, Didles JA. Mechanics of glenohumeral instability. In: Hawkins RJ, ed. *Clinics in Sports Medicine: Basic Science and Clinical Application in the Athlete's Shoulder.* Philadelphia: Saunders; 1991.

Mazzocca AD, Brown FR, Carreira DS, et al. Arthroscopic shoulder stabilization in collision and contact athletes. *Am J Sports Med.* 2005;33(1):52-60.

Mileski RA, Snyder SJ. Superior labral lesions in the shoulder: patho-anatomy and surgical management. *J Am Acad Orthop Surg.* 1998;6:121-131.

Miller SL, Gladstone JN, Cleeman E, et al. Anatomy of the posterior rotator interval: implications for cuff mobilization. *Clin Orthop Relat Res.* 2003;408:152-156.

Moore KL. *Clinically Oriented Anatomy.* Baltimore: Williams & Wilkins; 1980.

Morrey BF, An KN. Biomechanics of the shoulder. In: Rockwood CA, Matsen FA, eds. *The Shoulder.* Philadelphia: Saunders; 1990:235.

Moseley HF. The clavicle: its anatomy and function. *Clin Orthop.* 1968;58:17-27.

Moseley HF, Overgaard B. The anterior capsular mechanism in recurrent anterior dislocation of the shoulder: morphological and clinical studies with special reference to the glenoid labrum and the gleno-humeral ligaments. *J Bone Joint Surg Br.* 1962;44:913-927.

Nicholson GP, Goodman DA, Flatow EL. The acromion: morphologic condition and age-related changes. A study of 420 scapulas. *J Shoulder Elbow Surg.* 1996;5:1-11.

Nobuhara K, Ikeda H. Rotator interval lesion. *Clin Orthop.* 1987;223:44-50.

Norkin C, Levangie P. *Joint Structure and Function: A Comprehensive Analysis.* Philadelphia: Davis; 1983.

O'Brien SJ, Neeves MC, Arnoczky SN, et al. The anatomy and histology of the inferior glenohumeral ligament complex of the shoulder. *Am J Sports Med.* 1990;18:449-456.

O'Brien SJ, Pagnani MJ, Fealy S, McGlynn SR, Wilson JB. The active compression test: a new and effective test for diagnosing labral tears and acromioclavicular joint abnormality. *Am J Sports Med.* 1998;26(5):610-613.

Osbahr DC, Cannon DL, Speer KP. Retroversion of the humerus in the throwing shoulder of college baseball players. *Am J Sports Med.* 2002;3:347-353.

Ovesen J, Nielsen S. Anterior and posterior shoulder instability: a cadaver study. *Acta Orthop Scand.* 1986a;57:324-327.

Ovesen J, Nielsen S. Posterior instability of the shoulder: a cadaver study. *Acta Orthop Scand.* 1986b;57:436-439.

Perry J. Normal upper extremity kinesiology. *Phys Ther.* 1973;58:265.

Perry J. Anatomy and biomechanics of the shoulder in throwing, swimming, gymnastics, and tennis. *Clin Sports Med.* 1983;2:247-270.

Petersson CJ, Redlund-Johnell I. The subacromial space in normal shoulder radiographs. *Acta Orthop Scand.* 1984;55:57-58.

Pieper HG. Humeral torsion in the throwing arm of handball players. *Am J Sports Med.* 1998;26:247-253.

Poppen NK, Walker PS. Forces at the glenohumeral joint in abduction. *Clin Orthop.* 1978;135:165-170.

Posner M, Cameron KL, Wolf JM, et al. Epidemiology of major league baseball injuries. *Am J Sports Med.* 2011;39(8):1676-1680.

Randelli M, Gambrioli PL. Glenohumeral osteometry by computed tomography in normal and unstable shoulders. *Clin Orthop.* 1986;208:151-156.

Rathbun JB, Macnab I. The microvascular pattern of the rotator cuff. *J Bone Joint Surg Br.* 1970;52:540.

Reagan KM, Meister K, Horodyski MB, et al. Humeral retroversion and its relationship to glenohumeral rotation in the shoulder of college baseball players. *Am J Sports Med.* 2002;30:354360.

Reeves B. Experiments on the tensile strength of the anterior capsular structures of the shoulder in man. *J Bone Joint Surg Br.* 1968;50:858-865.

Resch H, Golser K, Thoeni H. Arthroscopic repair of superior glenoid labral detachment (the SLAP lesion). *J Shoulder Elbow.* 1993;2:147-155.

Rothman RH, Marvel JP, Heppenstall RB. Anatomic considerations in the glenohumeral joint. *Orthop Clin North Am.* 1975;6:341-352.

Rothman RH, Parke WW. The vascular anatomy of the rotator cuff. *Clin Orthop.* 1965;41:176-186.

Rowe CR, Zarins B. Recurrent transient subluxation of the shoulder. *J Bone Joint Surg.* 1981;63A:863-872.

Saha AK. Dynamic stability of the glenohumeral joint. *Acta Orthop Scand.* 1971;42:491.

Saha AK. Mechanics of elevation of glenohumeral joint: its application in rehabilitation of flail shoulder in upper brachial plexus injuries and poliomyelitis and in replacement of the upper humerus by prosthesis. *Acta Orthop Scand.* 1973;44:668-678.

Saha AK. Mechanism of shoulder movements and a plea for the recognition of "zero position" of the glenohumeral joint. *Clin Orthop.* 1983;173:3-10.

Sarrafian SK. Gross and functional anatomy of the shoulder. *Clin Orthop.* 1983;173:11-19.

Schwartz E, Warren RF, O'Brien SJ, et al. Posterior shoulder instability. *Orthop Clin North Am.* 1987;18:409-419.

Simonet WT, Cofield RH. Prognosis in anterior shoulder dislocation. *Am J Sports Med.* 1984;12:19-24.

Steindler A. *Kinesiology of Human Body Under Normal and Pathological Conditions.* Springfield, IL: Charles C Thomas; 1955.

Turkel SJ, Panio MW, Marshall JL, Girgis FG. Stabilizing mechanisms preventing anterior dislocation of the glenohumeral joint. *J Bone Joint Surg Am.* 1981;63:1208-1217.

Vare AM, Indurak GM. Some anomalous findings in the axillary muscles. *J Anat Soc India.* 1965;14:34.

Walch G, Edwards TB, Boulahia A, et al. Arthroscopic tentomy of the long head of the biceps in the treatment of rotator cuff tears: clinical and radiographic results of 307 cases. *J Shoulder Elbow Surg.* 2005;14:238-246.

Warwick R, Williams P, eds. *Gray's Anatomy.* 35th ed. London: Longman; 1973.

Weiner DS, Macnab I. Superior migration of the humeral head: a radiological aid in the diagnosis of tears of the rotator cuff. *J Bone Joint Surg Br.* 1970;52:524-537

Wilk KE, Arrigo C. Current concepts in the rehabilitation of the athletic shoulder. *J Orthop Sports Phys Ther.* 1993;18:365-78.

Wilk KE. Rehabilitation after shoulder stabilization surgery. In: Warren RF, Craig EV, Altchek DW, eds. *The Unstable Shoulder.* Philadelphia: Lippincott-Raven; 1999:367-402.

Wulker N, Rossig S, Korell M, Thren K. Dynamic stability of the glenohumeral joint. A biomechanical study. *Sportverletz Sportschaden.* 1995;9:1-8.

Chapter 2

Alyas F, Turner M, Connell D. MRI findings in the lumbar spines of asymptomatic adolescent elite tennis players. *Br J Sports Med.* 2007;41:836-841.

Atwater AE. Biomechanics of overarm throwing movements and of throwing injuries. *Exerc Sport Sci Rev.* 1979;7:43-85.

Bagg SD, Forrest WJ. A biomechanical analysis of scapular rotation during arm abduction in the scapular plane. *Am J Phys Med Rehabil.* 1988;67(6):238-245.

Bahamonde RE. Joint power production during flat and slice tennis serves. In: Wilkerson JD, Ludwig KM, Zimmerman WJ, eds. *Proceedings of the 15th International Symposium on Biomechanics in Sports.* Denton, TX: Texas Woman's University; 1997:489-494.

Bahamonde RE, Knudson D. Ground reaction forces of two types of stances and tennis serves. *Med Sci Sports Exerc.* 2001;33:S102.

Bak K. Nontraumatic glenohumeral instability and coracoacromial impingement in swimmers. *Scand J Med Sci Sports.* 1996;6(3):132-144.

Barrentine S, Fleisig G, Whiteside J, Escamilla RF, Andrews JR. Biomechanics of windmill softball pitching with implications about injury mechanisms at the shoulder and elbow. *J Orthop Sports Phys Ther.* 1998a;28:405-415.

Barrentine SW, Matuso T, Escamillia RF, Fleisig GS, Andrews JR. Kinematic analysis of the wrist and forearm during baseball pitching. Journal of Applied Biomechanics 1998b;14:24-39.

Bigliani LU, Codd TP, Connor WP, et al. Shoulder motion and laxity in the professional baseball player. *Am J Sports Med.* 1997;25:609-613.

Blackburn TA. Shoulder injuries in baseball. In: Donatelli R, ed. *Physical Therapy of the Shoulder.*

2nd ed. New York: Churchill Livingstone; 1991:239-245.

Bradley JP. Electromyographic analysis of muscle action about the shoulder. *Clin Sports Med.* 1991;10:789-805.

Briner WW Jr, Kaemar I. Common volleyball injuries: mechanisms of injury, prevention and rehabilitation. *Sports Med.* 1997;24(1):65-71.

Brose DE, Hanson DL. Effects of overload training on velocity and accuracy of throwing. *Res Q.* 1967;38:528.

Brown LP, Niehues SL, Harrah A. Upper extremity range of motion and isokinetic strength of internal and external shoulder rotators in major league baseball players. *Am J Sports Med.* 1988;16:577-585.

Burkhart SS, Morgan CD, Kibler WB. The disabled throwing shoulder: spectrum of pathology Part I: pathoanatomy and biomechanics. *Arthroscopy.* 2003;19(4):404-420.

Cain PR. Anterior stability of the glenohumeral joint. *Am J Sports Med.* 1987;15:144-148.

Campbell KR, Hagood SS, Takagi Y, et al. Kinetic analysis of the elbow and shoulder in professional and little league pitchers. *Med Sci Sports Exerc.* 1994;26:S175.

Chow JW, Carleton LG, Lim YT. Comparing the pre- and post-impact ball and racquet kinematics of elite tennis players' first and second serves: a preliminary study. *J Sports Sci.* 2003;21(7):529-537.

Chow JW, Park S, Tillman MD. Lower trunk kinematics and muscle activity during different types of tennis serves. *Sports Med Arthosc Rehabil Ther Technol.* 2009;1(24):1-24.

Cools AM, Witvrouw EE, Mahieu NN, et al. Isokinetic scapular muscle performance in overhead athletes with and without impingement symptoms. *J Athl Train* 2005;40:104–10.

Cordo PJ, Nasher LM. Properties of postural adjustments associated with rapid arm movements. *J Neurophysiol.* 1982;47:287-308.

Cosgarea AJ, Campbell KR, Hagood SS, et al. Comparative analysis of throwing kinematics from the little league to professional baseball pitchers. *Med Sci Sports Exerc.* 1993;25:S131.

Costill DL, Maglischo EW, Richardson AB. *Swimming (Handbook of Sports Medicine and Science).* Champaign IL: Human Kinetics; 1992.

Counsilman JE. *The New Science of Swimming.* 2nd ed. Englewood Cliffs, NJ: Prentice Hall; 1994.

Davies GJ. *A Compendium of Isokinetics in Clinical Usage.* La Crosse, WI: S & S Publishers; 1992.

Davies GJ, Matheson JW, Ellenbecker TS, Manske R. The shoulder in swimming. In: Wilk KE, Reinold MM, Andrews JR, eds. *The Athlete's Shoulder.* 2nd ed. Philadelphia: Churchill Livingstone Elsevier; 2009.

Davis JT, Limpivasti O, Fluhme D, et al. The effect of pitching biomechanics on the upper extremity in youth and adolescent baseball pitchers. *Am J Sports Med.* 2009;37:1484-1491.

DeRenne C, House T. *Power Baseball.* New York: West; 1993:202.

DiGiovine NM. An electromyographic analysis of the upper extremity in pitching. *J Shoulder Elbow Surg.* 1992;1:15-25.

Dillman CJ. Proper mechanics of pitching. *Sports Med Update.* 1990;5:15-18.

Dillman CJ, Fleisig GS, Andrews JR. Biomechanics of pitching with emphasis upon shoulder kinematics. *J Orthop Sports Phys Ther.* 1993;18:402-408.

Douoguhi WA, Dolce DL, Lincoln AE. Early cocking phase mechanics and upper extremity surgery risk in starting professional baseball pitchers. *Orthop J Sports Med.* 2015;3(4):1-5.

Ellenbecker TS. A total arm strength isokinetic profile of highly skilled tennis players. *Isokinet Exerc Sci.* 1991;1:9-21.

Ellenbecker TS. Shoulder internal and external rotation strength and range of motion in highly skilled tennis players. *Isokinet Exerc Sci.* 1992;2:1-8.

Ellenbecker TS. Rehabilitation of shoulder and elbow injuries in tennis players. *Clin Sports Med.* 1995;14(1):87-110.

Ellenbecker TS. *Shoulder Rehabilitation: Non-Operative Treatment.* New York: Thieme; 2006.

Ellenbecker TS, Cools A. Rehabilitation of shoulder impingement syndrome and rotator cuff injuries: an evidenced based review. *Br J Sports Med.* 2010;44:319-327.

Ellenbecker TS, Ellenbecker GA, Roetert EP, Silva RT, Keuter G, Sperling F. Descriptive profile of hip rotation range of motion in elite tennis players and professional baseball pitchers. *Am J Sports Med.* 2007;35(8):1371-6.

Ellenbecker TS, Reinold MM, Nelson CO. Clinical concepts for treatment of the elbow in the adolescent overhead athlete. *Clin Sports Med.* 2010;29(4):705-724.

Ellenbecker TS, Roetert EP. Age specific isokinetic glenohumeral internal and external rotation strength in elite junior tennis players. *J Sci Med Sport.* 2003;6(1):63-70.

Ellenbecker TS, Roetert EP, Baillie DS, Davies GJ, Brown SW. Glenohumeral joint total rotation range of motion in elite tennis players and baseball pitchers. *Med Sci Sports Exerc.* 2002;34(12):2052-2056.

Ellenbecker TS, Roetert EP, Kibler WB, Kovacs MS. Applied biomechanics of tennis. In: Magee DJ, Manske RC, Zachazewski JE, Quillen WS, *Athletic and Sport Issues in Musculoskeletal Rehabilitation.* St. Louis: Saunders; 2010.

Elliott BC. Biomechanics of tennis. In: Renstrom P, ed. *Tennis.* Oxford, UK: Blackwell; 2002:1-28.

Elliott B, Fleisig GS, Nicholls R, Escamilla R. Technique effects on upper limb loading in the tennis serve. *J Sci Med Sport.* 2003;6(1):76-87.

Elliott BC, Marhs T, Blanksby B. A three-dimensional cinematographical analysis of the tennis serve. *Int J Sport Biomech.* 1986;2:260-270.

Elliott BC, Marshall RN, Noffal GJ. Contributions of upper limb segment rotations during the power serve in tennis. *J Appl Biomech.* 1995;11:433-442.

Elliott BC, Wood GA. The biomechanics of the foot-up and foot-back tennis service techniques. *Aust J Sports Sci.* 1983;3:3-6.

Escamilla R, Fleisig G, Barrentine S, Andrews J, Moorman C III. Kinematic and kinetic comparisons between American and Korean professional baseball pitchers. *Sports Biomech.* 2002;1(2):213-28.

Escamilla R. Electromyographic activity during upper extremity sports. In: Wilk KE, Reinold MM, Andrews JR, eds. *The Athlete's Shoulder.* 2nd ed. Philadelphia: Churchill Livingstone Elsevier; 2009.

Escamilla RF, Fleisig GS, Barrentine SW, et al. Kinematic comparisons of throwing different types of baseball pitches. *J Appl Biomech.* 1998;14:1-23.

Feltner ME, Dapena J. Three-dimensional interactions in a two-segment kinetic chain. Part I: General model. *Int J Sport Biomech.* 1989a;5:403-419.

Feltner ME, Dapena J. Three-dimensional interactions in a two-segment kinetic chain. Part II: Application to throwing arm in baseball pitching. *Int J Sport Biomech.* 1989b;5:420-450.

Feltner, M., & Dapena, J. Dynamics of the shoulder and elbow joints of the throwing arm during the baseball pitch. *Int J Sport Biomech* . 1986;2:235-259.

Flatow EL, Soslowsky LJ, Ticker JB, et al. Excursion of the rotator cuff under the acromion. Patterns of subacromial contact. *Am J Sports Med.* 1994;22(6):779-788.

Fleisig GS, Andrews JR, Cutter GR, et al. Risk of serious injury for young baseball pitchers: a 10 year prospective study. *Am J Sports Med.* 2011a;39:253-257.

Fleisig GS, Andrews JR, Dillman CJ, Escamilla RF. Kinetics of baseball pitching with implications about injury mechanisms. *Am J Sports Med.* 1995;23:233-239.

Fleisig GS, Barrentine SW, Zheng N, Escamilla RF, Andrews J. Kinematic and kinetic comparison of baseball pitching among various levels of development. *J Biomech.* 1999;32:1371-1375.

Fleisig GS, Dillman CJ, Andrews JR. Biomechanics of the shoulder during throwing. In: Andrews JR, Wilk KE, eds. *The Athlete's Shoulder.* New York: Churchill Livingstone; 1993:355.

Fleisig GS, Escamilla RF, Andrews JR, et al. Kinematic and kinetic comparison between baseball pitching and football passing. *J Appl Biomech.* 1996;12:207-224.

Fleisig GS, Escamilla RF, Andrews JR. Applied biomechanics of baseball pitching. In: Magee DJ, Manske RC, Zachazewski JE, Qiullen WS, eds. *Athletic and Sport Issues in Musculoskeletal Rehabilitation.* St. Louis: Elsevier; 2011b.

Fleisig GS, Jameson EG, Dillman CJ, et al. Biomechanics of overhead sports. In: Garrett WE, Kirkendall DT, eds. *Exercise and Sport Science.* Philadelphia: Lippincott Williams & Wilkins; 2000:563-584.

Fleisig GS, Kingsley DS, Loftice JW, et al. Kinetic comparison among fastball, curveball, change-up, and slider in collegiate baseball pitchers. *Am J Sports Med.* 2006;34:423-430.

Fleisig G, Nicholls R, Elliott B, Escamilla R. Kinematics used by world class tennis players to produce high-velocity serves. *Sports Biomech.* 2003;2(1):51-71.

Fleisig GS, Weber A, Hassell N, Andrews JR. Prevention of elbow injuries in youth baseball pitchers. *Curr Sports Med Rep.* 2009;8:250-254.

Girard O, Micallef JP, Millet GP. Lower-limb activity during the power serve in tennis: effects of performance level. *Med Sci Sports Exerc.* 2005;37(6):1021-1029.

Gowan ID, Jobe FW, Tibone JE, Perry J, Moynes DR. A comparative electromyographic analysis of the shoulder during pitching. Professional versus amateur pitchers. *Am J Sports Med.* 1987;15(6):586-90.

Groppel JL. *Tennis for Advanced Players and Those Who Would Like to Be.* Champaign, IL: Human Kinetics; 1984.

Groppel JL. *High Tech Tennis.* 2nd ed. Champaign, IL: Human Kinetics; 1992.

Harryman DT, Sidles JA, Clark JM, Mcquade KJ, Gibb TD, Matsen FA. Translation of the humeral head on the glenoid with passive glenohumeral joint motion. *J Bone Joint Surg.* 1990;72A(9):1334-1343.

Inman VT, Saunders JB, Abbott LC. Observations on the function of the shoulder joint. *J Bone Joint Surg.* 1944;26(1):1-30.

Jacobs P. The overhand baseball pitch: a kinesiological analysis and related Strength-conditioning programming. *Natl Cond Strength Assoc J.* 1987;9:5-13.

Jobe FW, Moynes DR, Anotonelli DJ. Rotator cuff function during a golf swing. *Am J Sports Med.* 1986;14(5):388-392.

Jobe FW, Moynes DR, Tibone JE, et al. An EMG analysis of the shoulder in pitching: a second report. *Am J Sports Med.* 1984;12:218-220.

Jobe FW, Tibone JE, Perry J, Moynes D. An EMG analysis of the shoulder in throwing and pitching: a preliminary report. *Am J Sports Med.* 1983;11(1):3-5.

Johnson JE, Sim FH, Scott SG. Musculoskeletal injuries in competitive swimmers. *Mayo Clin Proc.* 1987;62(4):289-304.

Kao JT, Pink M, Jobe FW. Electromyographic analysis of the scapular muscles during a golf swing. *Am J Sports Med.* 1995;23(1):19-23.

Kapandji IA. *The Physiology of the Joints. Upper Extremity.* Philadelphia: Churchill Livingstone; 1985.

Kibler WB. Role of the scapula in the overhead throwing motion. *Contemp Orthop.* 1991;22:525.

Kibler WB. Biomechanical analysis of the shoulder during tennis activities. *Clin Sports Med.* 1995;14(1):79-85.

Kibler WB. The role of the scapula in athletic shoulder function. *Am J Sports Med.* 1998; 26(2):325-337.

Kibler WB. The 4000-watt tennis player: power development for tennis. *Med Sci Tennis.* 2009;14(1):5-8.

Kibler WB, Chandler TJ. Range of motion in junior tennis players participating in an injury risk modification program. *J Sci Med Sport.* 2003;6(1):51-62.

Kibler WB, Chandler TJ, Livingston BP, Roetert EP. Shoulder range of motion in elite tennis players. *Am J Sports Med.* 1996;24(3):279-285.

Kovacs M, Ellenbecker TS. An 8-stage model for evaluating the tennis serve: implications for performance enhancement and injury prevention. *Sports Health.* 2011;3(6):504-513.

Kovacs M, Ellenbecker TS, Kibler WB, Roetert EP, Lubbers P. Injury trends in American competitive junior tennis players. *J Sci Med Tennis.* 2014;19(1):19-23.

Litwhiler D, Hamm L. Overload: effect on throwing velocity and accuracy. *Athl Train J.* 1973;53:64.

Lyman S, Fleisig GS, Andrews JR, Osinski ED. Effect of pitch type, pitch count, and pitching mechanics on risk of elbow and shoulder pain in youth baseball pitchers. *Am J Sports Med.* 2002;30:463-468.

Maffet MS, Jobe FW, Pink MM, et al. Shoulder muscle firing patterns during the windmill softball pitch. *Am J Sports Med.* 1994;25:369-374.

Mallon WJ. Golf. In: Hawkins RJ, Misamore GW, eds. *Shoulder Injuries in the Athlete.* New York: Churchill Livingstone; 1996.

Manske RC, Meschke M, Porter A, Smith B, Reiman M. A randomized controlled single-blinded comparison of stretching versus stretching and joint mobilization for posterior shoulder tightness measured by internal rotation loss. *Sports Health.* 2010;2(2):94-100.

Matsuo T, Escamilla RF, Fleisig GS, Barrentine SW, Andrews JR. Original research comparison of kinematic and temporal parameters between different pitch velocity groups. *Journal Of Applied Biomechanics.* 2001;17:1-13.

Matsuo T, Matsumoto T, Takada Y, Mochizuki Y. Influence of lateral trunk tilt on throwing arm kinetics during baseball pitching. In: Hong Y, Johns DP, eds. *Proceedings of XVIII International Symposium on Biomechanics in Sports.* Hong Kong: The Chinese University of Hong Kong; 2000a:882-886.

Matsuo T, Takada Y, Matsumoto T, Saito K. Biomechanical characteristics of sidearm and underhand baseball pitching: comparison with those of overhand and three-quarter-hand pitching. *Jpn J Biomech Sports Exerc.* 2000b;4:243-252.

McClure P, Balaicuis J, Heiland D, Broersma ME, Thorndike CK, Wood A. A randomized controlled comparison of stretching procedures for posterior shoulder tightness. *J Orthop Sports Phys Ther.* 2007;37:108-114.

McCulloch PC, Patel JK, Ramkumar PN, Noble PC, Lintner DM. Asymmetric hip rotation in professional baseball pitchers. *Orthop J Sports Med.* 2014;2(2):1-6. doi: 10.1177/2325967114521575.

McLeod WD. The pitching mechanism. In: Zarin B, Andrews JR, Carson WR, eds. *Injuries to the Throwing Arm.* Philadelphia: Saunders; 1985:22.

McMahon PJ, Jobe FW, Pink MM, Brault JR, Perry J. Comparative electromyographic analysis of shoulder muscles during planar motions: anterior glenohumeral instability versus normal. *J Shoulder Elbow Surg.* 1996;5(2 Pt 1):118-23.

McMaster WC, Troup J. A survey of interfering shoulder pain in United States competitive swimmers. *Am J Sports Med.* 1993;21(1):67-70.

Michaud T. Biomechanics of unilateral overhead throwing motion: an overview. *Chiropr Sports Med.* 1990;4:13-16.

Mihata T, Gates J, McGarry MH, Neo M, Lee TQ. Effect of posterior shoulder tightness on internal impingement in a cadaveric model of throwing. *Knee Surg Sports Traumatol Arthrosc.* 2015;23:548-554.

Mihata T, McGarry MH, Kinoshita M, Lee TQ. Excessive glenohumeral horizontal abduction as occurs during the late cocking phase of the throwing motion can be critical for internal impingement. *Am J Sports Med.* 2010;38(2):369-374.

Miyashita M, Tsundoda T, Sakurai S, Nishizona H, Mizunna T. Muscular activities in the tennis serve and overhead throwing. *Scand J Sport Sci.* 1980;2:52-58.

Monad H. Contractivity of muscle during prolonged and static and repetitive activity. *Ergonomics.* 1985;28:81-89.

Mones DR, Perry J, Antonelli DJ, Jobe FW. Electromyography and motion analysis of the upper extremity in sports. *Phys Ther.* 1986;66(12):1905-11.

Nagano A, Gerritsen KGM. Effects of neuromuscular strength training on vertical jumping performance—a computer simulation study. *J Appl Biomech.* 2001;17:113-128.

Neumann DA. *Kinesiology of the Musculoskeletal System: Foundations for Physical Rehabilitation.* St. Louis: Mosby; 2002.

Nissen CW, Westwell M, Ounpuu S, et al. A biomechanical comparison of the fastball and curveball in adolescent baseball pitchers. *Am J Sports Med.* 2009;37:1492-1498.

Penny JN, Smith C. The prevention and treatment of swimmer's shoulder. *Can J Appl Sport Sci.* 1980;5(3):195-202.

Perry J, Gousman R. Biomechanics of throwing. In: Nicholas JA, Hershman EB, eds. *The Upper Extremity in Sports Medicine.* St. Louis: Mosby; 1990:735.

Pink M, Jobe FW, Perry J. Electromyographic analysis of the shoulder during a golf swing. *Am J Sports Med.* 1990;18(2):137-140.

Pink M, Perry J, Browne A, et al. The normal shoulder during freestyle swimming: an electromyographic and cinematographic analysis of twelve muscles. *Am J Sports Med.* 1991;19(6):569-576.

Pink M, Perry J, Jobe FW. Electromyographic analysis of the trunk in golfers. *Am J Sports Med.* 1993;21(3):385-388.

Pluim BM, Staal JB, Windler GE, Jayanthi N. Tenis injuries: occurence, aetiology, and prevention. *Br J Sports Med.* 2006;40:415-423.

Reece LA, Fricker PA, Maguire KF. Injuries to elite young tennis players at the Australian Institute of Sport. *Aust J Sci Med Sports.* 1986;18:11-15.

Reeser JC, Fleisig GS, Bolt B, Ruan M. Upper limb biomechanics during the volleyball serve and spike. *Sports Health.* 2010;2(5):368-374.

Reid M, Elliott B, Alderson J. Lower-limb coordination and shoulder joint mechanics in the tennis serve. *Med Sci Sports Exerc.* 2008;40(2):308-315.

Richardson AB, Jobe FW, Collins HR. The shoulder in competitive swimming. *Am J Sports Med.* 1980;8(3):159-163.

Roetert EP, Ellenbecker TS. *Complete Conditioning for Tennis.* Champaign, IL: Human Kinetics; 2007.

Roetert EP, Ellenbecker TS, Brown SW. Shoulder internal and external rotation range of motion in nationally ranked junior tennis players: a longitudinal analysis. *J Strength Cond Res.* 2000;14(2):140-143.

Roetert EP, Groppel JL. Mastering the kinetic chain. In: Roetert EP, Groppel JL, eds. *World Class Tennis Technique.* Champaign, IL: Human Kinetics; 2001:99-113.

Roetert EP, Kovacs MS. *Tennis Anatomy.* Champaign, IL: Human Kinetics; 2011.

Rokito AS, Jobe FW, Pink MM, Brault J. Electromyographic analysis of shoulder function during the volleyball serve and spike. *J Shoulder Elbow Surg.* 1998;7(3):256-263.

Ryu KN, McCormick FW, Jobe FW, Moynes DR, Antonell DJ. An electromyographic analysis of shoulder function in tennis players. *Am J Sports Med.* 1988;16:481-485.

Saha AK. Mechanism of shoulder movements and a plea for the recognition of "zero position" of glenohumeral joint. *Clin Orthop.* 1983;173:3-10.

Scovazzo ML, Browne A, Pink M, et al. The painful shoulder during freestyle swimming. An electromyographic cinematographic analysis of twelve muscles. *Am J Sports Med.* 1991;19(6):577-582.

Segal DK. *Tenis. Sistema Biodinamico.* Buenos Aires: Tennis Club Argentino; 2002.

Sisto DJ, Jobe FW, Moynes DR, Antonelli DJ. An electromyographic analysis of the elbow in pitching. *Am J Sports Med.* 1987 May-Jun;15(3):260-3.

Stocker D, Pink M, Jobe FW. Comparison of shoulder injury in collegiate and masters' level swimmers. *Clin J Sports Med.* 1995;5(1):4-8.

Toyoshima S, et al. Contribution of the body parts to throwing performance. *Biomechanics IV.* Baltimore: University Park Press; 1974:169-174.

Tullos HS, King JW. Lesions of the pitching arm in adolescents. *JAMA.* 1972; 220:264-721.

Van Gheluwe B, Hebbelinck M. Muscle actions and ground reaction forces in tennis. *Int J Sport Biomech.* 1986;2:88-99.

Watkins RG, Dennis S, Dillin WH, Schnebel B, Schneiderman G, Jobe F, Farfan H, Perry J, Pink M. Dynamic EMG analysis of torque transfer in professional baseball pitchers. *Spine.* 1989;14(4):404-408.

Weiner DS, MacNab I. Superior migration of the humeral head. *J Bone Joint Surg Br.* 1970;52:524-527.

Werner SL, Fleisig GS, Dillman CJ, et al. Biomechanics of the elbow during baseball pitching. *J Orthop Sports Ther.* 1993;17:274-278.

Werner SL, Jones DG, Guido JA, Brunet ME. Kinematics and kinetics of elite windmill softball pitching. *Am J Sport Med.* 2006;34(4):597-603.

Wilk KE. Conditioning and training techniques. In: Hawkins RJ, Misamore GW, eds. *Shoulder Injuries in the Athlete.* New York: Churchill Livingstone; 1996:339-364.

Wilk KE. Physiology of baseball. In: Garrett WE, Kirkendall DT, eds. *Exercise and Sport Science.* Philadelphia: Lippincott Williams & Wilkins; 2000:709-731.

Wilk KE, Andrews JR, Arrigo CA, et al. *Preventive and Rehabilitative Exercises for the Shoulder and Elbow.* 5th ed. Birmingham, AL: American Sports Medicine Institute; 2007.

Wilk KE, Meister K, Andrews JR. Current concepts in the rehabilitation of the overhead throwing athlete. *Am J Sports Med.* 2002;30:136-151.

Wilk KE, Obma P, Simpson CD, et al. Shoulder injuries in the overhead athlete. *J Orthop Sports Phys Ther.* 2009a;39:38-54.

Wilk KE, Reinold MM, Macrina LC, et al. Glenohumeral internal rotation measurements differ depending on stabilization techniques. *Sports Health.* 2009b;1(2):131-136.

Wilk KE, Yenchak AJ, Arrigo CA, Andrews JR. The advanced throwers ten program: a new exercise series for enhanced dynamic shoulder control in the overhead throwing athlete. *Phys Sportsmed.* 2011;39:90-97.

Wilson FD, Andrews JR, Blackburn TA, McCluskey G. Valgus extension overload in the pitching elbow. *Am J Sports Med.* 1983 Mar-Apr;11(2):83-8.

Wuelker N, Korell M, Thren K. Dynamic glenohumeral joint stability. *J Shoulder Elbow Surg.* 1998;7:43-52.

Zattara M, Bouisset S. Posturo-kinetic organization during the early phase of voluntary upper-limb movement. *J Neurol Neurosurg Psychol.* 1988;51:956-965.

Chapter 3

Altchek DW, Dines DW. The surgical treatment of anterior instability: selective capsular repair. *Oper Tech Sports Med.* 1993;1:285-292.

Altchek DW, Warren RF, Wickiewicz TL, Ortiz G. Arthroscopic labral debridement: a three year follow-up study. *Am J Sports Med.* 1992;20(6):702-706.

Andrews JR, Gillogly S. Physical examination of the shoulder in throwing athletes. In: Zarins B, Andrews JR, Carson WG, eds. *Injuries to the Throwing Arm.* Philadelphia: Saunders; 1985.

Bankart AS. Recurrent or habitual dislocation of the shoulder joint. *Br Med J.* 1923;2:1132-1133.

Bankart AS. The pathology and treatment of recurrent dislocation of the shoulder joint. *Br Med J.* 1938;26:23-29.

Bassett RW, Browne AO, Morrey BF, An KN. Glenohumeral muscle force and moment mechanics in a position of shoulder instability. *J Biomech.* 1994;23:405-415.

Beighton P, Horan F. Orthopaedic aspects of the Ehlers-Danlos syndrome. *J Bone Joint Surg Br.* 1969;51(3):444-453.

Bennet WF. Specificity of the Speeds test: arthroscopic technique for evaluating the biceps tendon at the level of the bicipital groove. *Arthroscopy.* 1998;14(8):789-796.

Bourne DA, Choo AMT, Regan WD, Macintyre DL, Oxland TR. Three dimensional rotation of the scapula during functional movements: an in-vivo study in healthy volunteers. *J Shoulder Elbow Surg.* 2007;16(2):150-162.

Burkhart SS, Morgan CD. The peel-back mechanism: its role in producing and extending posterior type II SLAP lesions and its effect on SLAP repair rehabilitation. *Arthroscopy.* 1998;14:637-640.

Burkhart SS, Morgan CD, Kibler WB. The disabled throwing shoulder: spectrum of pathology. Part I: pathoanatomy and biomechanics. *Arthroscopy.* 2003;19:404-420.

Byram IR, Bushnell BD, Dugger K, Charron K, Harrell FE Jr, Noonan TJ. Preseason shoulder strength measurements in professional baseball pitchers: identifying players at risk for injury. *Am J Sports Med.* 2010;38(7):1375-1382.

Cameron KL, Duffey ML, DeBerardino TM, Stoneman PD, Jones CJ, Owens BD. Association of generalized joint hypermobility with a history of glenohumeral joint instability. *J Athl Train.* 2010;45(3):253-258.

Carter C, Wilkinson J. Persistent joint laxity and congenital dislocation of the hip. *J Bone Joint Surg Br.* 1964;46:40-45.

Chandler TJ, Kibler WB, Uhl TL, Wooten B, Kiser A, Stone E. Flexibility comparisons of elite junior tennis players to other athletes. *Am J Sports Med.* 1990;18:134-136.

Cheng JC, Karzel RP. Superior labrum anterior posterior lesions of the shoulder: operative techniques of management. *Oper Tech Sports Med.* 1997;5(4):249-256.

Collins DR, Hedges PB. *A Comprehensive Guide to Sports Skills Tests and Measurement.* Springfield, IL: Charles C Thomas; 1978:330-333.

Cook C, Beaty S, Kissenberth MJ, Siffri P, Pill SG, Hawkins RJ. Diagnostic accuracy of five orthopedic clinical tests for diagnosis of superior labrum anterior posterior (SLAP) lesions. *J Shoulder Elbow Surg.* 2012 Jan;21(1):13-22. doi: 10.1016/j.jse.2011.07.012.

Daniels L, Worthingham C. *Muscle Testing: Techniques of Manual Examination.* 4th ed. Philadelphia: Saunders; 1980.

Davies GJ. *A Compendium of Isokinetics in Clinical Usage and Rehabilitation Techniques.* 4th ed. Onalaska, WI: S & S; 1992.

Davies GJ, DeCarlo MS. Examination of the shoulder complex. *Current Concepts in Rehabilitation of the Shoulder.* La Crosse, WI: Sports Physical Therapy Association; 1995.

Davies GJ, Dickhoff-Hoffman S. Neuromuscular testing and rehabilitation of the shoulder complex. *J Orthop Sports Phys Ther.* 1993;18:449-458.

Ellenbecker TS. Shoulder internal and external rotation strength and range of motion of highly skilled junior tennis players. *Isokinet Exerc Sci.* 1992:2:1-8.

Ellenbecker TS. Rehabilitation of shoulder and elbow injuries in tennis players. *Clin Sports Med.* 1995;14:87.

Ellenbecker TS. Muscular strength relationship between normal grade manual muscle testing and isokinetic measurement of the shoulder internal and external rotators. *Isokinet Exerc Sci.* 1996;6:51-56.

Ellenbecker TS. *Clinical Examination of the Shoulder.* St. Louis: Elsevier Saunders; 2004a.

Ellenbecker TS. Etiology and evaluation of rotator cuff pathologic conditions and rehabilitation. In: Donatelli RA, ed. *Physical Therapy of the Shoulder.* 4th ed. Philadelphia: Churchill Livingstone; 2004b:337-358.

Ellenbecker TS, Bailie DS, Mattalino AJ, et al. Intrarater and interrater reliability of a manual technique to assess anterior humeral head translation of the glenohumeral joint. *J Shoulder Elbow Surg.* 2002;11(5):470-475.

Ellenbecker TS, Davies GJ. The application of isokinetics in testing and rehabilitation of the shoulder complex. *J Athl Train.* 2000;35(3):338-350.

Ellenbecker TS, Kibler WB, Caplinger R, Davies GJ, Riemann BL. Reliability of scapular classification in examination of professional baseball players. *Clin Orthop Rel Res.* 2012;470(6):1540-1544.

Ellenbecker TS, Kovacs M. Bilateral comparison of shoulder horizontal adduction range of motion in elite tennis players. *J Orthop Sports Phys Ther.* 2013;43(1):A51-A52.

Ellenbecker TS, Mattalino AJ. *The Elbow in Sport.* Champaign, IL: Human Kinetics; 1997.

Ellenbecker TS, Mattalino AJ. Concentric isokinetic shoulder internal and external rotation strength in professional baseball pitchers. *J Orthop Sports Phys Ther.* 1999;25:323-328.

Ellenbecker TS, Mattalino AJ, Elam EA, Caplinger RA. Medial elbow laxity in professional baseball pitchers: a bilateral comparison using stress radiography. *Am J Sports Med.* 1998;26(3):420-424.

Ellenbecker TS, Roetert EP. Age specific isokinetic glenohumeral internal and external rotation strength in elite junior tennis players. *J Sci Med Sport.* 2003;6(1):63-70.

Ellenbecker TS, Roetert EP, Bailie DS, Davies GJ, Brown SW. Glenohumeral joint total rotation range of motion in elite tennis players and baseball pitchers. *Med Sci Sports Exerc.* 2002;34(12):2052-2056.

Ellenbecker TS, Roetert EP, Piorkowski P. Shoulder internal and external rotation range of motion of elite junior tennis players: a comparison of two protocols [abstract]. *J Orthop Sports Phys Ther.* 1993;17:A65.

Elliott B, Marsh T, Blanksby B. A three dimensional cinematographic analysis of the tennis serve. *Int J Sports Biomech.* 1986;2:260-271.

Fleisig G, Nicholls R, Elliott B, Escamilla R. Kinematics used by world class tennis players to produce high-velocity serves. *Sports Biomech.* 2003;2(1):51-71.

Gerber C, Ganz R. Clinical assessment of instability of the shoulder with special reference to anterior and posterior drawer tests. *J Bone Joint Surg Br.* 1984;66(4):551-556.

Gerber C, Krushell RJ. Isolated rupture of the tendon of the subscapularis muscle. Clinical features in 16 cases. *J Bone Joint Surg Br.* 1991;73:389-394.

Gill TJ, Micheli LJ, Gebhard F, Binder C. Bankart repair for anterior instability of the shoulder. *J Bone Joint Surg Am.* 1997;79:850-857.

Goldbeck TG, Davies GJ. Test-retest reliability of the closed kinetic chain upper extremity stability test: a clinical field test. *J Sport Rehabil.* 2000;9:35-45.

Gould JA. The spine. In: Gould JA, Davies GJ, eds. *Orthopaedic and Sports Physical Therapy.* St. Louis: Mosby; 1985.

Grossman MG, Tibone JE, McGarry MH, Schneider DJ, Veneziani S, Lee TQ. A cadaveric model of the throwing shoulder: a possible etiology of superior labrum anterior-to-posterior lesions. *J Bone Joint Surg Am.* 2005;87(4):824-831.

Hamner DL, Pink MM, Jobe FW. A modification of the relocation test: arthroscopic findings associated with a positive test. *J Shoulder Elbow Surg.* 2000;9:263-267.

Harryman DT 2nd, Sidles JA, Clark JM, McQuade KJ, Gibb TD, Matsen FA 3rd. Translation of the humeral head on the glenoid with passive glenohumeral joint motion. *J Bone Joint Surg Am.* 1990;72:1334-1343.

Harryman DT, Sidles JA, Harris SL, Matsen FA. Laxity of the normal glenohumeral joint: in-vivo assessment. *J Shoulder Elbow Surg.* 1992;1:66-76.

Hawkins RJ, Kennedy JC. Impingement syndrome in athletes. *Am J Sports Med.* 1980;8:151-158.

Hawkins RJ, Mohtadi NGH. Clinical evaluation of shoulder instability. *Clin J Sports Med.* 1991;1:59-64.

Hawkins RJ, Schulte JP, Janda DH, Huckell GH. Translation of the glenohumeral joint with the patient under anesthesia. *J Shoulder Elbow Surg.* 1996;5:286-292.

Hegedus EJ, Goode A, Campbell S, et al. Physical examination tests of the shoulder: a systematic review with meta-analysis of individual tests. *Br J Sports Med.* 2008;42:80-92.

Hegedus EJ, Goode AP, Cook CE, et al. Which physical examination tests provide clinicians with the most value when examining the shoulder? Update of a systematic review with meta-analysis of individual tests. *Br J Sports Med.* 2012;46(14);964-978.

Hoppenfeld S. *Physical Examination of the Spine and Extremities.* Norwalk, CT: Prentice Hall; 1976.

Itoi E, Kido T, Sano A, Urayama M, Sato K. Which is more useful, the "full can test" or the "empty can test" in detecting the torn supraspinatus tendon? *Am J Sports Med.* 1999;27(1):65-68.

Jaeschke R, Guyatt GH, Sackett DL. Users' guides to the medical literature: III, how to use an article about a diagnostic test. B, What are the results and will they help me in caring for my patients? The Evidence Based Working Group. *JAMA.* 1994;271(9):703-707.

Jee WH, McCauley TR, Katz LD, Matheny JM, Ruwe PA, Daigneault JP. Superior labral anterior posterior (SLAP) lesions of the glenoid labrum. Reliability and accuracy of MR arthrography for diagnosis. *Radiology.* 2001;218:127-132.

Jenp YN, Malanga BA, Gowney ES, An KN. Activation of the rotator cuff in generating isometric shoulder rotation torque. *Am J Sports Med.* 1996;24:477-485.

Jobe FW, Bradley JP. The diagnosis and nonoperative treatment of shoulder injuries in athletes. *Clin Sports Med.* 1989;8:419-437.

Juul-Kristensen B, Rogind H, Jensen DV, Remvig L. Inter-examiner reproducibility of tests and criteria for generalized joint hypermobility and benign joint hypermobility syndrome. *Rheumatology (Oxford).* 2007;46(12):1835-1841.

Kawasaki T, Yamakawa J, Kaketa T, Kobayahsi H, Kaneko K. Does scapular dyskinesis affect top rugby players during a game season? *J Shoulder Elbow Surg.* 2012;21(6):709-714.

Kelley MJ, Kane TE, Leggin BG. Spinal accessory nerve palsy: associated signs and symptoms. *J Orthop Sports Phys Ther.* 2008;38(2):78-86.

Kelly BT, Kadrmas WH, Speer KP. The manual muscle examination for rotator cuff strength. An electromyographic investigation. *Am J Sports Med.* 1996;24:581-588.

Kendall FD, McCreary EK. *Muscle Testing and Function.* 3rd ed. Baltimore: Williams & Wilkins; 1983.

Kibler WB. Role of the scapula in the overhead throwing motion. *Contemp Orthop.* 1991;22:525.

Kibler WB. The role of the scapula in athletic shoulder function. *Am J Sports Med.* 1998;26:325-337.

Kibler WB. Specificity and sensitivity of the anterior slide test in throwing athletes with superior glenoid labral tears. *Arthroscopy.* 1995 Jun;11(3):296-300.

Kibler WB, Chandler J, Livingston BP, Roetert EP. Shoulder range of motion in elite tennis players: effect of age and years of tournament play. *Am J Sports Med.* 1996;24(3):279-285.

Kibler WB, Sciascia A, Dome D. Evaluation of apparent and absolute supraspinatus strength in patients with shoulder injury using the scapular retraction test. *Am J Sports Med.* 2006;34(10):1643-1647.

Kibler WB, Uhl TL, Cunningham TJ. The effect of the scapular assistance test on scapular kinematics in the clinical exam. *J Orthop Sports Phys Ther.* 2009;39(11):A12.

Kibler WB, Uhl TL, Maddux JW, Brooks PV, Zeller B, McMullen J. Qualitative clinical evaluation of scapular dysfunction: a reliability study. *J Shoulder Elbow Surg.* 2002;11:550-556.

Kim SH, Ha KI, Ahn JH et al. The biceps load test II: a clinical test for SLAP lesions of the shoulder. *Arthroscopy.* 2001;17(2):160-164.

Knops JE, Meiners TK, Davies GJ, et al. Isokinetic test retest reliability of the modified neutral shoulder test position. Unpublished master's thesis. La Crosse, WI: University of Wisconsin-La Crosse, 1998.

Koffler KM, Bader D, Eager M, et al. The effect of posterior capsular tightness on glenohumeral translation in the late-cocking phase of pitching: a cadaveric study [Abstract SS-15]. Presented at the annual meeting of the Arthroscopy Association of North America, Washington, DC, 2001.

Kuhn JE, Bey MJ, Huston LJ, Blasier RB, Soslowsky LJ. Ligamentous restraints to external rotation in the humerus in the late-cocking phase of throwing: a cadaveric biomechanical investigation. *Am J Sports Med.* 2000;28:200-205.

Kurokawa D, Sano H, Nagamoto H, Omi R, Shinozaki N, Watanuki S, Kishimoto KN, Yamamoto N, Hiraoka K, Tashiro M, Itoi E. Muscle activity pattern of the shoulder external rotators differs in adduction and abduction: an analysis using positron emission tomography. *J Shoulder Elbow Surg.* 201 4 May;23(5):658-64. doi: 10.1016/j.jse.2013.12.021.

Laudner KG, Moline MT, Meister K. The relationship between forward scapular posture and posterior shoulder tightness among baseball players. *Am J Sports Med.* 2010;38(10):2106-2112.

Leroux JL, Codine P, Thomas E, Pocholle M, Mailhe D, Flotman F. Isokinetic evaluation of rotational strength in normal shoulders and shoulders with impingement syndrome. *Clin Orthop.* 1994;304:108-115.

Liu SH, Henry MH, Nuccion S. A prospective evaluation of a new physical examination in predicting glenoid labrum tears. *Am J Sports Med.* 1996;24(6):721-725.

Magee DJ. *Orthopaedic Physical Assessment.* 3rd ed. Philadelphia: Saunders; 1997.

Magee DJ. *Orthopaedic Physical Assessment.* 5th ed. St. Louis: Saunders; 2009.

Magee DJ, Manske RC, Zachezewski JE, Quillen WS. *Athletic and Sport Issues in Musculoskeletal Rehabilitation.* St. Louis: Elsevier Saunders; 2011.

Malanga GA, Jemp YN, Growney E, An K. EMG analysis of shoulder positioning in testing and strengthening the supraspinatus. *Med Sci Sports Exerc.* 1996;28:661-664.

Manske RM, Wilk KE, Davies GJ, Ellenbecker TS, Reinold M. Glenohumeral motion deficits: friend or foe? *Int J Sports Phys Ther.* 2013;8(5):537-553.

Matsen FA III, Artnz CT. Subacromial impingement. In: Rockwood CA Jr, Matsen FA III, eds. *The Shoulder.* Philadelphia: Saunders; 1990.

Matsen FA, Harryman DT, Sidles JA. Mechanics of glenohumeral instability. *Clin Sports Med.* 1991;10:783-788.

McClure PW, Tate AR, Kareha S, Irwin D, Zlupko E. A clinical method for identifying scapular dyskinesis, part 1: reliability. *J Athl Train.* 2009;44:160-164.

McFarland EG. *Examination of the Shoulder: The Complete Guide.* New York: Theime; 2006.

McFarland EG, Torpey BM, Carl LA. Evaluation of shoulder laxity. *Sports Med.* 1996;22:264-272.

Michener LA, Doukas WC, Murphy KP, Walsworth MK. Diagnostic accuracy of history and physical examination of superior labrum anterior-posterior lesions. *J Athl Train.* 2011;46(6):343-348.

Mihata T, McGarry MH, Kinoshita M, Lee TQ. Excessive glenohumeral horizontal abduction as occurs during the late cocking phase of the throwing motion can be critical for internal impingement. *Am J Sports Med.* 2010;38(2):369-374.

Moen MH, de Vos RJ, Ellenbecker TS, Weir A. Clinical tests in shoulder examination: how to perform them. *Br J Sports Med.* 2010;44:370-375.

Morgan CD, Burkhart SS, Palmeri M, Gillespie M. Type II SLAP lesions: three subtypes and their relationships to superior instability and rotator cuff tears. *Arthroscopy.* 1998;14:553-565.

Morrey B, An KN. Articular and ligamentous contributions to the stability of the elbow joint. *Am J Sports Med.* 1983;11:315-319.

Muraki T, Yamamoto N, Zhao KD, et al. Effect of posterior inferior capsule tightness on contact pressure and area beneath the coracoacromial arch during the pitching motion. *Am J Sports Med.* 2010;38(3):600-607.

Myers JP, Laudner KG, Pasquale MR, Bradley JP, Lephart SM. Glenohumeral range of motion deficits and posterior shoulder tightness in throwers with pathologic internal impingement. *Am J Sports Med.* 2006;34(3):385-391.

Myers TH, Zemanovic JR, Andrews JR. The resisted supination external rotation test: a new test for the diagnosis of superior labral anterior posterior lesions. *Am J Sports Med.* 2005;33(9):1315-1320.

Neer CS, Welsh RP. The shoulder in sports. *Orthop Clin North Am.* 1977;8:583-591.

Nirschl RP, Ashman ES. Tennis elbow tendinosis (epicondylitis). *Instr Course Lect.* 2004;53:587-598.

O'Brien SJ, Neves MC, Arnvoczky SP, et al. The anatomy and histology of the inferior glenohumeral ligament complex of the shoulder. *Am J Sports Med.* 1990;18:449-456.

O'Brien SJ, Pagnani MJ, Fealy S, McGlynn SR, Wilson JB. The active compression test: a new and effective test for diagnosing labral tears and acromioclavicular joint abnormality. *Am J Sports Med.* 1998;26(5):610-613.

Pagnani MJ, Warren RF. Stabilizers of the glenohumeral joint. *J Shoulder Elbow Surg.* 1994;3:73-90.

Pandya NK, Colton A, Webner D, Sennett B, Huffman GR. Physical examination and magnetic resonance imaging in the diagnosis of superior labrum anterior-posterior lesions of the shoulder: a sensitivity analysis. *Arthroscopy.* 2008;24(3):311-317.

Patte D, Goutallier D, Monpierre H, Debeyre J. Over-extension lesions. *Rev Chir Orthop.* 1988;74:314-318.

Pennock AT, Pennington WW, Torry MR, et al. The influence of arm and shoulder position on the bear-hug, belly-press, and lift-off tests: an electromyographic study. *Am J Sports Med.* 2011;39:2338-2346.

Perthes G. Ueber operationen der habituellen schulterluxation. *Deutsche Ztschr Chir.* 1906;85:199.

Piatt BE, Hawkins RJ, Fritz RC, Ho CP, Wolf E, Schickendantz M. Clinical evaluation and treatment of spinoglenoid notch ganglion cysts. *J Shoulder Elbow Surg.* 2002;11:600-604.

Portney LG, Watkins MP. *Foundations of Clinical Research: Applications to Practice.* Stamford, CT: Appleton and Lange; 1993.

Priest JD, Nagel DA. Tennis shoulder. *Am J Sports Med.* 1976;4(1):28-42.

Rabin A, Irrgang JJ, Fitzgerald GK, Eubanks A. The intertester reliability of the Scapular Assistance Test. *J Orthop Sports Phys Ther.* 2006;36(9):653-660.

Rankin SA, Roe JR. Test-retest reliability analysis of Davies clinically oriented functional throwing performance index (FTPI) over extended time intervals. Unpublished master's thesis. Lexington, KY: University of Kentucky; 1996.

Reiman MP, Manske RC. *Functional Testing in Human Performance.* Champaign, IL: Human Kinetics; 2009.

Reuss BL, Schwartzberg R, Ziatkin MB, Cooperman A, Dixon JR. Magnetic imaging accuracy for the diagnosis of superior labrum anterior-posterior lesions in the community setting. Eighty-three arthroscopically confirmed cases. *J Shoulder Elbow Surg.* 2006;15:580-585.

Riemann BL, Davies GJ, Ludwig L, Gardenhour H. Hand-held dynamometer testing of the internal and external rotator musculature based on selected positions to establish normative data and unilateral ratios. *J Shoulder Elbow Surg.* 2010;19(8):1175-1183.

Roetert EP, Ellenbecker TS, Brown SW. Shoulder internal and external rotation range of motion in nationally ranked junior tennis players: a longitudinal analysis. *J Strength Cond Res.* 2000;14(2):140-143.

Safran M. Nerve injury about the shoulder in athletes. Part 1: suprascapular nerve and axillary nerve. *Am J Sports Med.* 2004;32(3):803-819.

Saha AK. Mechanism of shoulder movements and a plea for the recognition of "zero position" of the glenohumeral joint. *Clin Orthop.* 1983;173:3-10.

Seitz AL, McClure PW, Lynch SS, Ketchum JM, Michener LA. Effects of scapular dyskinesis and scapular assistance test on subacromial space during static arm elevation. *J Shoulder Elbow Surg.* 2012;21(5):631-640.

Shanley E, Rauh MJ, Michener LA, Ellenbecker TS, Garrison JC, Thigpen CA. Shoulder range of motion measures as risk factors for shoulder and elbow injuries in high school softball and baseball players. *Am J Sports Med.* 2011;39:1997-2006.

Snyder SJ, Karzel RP, Del Pizzo W, Ferkel RD, Friedman MJ. SLAP lesions of the shoulder. *Arthroscopy.* 1990;6:274-279.

Speer KP, Hannafin KP, Altchek DW, Warren RF. An evaluation of the shoulder relocation test. *Am J Sports Med.* 1994;22(2):177-183.

Stefko JM, Jobe FW, VanderWilde RS, Carden E, Pink M. Electromyographic and nerve block analysis of the subscapularis liftoff test. *J Shoulder Elbow Surg.* 1997;6:347-355.

Stetson WB, Templin K. The crank test, the O'Brien test, and routine magnetic resonance imaging scans in the diagnosis of labral tears. *Am J Sports Med.* 2002;30(6):806-809.

Tate AR, McClure P, Kareha S, Irwin D, Barbe MF. A clinical method for identifying scapular dyskinesis, part 2. Validity. *J Athl Train.* 2009;44:165-173.

T'Jonck L, Lysens R, Gunther G. Measurement of scapular position and rotation: a reliability study. *Physiother Res Int.* 1996;1(3):148-158.

Tong HC, Haig AJ, Yamakawa K. The Spurling test and cervical radiculopathy. *Spine.* 2002;27(2):156-159.

Tyler TF, Nicholas SJ, Lee SJ, Mullaney M, McHugh MP. Correction of posterior shoulder tightness is associated with symptom resolution in patients with internal impingement. *Am J Sports Med.* 2010;38(1):114-119.

Uhl TL, Cunningham TJ, Kibler WB. Kinematic and neuromuscular actions during the scapular retraction test (SRT). *J Orthop Sports Phys Ther.* 2009a;39(11):A12.

Uhl TL, Kibler WB, Grecewich B, Tripp BL. Evaluation of clinical assessment methods for scapular dyskinesis. *Arthroscopy.* 2009b;11:1240-1248.

Valadie AL 3rd, Jobe CM, Pink MM, Ekman EF, Jobe FW. Anatomy of provocative tests for impingement syndrome of the shoulder. *J Shoulder Elbow Surg.* 2000;9(1):36-46.

Walch F, Boulahia A, Calderone S, Robinson AH. The "dropping" and "hornblower's" signs in evaluation of rotator cuff tears. *J Bone Joint Surg Br.* 1998;80(4):624-628.

Warner JJP, Micheli LJ, Arslanian LE, Kennedy J, Kennedy R. Patterns of flexibility, laxity, and strength in normal shoulders and shoulders with instability and impingement. *Am J Sports Med.* 1990;18:366.

Wilk KE, Andrews JR, Arrigo CA, Keirns MA, Erber DJ. The strength characteristics of internal and external rotator muscles in professional baseball pitchers. *Am J Sports Med.* 1993;21:61-66.

Wilk KE, Macrina LC, Arrigo C. Passive range of motion characteristics in the overhead baseball pitcher and their implications for rehabilitation. *Clin Orthop Rel Res.* 2012;470(6):1586-1594.

Wilk KE, Macrina LC, Fleisig GS, et al. Correlation of glenohumeral internal rotation deficit and total rotational motion to shoulder injuries in professional baseball pitchers. *Am J Sports Med.* 2011;39:329-335.

Wilk KE, Reinold MM, Macrina LC, et al. Glenohumeral internal rotation measurements differ depending on stabilization techniques. *Sports Health.* 2009;1(2):131-136.

Yocum LA. Assessing the shoulder. *Clin Sports Med.* 1983;2:281-289.

Chapter 4

Andrews JR, Alexander EJ. Rotator cuff injury in throwing and racquet sports. *Sports Med Arthrosc.* 1995;3:30-38.

Andrews JR, Carson WG, McLeod WD. The arthroscopic treatment of glenoid labrum tears in the throwing athlete. *Am J Sports Med.* 1985;13:337-341.

Bankart AS. Recurrent or habitual dislocation of the shoulder joint. *Br Med J.* 1923;2:1132-1133.

Bankart AS. The pathology and treatment of recurrent dislocation of the shoulder joint. *Br Med J.* 1938;26:23-29.

Beaton D, Richards RR. Assessing the reliability and responsiveness of 5 shoulder questionnaires. *J Shoulder Elbow Surg.* 1998;7:565-572.

Bigliani LU, Ticker JB, Flatow EL, Soslowsky LJ, Mow VC. The relationship of acromial architecture to rotator cuff disease. *Clin Sports Med.* 1991;10:823-828.

Borsa PA, Sauers EL, Herling DE. In vivo assessment of AP laxity in healthy shoulders using an instrumented arthrometer. *J Sports Rehabil.* 1999;8:157-170.

Burkhart SS, Morgan CD. The peel-back mechanism: its role in producing and extending posterior type II SLAP lesions and its effect on SLAP repair rehabilitation. *Arthroscopy.* 1998;14:637-640.

Cave EF, Burke JF, Boyd RJ. *Trauma Management.* Chicago: Year Book Medical; 1974:437.

Cofield R. Rotator cuff disease of the shoulder. *J Bone Joint Surg Am.* 1985;67:974-979.

Cotton RE, Rideout DF. Tears of the humeral rotator cuff: a radiological and pathological necropsy survey. *J Bone Joint Surg Br.* 1964;46:314-328.

Field LD, Savoie FH. Arthroscopic suture repairs of superior labral lesions of the shoulder. *Am J Sports Med.* 1993;21:783-790.

Fleisig GS, Andrews JR, Dillman CJ, Escamilla RF. Kinetics of baseball pitching with implications about injury mechanisms. *Am J Sports Med.* 1995;23:233-239.

Gartsman GH, Hammerman SM. Superior labrum, anterior and posterior lesions. When and how to treat them. *Clin Sports Med.* 2000;19:115-124.

Gill TJ, Micheli LJ, Gebhard F, Binder C. Bankart repair for anterior instability of the shoulder. *J Bone Joint Surg Am.* 1997;79:850-857.

Glousman RE, Jobe FW, Tibonne JE, Moynes D, Antonelli D, Perry J. Dynamic electromyographic analysis of the throwing shoulder with glenohumeral instability. *J Bone Joint Surg.* 1988;70:220-226.

Golding FC. The shoulder: the forgotten joint. *Br J Radiol.* 1962;35:149.

Halbrecht JL, Tirman P, Atkin D. Internal impingement of the shoulder: comparison of findings between the throwing and nonthrowing shoulders of college baseball players. *Arthroscopy.* 1999;15(3):253-258.

Handelberg F, Willems S, Shahabpour M, Huskin JP, Kute J. SLAP lesions: a retrospective study. *Arthroscopy.* 1998;14:856-862.

Hawkins RJ, Mohtadi NGH. Clinical evaluation of shoulder instability. *Clin J Sports Med.* 1991;1:59-64.

Hawkins RJ, Neer CS, Pianta R, Mendoza FX. Locked posterior dislocation of the shoulder. *J Bone Joint Surg.* 1987;69(A):9-18.

Jobe CM. Posterior superior glenoid impingement: expanded spectrum. *Arthroscopy.* 1995;11:530-536.

Jobe FW, Bradley JP. The diagnosis and nonoperative treatment of shoulder injuries in athletes. *Clin Sports Med.* 1989;8:419-437.

Jobe FW, Kivitne RS, Giangarra CE. Shoulder pain in the overhand or throwing athlete: the relationship of anterior instability and rotator cuff impingement. *Orthop Rev.* 1989;28:963-975.

Jobe FW, Pink M. The athlete's shoulder. *J Hand Ther.* 1994;7:107-110.

Kazar B, Relovszky E. Prognosis of primary dislocation of the shoulder. *Acta Orthop Scand.* 1969;40:216.

Kim S-H, Ha K-I, Ahn J-H, Kim S-H, Choi H-J. Biceps load test II: a clinical test for SLAP lesions of the shoulder. *Arthroscopy.* 2001;17:160-164.

Kim TK, Queale WS, Cosgarea AJ, McFarland EG. Clinical features of the different types of SLAP lesions: an analysis of one hundred and thirty-nine cases. *J Bone Joint Surg.* 2003;85A:66-71.

Kraeutler MJ, Ciccotti MG, Dodson CC, Frederick RW, Cammarota B, Cohen SB. Kerlan-Jobe Orthopaedic Clinic overhead athlete scores in asymptomatic professional baseball pitchers. *J Shoulder Elbow Surg.* 2013;22:329-332.

Kraushaar BS, Nirschl RP. Tendinosis of the elbow (tennis elbow). Clinical features and findings of histological, immunohistochemical, and electron microscopy studies. *J Bone Joint Surg Am.* 1990;81(2):259-278.

Kuhn JE, Lindholm SR, Huston LJ, Soslowsky LJ, Blasier RB. Failure of the biceps superior labral complex: a cadaveric biomechanical investigation comparing the late cocking and early deceleration positions of throwing. *Arthroscopy.* 2003;19:373-379.

Kuhn JE, Dunn WR, Sanders R, et al. Effectiveness of physical therapy in treating atraumatic full-thickness rotator cuff tears: a multi-center prospective cohort study. *J Shoulder Elbow Surg.* 2013;22:1371-1379.

Maffet MW, Gartsman GM, Moseley B. Superior labrum-biceps tendon complex lesions of the shoulder. *Am J Sports Med.* 1995;23:93-98.

Matsen FA, Fu FH, Hawkins RJ. *The Shoulder: A Balance of Mobility and Stability.* Park Ridge, IL: American Academy of Orthopaedic Surgeons; 1992.

Matsen FA, Harryman DT, Sidles JA. Mechanics of glenohumeral instability. *Clin Sports Med.* 1991;10:783.

Matsen FA, Lippittt SB, Sidles JA, Harryman DT. *Practical Evaluation and Management of the Shoulder.* Philadelphia: Saunders; 1994.

Matsen FA, Thomas SC, Rockwood CA, Wirth MA. Glenohumeral instability. In: Rockwood CA, Matsen FA, eds. *The Shoulder.* Philadelphia: Saunders; 1998.

McFarland EG, Torpey BM, Carl LA. Evaluation of shoulder laxity. *Sports Med.* 1996;22:264-272.

Mihata T, McGarry MH, Kinoshita M, Lee TQ. Excessive glenohumeral horizontal abduction as occurs during the late cocking phase of the throwing motion can be critical for internal impingement. *Am J Sports Med.* 2010;38(2):369-374.

Morgan CD, Burkhart SS, Palmeri M, Gillespie M. Type II SLAP lesions: three subtypes and their relationships to superior instability and rotator cuff tears. *Arthroscopy.* 1998;14:553-565.

Moseley HF, Overgaard B. The anterior capsular mechanism in recurrent anterior dislocation of the shoulder: morphological and clinical studies with special reference to the glenoid labrum and gleno-humeral ligaments. *J Bone Joint Surg.* 1962;443(4):913-927.

Neer CS. Anterior acromioplasty for the chronic impingement syndrome in the shoulder. *J Bone Joint Surg Am.* 1972;54:41-50.

Neer CS. Impingement lesions. *Clin Orthop.* 1983;173:70-77.

Neer CS, Foster CR. Inferior capsular shift for involuntary inferior and multidirectional instability of the shoulder: a preliminary report. *J Bone Joint Surg.* 1980;62A:897.

Nirschl RP. Shoulder tendonitis. In: Pettrone FP, ed. *Upper Extremity Injuries in Athletes.* American Academy of Orthopaedic Surgeons Symposium, Washington, DC. St. Louis: Mosby; 1988.

O'Brien SJ, Beves MC, Arnoczky SJ, et al. The anatomy and histology of the inferior glenohumeral ligament complex of the shoulder. *Am J Sports Med.* 1990;18:449-456.

O'Brien SJ, Pagnani MJ, Fealy S, McGlynn SR, Wilson SB. The active compression test: a new effective test for diagnosing labral tears and acromioclavicular joint abnormality. *Am J Sports Med.* 1998;26:610-613.

Pagnani MJ, Deng XH, Warren RF, Torzilli PA, Altchek DW. Effect of lesions of the superior portion of the glenoid labrum on glenohumeral translation. *J Bone Joint Surg Am.* 1995a;77:1003-1010.

Pagnani MJ, Speer KP, Altchek DW, Warren RF, Dines DW. Arthroscopic fixation of superior labral lesions using a biodegradable implant: a preliminary report. *Arthroscopy.* 1995b;11:194-198.

Paley KJ, Jobe FW, Pink MM, Kvitne RS, ElAttrache NS. Arthroscopic findings in the overhand throwing athlete: evidence for posterior internal impingement of the rotator cuff. *Arthroscopy.* 2000;16(1):35-40.

Perthes G. Ueber operationen der habituellen schulterluxation. *Deutsche Ztschr Chir.* 1906;85:199.

Poppen NK, Walker PS. Forces at the glenohumeral joint in abduction. *Clin Orthop.* 1978;135:165-170.

Powell SE, Nord KD, Ryu RN. The diagnosis, classification, and treatment of SLAP lesions. *Oper Tech Sports Med.* 2012;20(1):45-56.

Pradham RL, Hoi E, Hatakeyama Y, Urayama M, Sato K. Superior labral strain during the throwing motion: a cadaveric study. *Am J Sports Med.* 2001;29:488-492.

Reinold MM, Wilk KE, Fleisig GS, et al. Electromyographic analysis of the rotator cuff and deltoid musculature during common shoulder external rotation exercises. *J Orthop Sports Phys Ther.* 2004;34(7):385-394.

Reinold MM, Wilk KE, Reed J, Crenshaw K, Andrews JR. Interval sport programs: guidelines for baseball, tennis and golf. *J Orthop Sports Phys Ther.* 2002;32(6):293-298.

Resch H, Golser K, Thoeni H. Arthroscopic repair of superior glenoid labral detachment (the SLAP lesion). *J Shoulder Elbow.* 1993;2:147-155.

Rowe CR. Acute and recurrent dislocations of the shoulder. *J Bone Joint Surg.* 1962;44A:998.

Shepard MF, Dugas JR, Zeng N, Andrews JR. Differences in the ultimate strength of the biceps anchor and the generation of Type II superior labral anterior posterior lesions in a cadaveric model. *Am J Sports Med.* 2004;32:1197-1201.

Snyder SJ, Banas MP, Karzel RP. An analysis of 140 consecutive injuries to the superior glenoid labrum. *J Shoulder Elbow Surg.* 1995;7:243-248.

Snyder SJ, Kollias LK. Labral tears. In: Timmerman JR, ed. *Diagnostic and Operative Arthroscopy.* Philadelphia: Saunders; 1997.

Speer KP, Hannafin KP, Altchek DW, Warren RF. An evaluation of the shoulder relocation test. *Am J Sports Med.* 1994;22(2):177-183.

Stetson WB, Templin K. The crank test, O'Brien test, and routine magnetic resonance imaging scans in the diagnosis of labral tears. *Am J Sports Med.* 2002;30:806-809.

Walch G, Boileau P, Noel E, Donell ST. Impingement of the deep surface of the supraspinatus tendon on the posterosuperior glenoid rim: an arthroscopic study. *J Shoulder Elbow Surg.* 1992;1:238-245.

Wilk KE, Reinold MM, Andrews JR. Postoperative treatment principles in the throwing athlete. *Sports Med Arthrosc Rev.* 2001;9:69-95.

Williams GN, Gangel TJ, Arciero RA, Uhorchak JM, Taylor DC. Comparison of the single assessment numeric evaluation method and two shoulder rating scales: outcomes measures after shoulder surgery. *Am J Sports Med.* 1999;27(2):214-221.

Williams MM, Snyder SJ, Buford D Jr. The Buford complex–the "cord-like" middle glenohumeral ligament and absent anterosuperior labrum complex: a normal anatomic capsulolabral variant. *Arthroscopy.* 1994;10:241-247.

Wuelker N, Plitz W, Roetman B. Biomechanical data concerning the shoulder impingement syndrome. *Clin Orthop.* 1994;303:242-249.

Zuckerman JD, Kummer FJ, Cuomo F, Simon J, Rosenblum S, Katz N. The influence of coracoacromial arch anatomy on rotator cuff tears. *J Shoulder Elbow Surg.* 1992;1:4-14.

Chapter 5

Altchek DW, Dines DW. The surgical treatment of anterior instability: selective capsular repair. *Oper Tech Sports Med.* 1993;1:285-292.

Awan R, Smith J, Boon AJ. Measuring shoulder internal rotation range of motion: a comparison of 3 techniques. *Arch Phys Med Rehabil.* 2002;83:1229-1234.

Ballantyne BT, O'Hare SJ, Paschall JL, et al. Electromyographic activity of selected shoulder muscles in commonly used therapeutic exercises. *Phys Ther.* 1993;73:668-677.

Basset RW, Browne AO, Morrey BF, An KN. GH muscle force and moment mechanics in a position of shoulder instability. *J Biomech.* 1994;23:405-415.

Bitter NL, Clisby EF, Jones MA, Magarey ME, Jaberzadeh S, Sandow MJ. Relative contributions of infraspinatus and deltoid during external rotation in healthy shoulders. *J Shoulder Elbow Surg.* 2007;16(5):563-568.

Blackburn TA, McLeod WD, White B, Wofford L. EMG analysis of posterior rotator cuff exercises. *Athl Train.* 1990;25:40-45.

Boon AJ, Smith J. Manual scapular stabilization: its effect on shoulder rotational range of motion. *Arch Phys Med Rehabil.* 2000;81(7):978-983.

Brown LP, Neihues SL, Harrah A, Yavorsky P, Hirshman HP. Upper extremity range of motion and isokinetic strength of the internal and external shoulder rotators in major league baseball players. *Am J Sports Med.* 1988;16:577-585.

Burkhart SS, Morgan CD, Kibler WB. The disabled throwing shoulder: spectrum of pathology part I: pathoanatomy and biomechanics. *Arthroscopy.* 2003a;19:404-420.

Burkhart SS, Morgan CD, Kibler WB. The disabled throwing shoulder. Spectrum of pathology. Part II: evaluation and treatment of SLAP lesions in throwers. *Arthroscopy.* 2003b;19:531-539.

Burkhart SS, Morgan CD, Kibler WB. The disabled throwing shoulder: spectrum of pathology part III: the SICK scapula, scapular dyskinesis, the kinetic chain, and rehabilitation. *Arthroscopy.* 2003c;19:641-661.

Byrum IR, Bushnell BD, Dugger K, Charron K, Harrell FE, Noonan TJ. Preseason shoulder strength measurements in professional baseball pitchers: identifying players at risk for injury. *Am J Sports Med.* 2010;38(7):1375-1382.

Carter AB, Kaminsky TW, Douex AT Jr, Knight CA, Richards JG. Effects of high volume upper extremity plyometric training on throwing velocity and functional strength ratios of the shoulder rotators in collegiate baseball players. *J Strength Cond Res.* 2007;21(1):208-215.

Castelein B, Cagnie B, Parlevliet, Cools A. Superficial and deep scapulothoracic muscle electromyographic activity during elevation exercises in the scapular plane. J Orthop Sports Phys Ther 2016; 46(3):184-193.

Chant CB, Litchfield R, Griffin S, Thain LM. Humeral head retroversion in competitive baseball players and its relationship to GH rotation range of motion. *J Orthop Sports Phys Ther.* 2007;37(9):514-520.

Crockett HC, Gross LB, Wilk KE, et al. Osseous adaptation and range of motion at the GH joint in professional baseball pitchers. *Am J Sports Med.* 2002;30:20-26.

Cyriax J. *Textbook of Orthopaedic Medicine.* 8th ed. London: Bailliere Tindall; 1982.

Davies GJ. *A Compendium of Isokinetics in Clinical Usage and Rehabilitation Techniques.* 4th ed. Onalaska, WI: S & S; 1992.

Decker MJ, Hintermeister RA, Faber KJ, Hawkins RJ. Serratus anterior muscle activity during selected rehabilitation exercises. *Am J Sports Med.* 1999;27:784-791.

Ebaugh DD, McClure PW, Karduna AR. Scapulothoracic and GH kinematics following an external rotation fatigue protocol. *J Orthop Sports Phys Ther.* 2006;36(8):557-571.

Ekstrom RA, Donatelli RA, Soderberg GL. Surface electromyographic analysis of exercises for the trapezius and serratus anterior muscles. *J Orthop Sports Phys Ther.* 2003;33:247-258.

Ellenbecker TS. Shoulder internal and external rotation strength and range of motion in highly skilled tennis players. *Isokinet Exerc Sci.* 1992;2:1-8.

Ellenbecker TS. Rehabilitation of shoulder and elbow injuries in tennis players. *Clin Sports Med.* 1995;14:87.

Ellenbecker TS. Musculoskeletal examination of elite junior tennis players. *Aspetar Sports Medicine Journal.* 2014 October;3(5):548-556.

Ellenbecker TS, Cools A. Rehabilitation of shoulder impingement syndrome and rotator cuff injuries: an evidence based review. *Br J Sports Med.* 2010;44(5):319-327.

Ellenbecker TS, Davies GJ. The application of isokinetics in testing and rehabilitation of the shoulder complex. *J Athl Train.* 2000;35(3):338-350.

Ellenbecker TS, Davies GJ. *Closed Kinetic Chain Exercise: A Comprehensive Guide to Multiple Joint Exercises.* Champaign, IL: Human Kinetics; 2001.

Ellenbecker TS, Davies GJ, Rowinski MJ. Concentric versus eccentric isokinetic strengthening of the rotator cuff: objective data versus functional test. *Am J Sports Med.* 1988;16:64-69.

Ellenbecker TS, Kovacs M. Bilateral comparison of shoulder horizontal adduction range of motion in elite tennis players. *J Orthop Sports Phys Ther.* 2013;43(1):A51-A52.

Ellenbecker TS, Manske RM, Sueyoshi T, Bailie DS. The acute effect of a contract/relax horizontal cross-body adduction stretch on shoulder internal rotation. J Orthop Sports Phys Ther 2016;46(1):A37 (Abstract)

Ellenbecker TS, Mattalino AJ. Concentric isokinetic shoulder internal and external rotation strength in professional baseball pitchers. *J Orthop Sports Phys Ther.* 1999;25:323-328.

Ellenbecker TS, Roetert EP. Age specific isokinetic GH internal and external rotation strength in elite junior tennis players. *J Sci Med Sport.* 2003;6(1):63-70.

Ellenbecker TS, Roetert EP, Bailie DS, Davies GJ, Brown SW. GH joint total rotation range of motion in elite tennis players and baseball pitchers. *Med Sci Sports Exerc.* 2002;34(12):2052-2056.

Ellenbecker TS, Roetert EP, Piorkowski PA, Schulz DA. GH joint internal and external rotation range of motion in elite junior tennis players. *J Orthop Sports Phys Ther.* 1996;24(6):336-341.

Ellenbecker TS, Sueyoshi T, Bailie DS. Muscular activation during plyometric exercises in 90° of glenohumeral joint abduction. Sports Health. 2015a Jan;7(1):75-9. doi: 10.1177/1941738114553165.

Ellenbecker TS, Windler G, Dines D, Renstrom R. Musculoskeletal profile of tennis players on the ATP world tour: results of a 9-year screening program. *Journal of Medicine and Science in Tennis.* 2015b;20(3):94-106.

Elliott B, Marsh T, Blanksby B. A three dimensional cinematographic analysis of the tennis serve. *Int J Sports Biomech.* 1986;2:260-271.

Englestad ED, Johnson RL, Jeno SHN, Mabey RL. An electromyographical study of lower trapezius muscle activity during exercise in traditional and modified positions [abstract]. *J Orthop Sports Phys Ther.* 2001;31(1):A29-A30.

Fleck SJ, Kraemer WJ. *Designing Resistance Training Programs.* 4th edition, Champaign IL: Human Kinetics; 2014.

Fleisig GS, Andrews JR, Dillman CJ, Escamilla RF. Kinetics of baseball pitching with implications about injury mechanisms. *Am J Sports Med.* 1995;23:233-239.

Gerber C, Ganz R. Clinical assessment of instability of the shoulder with special reference to anterior and posterior drawer tests. *J Bone Joint Surg Br.* 1984;66(4):551-556.

Graichen H, Hinterwimmer S, von Eisenhart-Roth R, Vogl T, Englmeier KH, Eckstein F. Effect of abducting and adducting muscle activity on GH translation, scapular kinematics and subacromial space width in vivo. *J Biomech.* 2005;38(4):755-760.

Happee R, VanDer Helm CT. The control of shoulder muscles during goal directed movements, an inverse dynamic analysis. *J Biomech.* 1995;28(10):1179-1191.

Hurd WJ, Kaplan KM, ElAttrache NS, Jobe FW, Morrey BF, Kaufman KR. A profile of GH internal and external rotation motion in the uninjured high school baseball pitcher: part I: motion. *J Athl Train.* 2011;46(3):282-288.

Ivey FM, Calhoun JH, Rusche K, Bierschenk J. Isokinetic testing of shoulder strength: normal values. *Arch Phys Med Rehabil.* 1985;66:384-386.

Izumi T, Aoki M, Muraki T, Hidaka E, Miyamoto S. Stretching positions for the posterior capsule of the GH joint: strain measurement using cadaveric measurements. *Am J Sports Med.* 2008;36:2014-2022.

Jensen BR, Sjogaard G, Bornmyr S, Arborelius M, Jørgensen K. Intramuscular laser-Doppler flowmetry in the supraspinatus muscle during isometric contractions. *Eur J Appl Physiol Occup Physiol.* 1995;71:373-378.

Kaltenborn FM. *Mobilization of the Extremity Joints. Examination and Basic Treatment Techniques.* Olaf Norlis Bokhandel; 1980.

Kibler WB. The role of the scapula in athletic shoulder function. *Am J Sports Med.* 1998;26:325-337.

Kibler WB, Sciascia AD, Uhl TL, Tambay N, Cunningham T. Electromyographic analysis of specific exercises for scapular control in the early phases of shoulder rehabilitation. *Am J Sports Med.* 2008;39(6):1789-1798.

Laudner KG, Sipes RC, Wilson JT. The acute effects of sleeper stretch on shoulder range of motion. *J Athl Train.* 2008;43(4):359-363.

Ludewig P, Cook T. Alterations in shoulder kinematics and associated muscle activity in people with symptoms of shoulder impingement. *Phys Ther.* 2000;80:276-291.

MacConaill MA. Movements of bones and joints: function of musculature. *J Bone Joint Surg.* 1949;31B:100-104.

Maitland GD. *Maitland's Vertebral Manipulations.* 6th ed. London: Butterworth-Heineman; 2000.

Malanga GA, Jemp YN, Growney E, An K. EMG analysis of shoulder positioning in testing and strengthening the supraspinatus. *Med Sci Sports Exerc.* 1996;28:661-664.

Manske R, Wilk KE, Davies G, Ellenbecker T, Reinold M. GH motion deficits: friend or foe? *Int J Sports Phys Ther.* 2013;8(5):537-553.

McCabe RA, Tyler TF, Nicholas SJ, McHugh M. Selective activation of the lower trapezius muscle in patients with shoulder impingement [abstract]. *J Orthop Sports Phys Ther.* 2001;31(1):A45.

McClure P, Balaicuis J, Heiland D, Broersma ME, Thorndike CK, Wood A. A randomized controlled comparison of stretching procedures in recreational athletes with posterior shoulder tightness [abstract]. *J Orthop Sports Phys Ther.* 2005;35(1):A5.

McFarland EG, Torpey BM, Carl LA. Evaluation of shoulder laxity. *Sports Med.* 1996;22:264-272.

Meister K, Day T, Horodyski MB, Kaminski TW, Wasik MP, Tillman S. Rotational motion changes in the GH joint of the adolescent little league baseball player. *Am J Sports Med.* 2005;33(5):693-698.

Moesley JB, Jobe FW, Pink M, Perry J, Tibone J. EMG analysis of the scapular muscles during a shoulder rehabilitation program. *Am J Sports Med.* 1992;20:128-134.

Moncrief SA, Lau JD, Gale JR, Scott SA. Effect of rotator cuff exercise on humeral rotation torque in healthy individuals. *J Strength Cond Res.* 2002;16(2):262-270.

Mont MA, Cohen DB, Campbell KR, Gravare K, Mathur SK. Isokinetic concentric versus eccentric training of the shoulder rotators with functional evaluation of performance enhancement in elite tennis players. *Am J Sports Med.* 1994;22:513-517.

Mulligan, BR. *Manual Therapy NAGS, SNAGS, MWMS etc.* 5th edition, New Zealand: Plane View Services Ltd.; 2016.

Myers JP, Laudner KG, Pasquale MR, Bradley JP, Lephart SM. GH range of motion deficits and posterior shoulder tightness in throwers with pathologic internal impingement. *Am J Sports Med.* 2006;34(3):385-391.

Niederbracht Y, Shim AL, Sloniger MA, Paternostro-Bayles M, Short TH. Effects of a shoulder injury prevention strength training program on eccentric external rotation muscle strength and GH joint imbalance in female overhead activity athletes. *J Strength Cond Res.* 2008;22(1):140-145.

Osbahr DC, Cannon DL, Speer KS. Retroversion of the humerus in the throwing shoulder of college baseball pitchers. *Am J Sports Med.* 2002;30(3):347-353.

Quincy RI, Davies GJ, Kolbeck KJ, Szymanski JL. Isokinetic exercise: the effects of training specificity on shoulder strength development. *J Athl Train.* 2000;35:S64.

Rathbun JB, Macnab I. The microvascular pattern of the rotator cuff. *J Bone Joint Surg.* 1970;52(3):540-553.

Reagan KM, Meister K, Horodyski MB, Werner DW, Carruthers C, Wilk K. Humeral retroversion and its relationship to GH rotation in the shoulder of college baseball players. *Am J Sports Med.* 2002;30(3):354-360.

Reeser JC, Joy EA, Porucznic CA, Berg RL, Colliver EB, Willick SE. Risk factors for volleyball-related shoulder pain and dysfunction. *Phys Med Rehabil.* 2012;2:27-36.

Reinold MM, Macrina LC, Wilk KE, et al. Electromyographic analysis of the supraspinatus and deltoid muscles during 3 common rehabilitation exercises. *J Athl Train.* 2007;42(4):464-469.

Reinold MM, Wilk KE, Fleisig GS, et al. Electromyographic analysis of the rotator cuff and deltoid musculature during common shoulder external rotation exercises. *J Orthop Sports Phys Ther.* 2004;34(7):385-394.

Saha AK. Mechanism of shoulder movements and a plea for the recognition of "zero position" of the GH joint. *Clin Orthop.* 1983;173:3-10.

Schulte-Edelmann JA, Davies GJ, Kernozek TW, Gerberding ED. The effects of plyometric training of the posterior shoulder and elbow. *J Strength Cond Res.* 2005;19(1):129-134.

Shanley E, Rauh MJ, Michener LA, Ellenbecker TS, Garrison JC, Thigpen CA. Shoulder range of motion measures as risk factors for shoulder and elbow injuries in high school softball and baseball players. *Am J Sports Med.* 2011;39:1997-2006.

Solem-Bertoft E, Thuomas K, Westerberg C. The influence of scapula retraction and protraction on the width of the subacromial space. *Clin Orthop.* 1993;266:99-103.

Sullivan PE, Markos PD, Minor MD. *An Integrated Approach to Therapeutic Exercise: Theory and Clinical Application.* Reston, VA: Reston; 1982.

Townsend H, Jobe FW, Pink M, Perry J. Electromyographic analysis of the GH muscles during a baseball rehabilitation program. *Am J Sports Med.* 1991;19:264-272.

Tsai NT, McClure PW, Karduna AR. Effects of muscle fatigue on 3-dimensional scapular kinematics. *Arch Phys Med Rehabil.* 2003;84:1000-1005.

Tsuruike M, Ellenbecker TS. Serratus anterior and lower trapezius muscle activities during multi-joint isotonic scapular exercises and isometric contractions. *J Athl Train.* 2015;50(2):199–210. doi: 10.4085/1062-6050-49.3.80

Uhl TL, Carver TJ, Mattacola CG, Mair SD, Nitz AJ. Shoulder musculature activation during upper extremity weight-bearing exercise. *J Orthop Sports Phys Ther.* 2003;33(3):109-117.

Vincenzino B, Hing W, Rivett D, Hall T. *Mobilisation with Movement: The art and the science.* Sydney: Elsevier; 2016.

Vossen JE, Kramer JE, Bruke DG, Vossen DP. Comparison of dynamic push-up training and plyometric push-up training on upper-body power and strength. *J Strength Cond Res.* 2000;14(3):248-253.

Warner JJP, Micheli LJ, Arslanian LE, Kennedy J, Kennedy R. Patterns of flexibility, laxity, and strength in normal shoulders and shoulders with instability and impingement. *Am J Sports Med.* 1990;18:366.

Wilk KE, Andrews JR, Arrigo CA, Keirns MA, Erber DJ. The strength characteristics of internal and external rotator muscles in professional baseball pitchers. *Am J Sports Med.* 1993;21:61-66.

Wilk KE, Meister K, Andrews JR. Current concepts in the rehabilitation of the overhead athlete. *Am J Sports Med.* 2002;30(1):136-151.

Wilk KE, Macrina LC, Arrigo C. Passive range of motion characteristics in the overhead baseball pitcher and their implications for rehabilitation. *Clin Orthop Rel Res.* 2012;470(6):1586-1594.

Wilk KE, Macrina LC, Fleisig GS, et al. Correlation of GH internal rotation deficit and total rotational motion to shoulder injuries in professional baseball pitchers. *Am J Sports Med.* 2011a;39:329-335.

Wilk KE, Macrina LC, Fleisig GS, et al. Correlation of shoulder range of motion and shoulder injuries in professional baseball pitchers: an 8 year prospective study. Presented at the *American Orthopaedic Society for Sports Medicine* annual conference, July 2013.

Wilk KE, Yenchak AJ, Arrigo CA, Andrews JR. The advanced throwers ten exercise program: a new exercise series for enhanced dynamic shoulder control in the overhead throwing athlete. *Phys Sportsmed.* 2011b;39(4):90-97.

Wuelker N, Plitz W, Roetman B. Biomechanical data concerning the shoulder impingement syndrome. *Clin Orthop.* 1994;303:242-249.

Zachezewski JE, Reischl S. Flexibility for the runner. Specific program considerations. *Top Acute Care Trauma Rehabil.* 1986;1:9-27.

Chapter 6

Altchek DW, Warren RF, Wickiewicz TL, Ortiz G. Arthroscopic labral debridement. A three year follow-up study. *Am J Sports Med.* 1992;20:702-706.

Andrews JR, Carson WG, McLeod WD. The arthroscopic treatment of glenoid labrum tears in the throwing athlete. *Am J Sports Med.* 1985;13:337-341.

Arndt J, Clavert P, Mielcarek P, et al. Immediate passive motion versus immobilization after endoscopic supraspinatus tendon repair. A prospective randomized study. *Orthop Truamatol Surg Res.* 2012;98 (suppl):S131-138.

Black KP, Lim TH, McGrady LM, Raasch W. In vitro evaluation of shoulder external rotation after a Bankart reconstruction. *Am J Sports Med.* 1997;25:449-453.

Brislin KJ, Field LD, Savoie FH III. Complications after arthroscopic rotator cuff repair. *Arthroscopy.* 2007;23:124-128.

Burkhart SS. A stepwise approach to arthroscopic rotator cuff repair based on biomechanical principles. *Arthroscopy.* 2000;16:82-90.

Burkhart SS, Danaceau SM, Pearce CE Jr. Arthroscopic rotator cuff repair: analysis of results by tear size and by repair technique: margin convergence versus direct tendon-to-bone repair. *Arthroscopy.* 2001;17:905-912.

Burkhart SS, Morgan CD. The peel-back mechanism: its role in producing and extending posterior type II SLAP lesions and its effect on SLAP repair rehabilitation. *Arthroscopy.* 1998;14:637-640.

Cuff DJ, Pupello DR. Prospective randomized study of arthroscopic rotator cuff repair using an early versus delayed postoperative physical therapy protocol. *J Shoulder Elbow Surgery.* 2012;21:1450-1455.

Davies MR, Dugas JR, Fleisig GS, Shepard MF, Andrews JR. The strength of the repaired Type II SLAP lesions in a cadaveric model. Proceedings of the American Sports Medicine Fellowship Society Symposium, Birmingham, AL, June 2004.

Donatelli RA, Ekstrom RA. Surface electromyographic analysis of exercises for the trapezius and serratus anterior muscles. *J Orthop Sports Phys Ther.* 2003;33(5):247-258.

Edwards SL, Lee JA, Bell JE, et al. Nonoperative treatment of superior labrum anterior posterior tears: improvements in pain, function, and quality of life. *Am J Sports Med.* 2010;38(7):1456-1461.

Ellenbecker TS. Etiology and evaluation of rotator cuff pathologic conditions and rehabilitation. In: Donatelli RA. *Physical Therapy of the Shoulder.* 4th ed. St. Louis: Churchill Livingstone; 2004.

Ellenbecker TS, Elmore EE, Bailie DS. Descriptive report of shoulder ROM and rotational strength 6 and 12 weeks following rotator cuff repair using a mini-open deltoid splitting technique. *J Orthop Sports Phys Ther.* 2006;36(5):326-335.

Ellenbecker TS, Mattalino AJ. Glenohumeral joint range of motion and rotator cuff strength following arthroscopic anterior stabilization with thermal capsulorraphy. *J Orthop Sports Phys Ther.* 1999 Mar;29(3):160-167.

Ellenbecker TS, Manske RC, Kelley MJ. *Current Concepts of Orthopaedic Physical Therapy.* 3rd edition, LaCrosse, WI: Orthopaedic Physical Therapy Association APTA; 2011.

Ellsworth AA, Mullaney M, Tyler TF, et al. Electromyography of selected shoulder musculature during un-weighted and weighted pendulum exercises. *N Am J Sports Phys Ther.* 2006;1(2):73-79.

Fealy S, Kingham P, Altchek DW. Mini-open rotator cuff repair using a 2 row fixation technique. Outcomes analysis in patients with small, moderate, and large rotator cuff tears. *Arthroscopy.* 2002;18:665-670.

Field LD, Savoie FH. Arthroscopic suture repairs of superior labral lesions of the shoulder. *Am J Sports Med.* 1993;21:783-790.

Flatow EL, Soslowski LJ, Ticker JB, et al. Excursion of the rotator cuff under the acromion: patterns of subacromial contact. *Am J Sports Med.* 1994;22(6):779-788.

Friedman LGM, Griesser MJ, Miniaci AA, Jones MH. Recurrent instability after revision anterior shoulder stabilization surgery. *Arthroscopy.* 2014;30(3):372-381.

Galatz LM, Ball CM, Teefey SA, Middleton WD, Yamaguchi K. The outcome and repair integrity of completely arthroscopically repaired large and massive rotator cuff tears. *J Bone Joint Surgery AM.* 2004;86:219-224.

Gartsman GH, Hammerman SM. Superior labrum, anterior and posterior lesions. When and how to treat them. *Clin Sports Med.* 2000;19:115-124.

Gill, TJ, Micheli, LJ, Gebhard F, et al. Bankart repair for anterior instability of the shoulder. *J Bone Joint Surg.* 1997;79A:850-857.

Hatakeyama Y, Itoi E, Urayama M, et al. Effect of superior capsule and coracohumeral ligament release on strain in the repaired rotator cuff tendon. *Am J Sports Med.* 2001;29:633-640.

Keener JD, Galatz LM, Stobbs-Cucchi G, Patton R, Yamaguchi K. Rehabilitation following arthroscopic rotator cuff repair. A prospective randomized trial of immobilization compared with early motion. *J Bone Joint Surgery AM.* 2014;96:11-19.

Kibler WB, et al. Electromyographic analysis of specific exercises for scapular control in early phases of shoulder rehabilitation. *Am J Sports Med.* 2008;36(9):1789-1798.

Kim YS, Chung SW, Kim JY, Ok JH, Park I, Oh JH. Is early passive motion exercise necessary after arthroscopic rotator cuff repair? *Am J Sports Med.* 2012;40:815-821.

Kuhn JE, Dunn WR, Sanders R, et al. Effectiveness of physical therapy in treating atraumatic full-thickness rotator cuff tears: a multi-center prospective cohort study. *J Shoulder Elbow Surg.* 2013;22:1371-1379.

Kukkonen J, Joukainen A, Lehtinen J, et al. Treatment of non-traumatic rotator cuff tears: a randomized controlled trial with one year clinical results. *J Bone Joint Surg.* 2014;96-B(1):75-81.

Lee SB, An KN. Dynamic GH stability provided by three heads of the deltoid muscle. *Clin Orthop Rel Res.* 2002;400:40-47.

Lee BG, Cho NS, Rhee YG. Effect of two rehabilitation protocols on range of motion and healing rates after arthroscopic rotator cuff repair: Aggressive versus limited early passive exercisers. *Arthroscopy.* 2012;28:34-42.

Lenters TL, Franta AK, Wolf FM, Leopold SS, Matsen FA. Arthroscopic compared with open repairs for recurrent anterior shoulder instability. *J Bone Joint Surg.* 2007;89:244-254.

Maffet MW, Gartsman GM, Moseley B. Superior labrum-biceps tendon complex lesions of the shoulder. *Am J Sports Med.* 1995;23:93-98.

Malanga GA, Jenp YN, Growney ES, et al. EMG analysis of shoulder positioning in testing and strengthening the supraspinatus. *Med Sci Sports Exerc.* 1996;28(6):661-664.

Malliou PC, Giannakopoulos K, Beneka AG, et al. Effective ways of restoring muscular imbalances of the rotator cuff muscle group: a comparative study of various training methods. *Br J Sports Med.* 2004;38(6):766-772.

McCann PD, Wooten ME, Kadaba MP, et al. A kinematic and electromyographic study of shoulder rehabilitation exercises. *Clin Orthop Rel Res.* 1993;288:178-189.

Mochizuki T, Sugaya H, Uomizu, M, et al. Humeral insertion of the supraspinatus and infraspinatus. New anatomical findings regarding the footprint of the rotator cuff surgical technique. *J Bone Joint Surg.* 2009;91:1-7.

Morgan CD, Burkhart SS, Palmeri M, Gillespie M. Type II SLAP lesions: three subtypes and their relationships to superior instability and rotator cuff tears. *Arthroscopy.* 1998;14:553-565.

Muraki T, Aoki M, Uchiyama E, et al. The effect of arm position on stretching of the supraspinatus, infraspinatus, and posterior portion of deltoid muscles: a cadaveric study. *Clin Biomech.* 2006;21(5):474-480.

Muraki T, Aoki M, Uchiyama E, Miyasaka T, Murakami G, Miyamoto S. Strain on the repaired supraspinatus tendon during manual traction and translational glide mobilization on the GH joint: a cadaveric biomechanics study. *Man Ther.* 2007;12(3):231-239.

Nam EK, Snyder SJ. The diagnosis and treatment of superior labrum, anterior and posterior (SLAP) lesions. *Am J Sports Med.* 2003;31(5):798-810.

Namdari S, Green A. Range of motion limitation after rotator cuff repair. *J Shoulder Elbow Surgery.* 2010;19:290-296.

Ozturk BY, Maak TG, Fabricant P, et al. Return to sports after arthroscopic anterior stabilization in patients aged younger than 25 years. *Arthroscopy.* 2013;29(12):1922-1931.

Pagnani MJ, Deng XH, Warren RF, Torzilli PA, Altchek DW. Effect of lesions of the superior portion of the glenoid labrum on GH translation. *J Bone Joint Surg Am.* 1995a;77:1003-1010.

Pagnani MJ, Speer KP, Altchek DW, Warren RF, Dines DW. Arthroscopic fixation of superior labral lesions using a biodegradable implant: a preliminary report. *Arthroscopy.* 1995b;11:194-198.

Park MC, ElAttrache NS, Tibone JE, Ahmad CS, Jun BJ, Lee TQ. Part I: footprint contact characteristics for a transosseous-equivalent rotator cuff repair technique compared with a double-row repair technique. *J Shoulder Elbow Surg.* 2007;16:461-468.

Penna J, Deramo D, Nelson CO, et al. Determination of anterior labral repair stress during passive arm motion in a cadaveric model. *Arthroscopy.* 2008;24(8):930-935.

Powell SE, Nord KD, Ryu RN. The diagnosis, classification, and treatment of SLAP lesions. *Oper Tech Sports Med.* 2012;20(1):45-56.

Reinold MM, Wilk KE, Fleisig GS, et al. Electromyographic analysis of the rotator cuff and deltoid musculature during common shoulder external rotation exercises. *J Orthop Sports Phys Ther.* 2004;34(7):385-394.

Reinold MM, Wilk KE, Hooks TR, Dugas JR, Andrews JR. Thermal-assisted capsular shrinkage of the GH joint in overhead athletes: a 15- to 47-month follow-up. *J Orthop Sports Phys Ther.* 2003;33(8):455-467.

Reinold MM, Wilk KE, Reed J, Crenshaw K, Andrews JR. Interval sport programs: guidelines for baseball, tennis and golf. *J Orthop Sports Phys Ther.* 2002;32(6):293-298.

Riboh JC, Garrigues GE. Early passive motion versus immobilization after arthroscopic rotator cuff repair. *Arthroscopy.* 2014;30:997-1005

Rodosky MW, Harner CD, Fu FH. The role of the long head of the biceps muscle and superior glenoid labrum in anterior stability of the shoulder. *Am J Sports Med.* 1994;22:121-130.

Saha AK. The classic. Mechanism of shoulder movements and a plea for the recognition of "zero position" of glenohumeral joint. *Clin Orthop Relat Res.* 1983 Mar;(173):3-10.

Shepard MF, Dugas JR, Zeng N, Andrews JR. Differences in the ultimate strength of the biceps anchor and the generation of Type II superior labral anterior posterior lesions in a cadaveric model. *Am J Sports Med.* 2004;32:1197-1201.

Snyder SJ, Banas MP, Karzel RP. An analysis of 140 consecutive injuries to the superior glenoid labrum. *J Shoulder Elbow Surg.* 1995;7:243-248.

Snyder SJ, Karzel RP, DelPizzo W, Ferkel RD, Friedman MJ. SLAP lesions of the shoulder. *Arthroscopy.* 1990;6:274-279.

Snyder SJ, Kollias LK. Labral tears. In: Timmerman JR, ed. *Diagnostic and Operative Arthroscopy.* Philadelphia: Saunders; 1997.

Speer KP, Hannafin JA, Altchek DW, et al. An evaluation of the shoulder relocation test. *Am J Sports Med.* 1994;22(2):177-183.

Stetson WB, Templin K. The crank test, O'Brien test, and routine magnetic resonance imaging scans in the diagnosis of labral tears. *Am J Sports Med.* 2002;30:806-809.

Tashjien RZ, Hollins AM, Kim HM, et al. Factors affecting healing rates after arthroscopic double row rotator cuff repair. *AM J Sports Med.* 2010;38:2435-2442.

Thigpen CA, Padua DA, Morgan N, Kreps C, Karas SG. Scapular kinematics during surpraspinatus rehabilitation exercise: a comparison of full can versus empty can techniques. *Am J Sports Med.* 2006;34(4):644-652.

Timmerman LA, Andrews JR, Wilk KE. Mini open repair of the rotator cuff. In: Andrews JR, Wilk KE. *The Athlete's Shoulder.* Philadelphia: Churchill Livingstone; 1994.

Vangsness CT Jr, Jurgenson SS, Watson T, et al. The origin of the long head of the biceps from the scapula and glenoid labrum: an anatomical study of 100 shoulders. *J Bone Joint Surg.* 1994;76B:951-954.

Walch G, Buileau P, Noel E, Donnell ST. Impingement of the deep surface of the supraspinatus tendon on the posterior glenoid rim: an arthroscopic study. *J Shoulder Elbow Surg.* 1992;1:238-245.

Wang CH, McClure P, Pratt NE, et al. Stretching and strengthening exercises: their effect on three-dimensional scapular kinematics. *Arch Phys Med Rehabil.* 1999;80:923-929.

Wilk KE. Rehabilitation after shoulder stabilization surgery. In: Warren RF, Craig EV, Altchek DW, eds. *The Unstable Shoulder.* Philadelphia: Lippincott-Raven; 1999:367-402.

Wilk KE, Andrews JR, Arrigo CA, et al. *Preventive and Rehabilitative Exercises for the Shoulder and Elbow.* 6th ed. Birmingham, AL: American Sports Medicine Institute; 2001a.

Wilk KE, Arrigo CA. Current concepts in the rehabilitation of the athletic shoulder. *J Orthop Sports Phys Ther.* 1993;18:365-378.

Wilk KE, Arrigo, CA, Andrews JR. Current concepts: the stabilizing structures of the GH joint. *J Orthop Sports Phys Ther.* 1997;25:364-379.

Wilk KE, Harrelson GL, Arrigo CA. Shoulder rehabilitation. In: Harrelson GL, Andrews JR, Wilk KE, eds. *Physical Rehabilitation of the Injured Athlete.* 3rd ed. Philadelphia: Saunders; 2004:513-589.

Wilk KE, Reinold MM, Andrews JR. Postoperative treatment principles in the throwing athlete. *Sports Med Arthrosc Rev.* 2001b;9:69-95.

Wilk KE, Reinold MM, Dugas JR, Andrews JR. Rehabilitation following thermal-assisted capsular shrinkage of the GH joint: current concepts. *J Orthop Sports Phys Ther.* 2002;32:268-292.

Williams MM, Snyder SJ, Buford D Jr. The Buford complex–the "cord-like" middle GH ligament and absent anterosuperior labrum complex: a normal anatomic capsulolabral variant. *Arthroscopy.* 1994;10:241-247.

Chapter 7

Bigliani LU, Codd TP, Connor PM, Levine WN, Littlefield MA, Hershon SJ. Shoulder motion and laxity in the professional baseball player. *Am J Sports Med.* 1997;25:609-613.

Brown LP, Niehues SL, Harrah A, Yavorsky P, Hirshman HP. Upper extremity range of motion and isokinetic strength of the internal and external shoulder rotators in major league baseball players. *Am J Sports Med.* 1988;16:577-585.

Burkhart SS, Morgan CD, Kibler WB. The disabled throwing shoulder: spectrum of pathology. Part II: evaluation and treatment of SLAP lesions in throwers. *Arthroscopy.* 2003;19:531-539.

Chant CB, Litchfield R, Griffin S, Thain LM. Humeral head retroversion in competitive baseball players and its relationship to glenohumeral rotation range of motion. *J Orthop Sports Phys Ther.* 2007;37:514-520.

Conte S, Requa RK, Garrick JG. Disability days in major league baseball. *Am J Sports Med.* 2009;29:431-436.

Crockett HC, Gross LB, Wilk KE, et al. Osseous adaptation and range of motion at the glenohumeral joint in professional baseball pitchers. *Am J Sports Med.* 2002;30:20-26.

Johnson L. Patterns of shoulder flexibility among college baseball players. *J Athl Train.* 1996;27:44-49.

Myers TH, Zemanovic JR, Andrews JR. The resisted supination external rotation test: a new test for the diagnosis of superior labral anterior lesions. *Am J Sports Med.* 2005;33:1315-1320.

Paine RM. The role of the scapula in the shoulder. In: Andrews JR. Wilk K, eds. *The Athlete's Shoulder.* New York: Churchill Livingstone; 1994:495-512.

Pieper HG. Humeral torsion in the throwing arm of handball players. *Am J Sports Med.* 1998;226:247-253.

Reagan KM, Meister K, Horodyski MB, Werner DW, Carruthers C, Wilk K. Humeral retroversion and its relationship to the shoulder of college baseball players. *Am J Sports Med.* 2002;30:354-360.

Wilk KE, Andrews JR, Arrigo CA. The abduction and adduction strength characteristics of professional baseball pitchers. *Am J Sports Med.* 1995;23:778.

Wilk KE, Andrews JR, Arrigo CA. The strength characteristics of internal and external rotator muscles in professional baseball pitchers. *Am J Sports Med.* 1993;21:61-66.

Wilk KE, Arrigo CA. Current concepts in the rehabilitation of the athletic shoulder. *J Orthop Phys Ther Clin N Am.* 1992;25:364-379.

Wilk KE, Meister K, Andrews JR. Current concepts in the rehabilitation of the overhead throwing athlete. *Am J Sports Med.* 2002;30(1):136-151.

Wilk KE, Obama P, Simpson II CD, Cain EL, Dugas J, Andrews JR. Shoulder injuries in the overhead athlete. *J Orthop Sports Phys Ther.* 2009;39(2):38-54.

Chapter 8

Ellenbecker TS, Kovacs M. Bilateral comparison of shoulder horizontal adduction range of motion in elite tennis players. *J Orthop Sports Phys Ther.* 2013;43(1):A51-A52.

Ellenbecker TS, Wilk KE, Reinold MM, Murphy TF, Paine RM. Use of interval return programs for shoulder rehabilitation. In: Ellenbecker TS. *Shoulder Rehabilitation: Non-Operative Treatment.* New York: Theime Medical; 2006.

Murphy TC. Shoulder injuries in swimming. In: Andrews JR, Wilk KE, eds. *The Athlete's Shoulder.* New York: Churchill Livingstone; 1994.

Reinold MM, Wilk KE, Reed J, Crenshaw K, Andrews JR. Interval sport programs: guidelines for baseball, tennis, and golf. *J Orthop Sports Phys Ther.* 2002;32(6):293-298.

Tovin BJ. Prevention and treatment of swimmer's shoulder. *N Am J Sports Phys Ther.* 2006 Nov;1(4):166-175.

Index

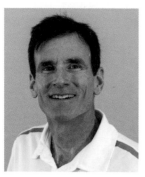

Todd S. Ellenbecker, DPT, MS, SCS, OCS, CSCS, is a physical therapist and clinic director for Physiotherapy Associates Scottsdale Sports Clinic in Scottsdale, Arizona, where he is also the national director of clinical research for Physiotherapy Associates. He is the vice president of medical services for the Association of Tennis Professionals (ATP) Tour and current member and past chairman of the United States Tennis Association (USTA) national sport science committee. He is also a certified United States Professional Tennis Association (USPTA) tennis teaching professional. He is a certified sports clinical specialist, orthopaedic clinical specialist, and strength and conditioning specialist.

Ellenbecker, who has more than 30 years of experience in physical therapy, has authored many books and articles in research journals and trade publications and is an international presenter on shoulder and elbow rehabilitation. He has also served on editorial boards for several journals.

Among many other honors, Ellenbecker was named the Sports Medicine Professional of the Year (2003) by the National Strength and Conditional Association and received the Ronald G. Peyton Lecture Award (2007) by the Sports Physical Therapy Section and the Samuel Hardy Educational Merit Award (2008) by the International Tennis Hall of Fame.

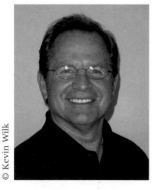

Kevin E. Wilk, PT, DPT, FAPTA, is the associate clinical director for Champion Sports Medicine in Birmingham, Alabama, as well as vice president of clinical education for Physiotherapy Associates. He is also the director of rehabilitative research at the American Sports Medicine Institute in Birmingham while also serving as the rehabilitation consultant for Major League Baseball's Tampa Bay Devil Rays.

Wilk, who has been a physical therapist, researcher, and educator for more than 30 years, has also published many books and articles and book chapters in various medical journals and industry publications. He is an adjunct assistant professor in the physical therapy program at Marquette University and has presented his work and research worldwide.

Wilk received the Catherine Worthingham Fellowship in 2012 by the American Physical Therapy Association, the Turner A. Blackburn Hall of Fame Lifetime Achievement Award in 2012 by the Sports Physical Therapy Section (SPTS), the Ronald G. Peyton Lecture Award in 2004 by SPTS, and the James R. Andrews, MD, Award for Excellence in Baseball Sports Medicine in 1999 by the American Sports Medicine Institute.

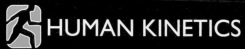
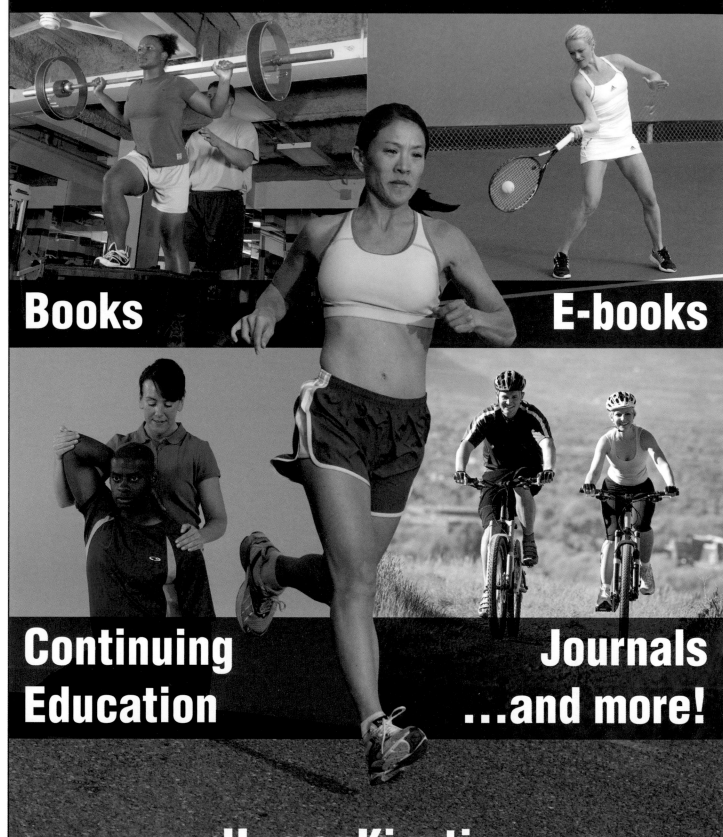